Urinary Tract Infection: Causes, Diagnosis and Clinical Management

Urinary Tract Infection: Causes, Diagnosis and Clinical Management

Editor: Cassian Cameron

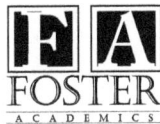

FA FOSTER
ACADEMICS

www.fosteracademics.com

www.fosteracademics.com

FA
FOSTER
ACADEMICS

Cataloging-in-Publication Data

Urinary tract infection : causes, diagnosis and clinical management / edited by Cassian Cameron.
    p. cm.
Includes bibliographical references and index.
ISBN 978-1-63242-694-9
1. Urinary tract infections. 2. Urinary tract infections--Etiology. 3. Urinary tract infections--Diagnosis.
4. Urinary tract infections--Treatment. I. Cameron, Cassian.
RC901.8 .U75 2019
616.6--dc3

Foster Academics,
118-35 Queens Blvd., Suite 400,
Forest Hills, NY 11375, USA

ISBN 978-1-63242-694-9 (Hardback)

Contents

Permissions

List of Contributors

Index

Preface

Every book is a source of knowledge and this one is no exception. The idea that led to the conceptualization of this book was the fact that the world is advancing rapidly; which makes it crucial to document the progress in every field. I am aware that a lot of data is already available, yet, there is a lot more to learn. Hence, I accepted the responsibility of editing this book and contributing my knowledge to the community.

A urinary tract infection (UTI) is an infection that affects either the lower or the upper urinary tract. The infection that affects the lower urinary tract is called bladder infection, whereas the one that affects the upper urinary tract is known as kidney infection. Escherichia coli, a bacterium of the genus Escherichia, is the primary cause of urinary tract infection. Some other forms of bacteria and fungi may also cause such infections. The diagnosis of urinary tract infection is based on a presentation of symptoms such as pain with urination, fever, constant need to urinate, flank pain, etc. and urine culture. In most cases, it can be treated with a course of antibiotics. In more complicated cases, intravenous antibiotics may be used. This book contains some path-breaking studies related to the causes, diagnosis and treatment of urinary tract infection. This book includes contributions of experts and doctors, which will provide innovative insights to readers.

While editing this book, I had multiple visions for it. Then I finally narrowed down to make every chapter a sole standing text explaining a particular topic, so that they can be used independently. However, the umbrella subject sinews them into a common theme. This makes the book a unique platform of knowledge.

I would like to give the major credit of this book to the experts from every corner of the world, who took the time to share their expertise with us. Also, I owe the completion of this book to the never-ending support of my family, who supported me throughout the project.

Editor

Concordance between European and US case definitions of healthcare-associated infections

Sonja Hansen[1*], Dorit Sohr[1], Christine Geffers[1], Pascal Astagneau[2], Alexander Blacky[3], Walter Koller[3], Ingrid Morales[4], Maria Luisa Moro[5], Mercedes Palomar[6], Emese Szilagyi[7], Carl Suetens[8] and Petra Gastmeier[1]

Abstract

Background: Surveillance of healthcare-associated infections (HAI) is a valuable measure to decrease infection rates. Across Europe, inter-country comparisons of HAI rates seem limited because some countries use US definitions from the US Centers for Disease Control and Prevention (CDC/NHSN) while other countries use European definitions from the Hospitals in Europe Link for Infection Control through Surveillance (HELICS/IPSE) project. In this study, we analyzed the concordance between US and European definitions of HAI.

Methods: An international working group of experts from seven European countries was set up to identify differences between US and European definitions and then conduct surveillance using both sets of definitions during a three-month period (March 1st -May 31st, 2010). Concordance between case definitions was estimated with Cohen's kappa statistic (κ).

Results: Differences in HAI definitions were found for bloodstream infection (BSI), pneumonia (PN), urinary tract infection (UTI) and the two key terms "intensive care unit (ICU)-acquired infection" and "mechanical ventilation". Concordance was analyzed for these definitions and key terms with the exception of UTI. Surveillance was performed in 47 ICUs and 6,506 patients were assessed. One hundred and eighty PN and 123 BSI cases were identified. When all PN cases were considered, concordance for PN was κ = 0.99 [CI 95%: 0.98-1.00]. When PN cases were divided into subgroups, concordance was κ = 0.90 (CI 95%: 0.86-0.94) for clinically defined PN and κ = 0.72 (CI 95%: 0.63-0.82) for microbiologically defined PN. Concordance for BSI was κ = 0.73 [CI 95%: 0.66-0.80]. However, BSI cases secondary to another infection site (42% of all BSI cases) are excluded when using US definitions and concordance for BSI was κ = 1.00 when only primary BSI cases, i.e. Europe-defined BSI with "catheter" or "unknown" origin and US-defined laboratory-confirmed BSI (LCBI), were considered.

Conclusions: Our study showed an excellent concordance between US and European definitions of PN and primary BSI. PN and primary BSI rates of countries using either US or European definitions can be compared if the points highlighted in this study are taken into account.

Keywords: Bloodstream infection, Pneumonia, Definitions, Healthcare-associated infections

Background

Implementation of surveillance of healthcare-associated infections (HAI) has been shown to result in decreasing HAI rates and contributes to the prevention of HAI [1–3]. Feedback of data on HAI rates to clinical staff has been shown to be a key factor reducing these rates [4–6].

Comparing HAI rates of one's own institution with reference data seems to be particularly successful. In the 1970s, the US Centers for Disease Control and Prevention (CDC) created the National Nosocomial Infection Surveillance System (NNIS) and published uniform surveillance definitions for nosocomial infections [7–9]. These definitions have been updated gradually for surgical site infection (SSI) [10], for ventilator-associated pneumonia (VAP) [11], primary bloodstream infection (BSI) [12] and in 2010 for urinary tract infection (UTI) [13]. Key terms such as "device-associated infection" or "intensive care unit

* Correspondence: sonja.hansen@charite.de
[1]Institute for Hygiene and Environmental Medicine, Charité – University Medicine Berlin, Campus Benjamin Franklin, Hindenburgdamm 27, D-12203, Berlin, Germany
Full list of author information is available at the end of the article

(ICU)-associated infection" were also defined [14]. This system is now integrated as part of the National Healthcare Safety Network (NHSN) [12].

In the 1980s and 1990s, many European countries performed national prevalence studies of HAI and established national surveillance systems using CDC definitions or a modified version of these definitions [15], while other countries developed their own surveillance definitions that better reflected European diagnostic practices. The first harmonization of national surveillance activities in Europe was performed by the Hospitals in Europe Link for Infection Control through Surveillance (HELICS) project, which was funded by the European Commission in the context of Decision 2119/98/EC of the European Parliament and of the Council on communicable disease surveillance and control in EU Member States [16].

The HELICS project (2000–2004) developed case definitions for surgical site infection (SSI), pneumonia (PN), bloodstream infection (BSI), catheter-related infection (CRI) and urinary tract infection (UTI) and recommended their use in EU Member States [17,18]. The work of HELICS was continued as a component of the European Commission-funded Improving Patient Safety in Europe (IPSE) network (2005–2008). The IPSE network aimed at contributing to European surveillance of HAI by describing HAI epidemiology, improving the understanding of inter-country variation of HAI rates and facilitating quality-of-care improvements in a multi-centre setting. In July 2008, the IPSE network was transferred to the European Centre for Disease Prevention and Control (ECDC) [19,20]. Since this date, HAI surveillance activities in Europe are coordinated by ECDC and the network was re-named the Healthcare-Associated Infections surveillance Network (HAI-Net). HAI-Net adopted the European (HELICS/IPSE) definitions for its HAI surveillance modules and for the ECDC point prevalence survey of HAI in European acute care hospitals. Comparisons of HAI rates between countries are essential to raising awareness about HAI and their prevention and control, but require a standardized methodology, including uniform definitions. Because they were implemented independently, national HAI surveillance systems in European countries decided to use either the US (CDC/NHSN) definitions [12–14] or the European (HELICS/IPSE) definitions [17,18] and questions have been raised about whether comparisons of HAI rates between national networks were indeed appropriate. While adoption of the European definitions is mandatory for newly implemented national HAI surveillance systems, changing definitions could interrupt continuity of reference data and require reorganization for an existing national surveillance system.

The present study was conducted to assess the concordance between US (CDC/NHSN) definitions and European (HELICS/IPSE) definitions of HAI for inter-country comparison of HAI rates. The study was initiated and sponsored by ECDC through a specific service contract (ECD.1781) with the Institute for Hygiene and Environmental Medicine, Charité – University Medicine Berlin, Germany.

Methods
Setting
The study was conducted in seven European countries (Austria, Belgium, France, Germany, Hungary, Italy and Spain) with existing networks for HAI surveillance. Network leaders and a senior expert from ECDC (CS) represented the international study working group responsible for the development and implementation of the study. Three meetings at the Institute of Hygiene, Charité – University Medicine, Berlin, were held to agree on the methodology, data collection and analysis.

A one-month study pre-test was performed in two countries to evaluate the feasibility of the study.

Surveillance
HAI surveillance was performed in intensive care units (ICUs) in all participating countries between March 1st and May 31st, 2010. Network leaders delivered study documents and trained the local surveillance personnel for both types of definitions by using standardized case studies. No validation phase was included in the study.

All patients aged one year or above that presented with symptoms for selected HAI were included in surveillance according to both types of definitions. The HAI did not necessarily need to be acquired in the participating ICU, and patients coming from another ward of the same hospital with symptoms of infection were also surveyed upon ICU admission.

Local surveillance personnel collected data by using both types of definitions simultaneously. A study case was defined as a patient with a HAI according to either type of definition. In addition to the definitions' criteria, the following data were obtained for further analysis: date of birth, date of admission to the ICU and to the hospital, date of onset of HAI, underlying cardiac or pulmonary diseases, and immunosuppression status. In addition, surveillance personnel assessed whether the infection was ICU-acquired, according to both sets of criteria. Association with a central line or with mechanical ventilation was also included according to the US and the European definitions. BSI cases that did not fulfill the criteria of US definitions for laboratory-confirmed bloodstream infection (LCBI) because signs and symptoms were related to an infection at another site, were recorded as "secondary BSI missed by US definitions".

Statistical analysis

Because the question remains open as to which set of definitions represents the gold standard, we could only assess, for each type of infection, the concordance (agreement) between the two types of definitions. To estimate the concordance between two case definitions, Cohen's kappa (κ) statistic [21,22] was chosen.

For sample size calculation, an incidence of HAI (BSI and PN) of 1–5 per 100 patients was assumed and a kappa value of 0.75-0.90 was anticipated according to previous HAI concordance studies [23–26]. Based on a kappa value of 0.75 and on an expected HAI incidence of 1%, we estimated a sample size of 98 cases per infection type.

Results

Differences in definitions

Both sets of definitions of HAI were reviewed by the working group. The group identified differences for the definitions of BSI, PN and UTI (Table 1).

BSI definitions varied since CDC/NHSN does not accept a positive blood culture with a microorganism related to an infection at another site. PN definitions were different concerning the microbiological diagnostic criteria: HELICS/IPSE includes more detailed categories according to the sampling procedure and the microbiology technique whereas CDC/NHSN definitions include additional age-dependent criteria and a specific subcategory for immunocompromised patients (PNU3). UTI definitions were identical until the end of 2009. Differences appeared when CDC/NHSN modified its UTI definitions to include the new subcategory "asymptomatic bacteremic UTI" in January 2010.

Definitions of the key term "ICU-acquired infection" varied because HELICS/IPSE defines it as an infection occurring later than 48 hours after admission to an ICU, whereas CDC/NHSN requires that there is no evidence that the infection was present or incubating at the time of admission to the ICU, without time restriction [12]. There were also differences for the key term "mechanical ventilation", which are described in Table 1.

The working group agreed to analyze concordance for the definitions of BSI and PN, and for the key terms "ICU-acquired infection" and "mechanical ventilation".

Table 1 Differences in HAI definitions (CDC/NHSN vs. HELICS/IPSE)

Type of HAI or key term	CDC/NHSN definitions	HELICS/IPSE definitions
Bloodstream infection (BSI) / Laboratory-confirmed bloodstream Infection (LCBI)	•LCBI (Positive blood culture with recognized pathogen or 2 blood cultures with skin contaminant incl. clinical symptoms. Organism cultured from blood is not related to an infection at another site) •CSEP (Clinical sepsis in patients ≤ 1 year)	•BSI-A (Positive blood culture with recognized pathogen or 2 blood culture with skin contaminant incl. clinical symptoms. Origin: "Catheter" (C), "Secondary to another site" (S) or "Unknown" (U))
Catheter-related infection (CRI)	-*	•CRI 1 (Local central venous catheter (CVC)-related infection) •CRI 2 (General CVC-related infection) • CRI 3 (CVC-related BSI) • CCO (Catheter colonisation)
Pneumonia (PNU/PN)	• PNU1 (Clinically defined pneumonia) • PNU2 (Pneumonia with specific laboratory findings) • PNU3 (Pneumonia in immunocompromised patients)	• PN 1 (Protected sample + quantitative culture) • PN 2 (Non-protected sample + quantitative culture) • PN 3 (Alternative microbiological criteria) • PN 4 (Sputum bacteriology or non-quantitative endotracheal aspirate (ETA)) • PN 5 (No microbiological criterion (only clinical criteria))
Urinary tract infection (UTI)	• SUTI (Symptomatic UTI) †/‡ • ASB (Asymptomatic bacteriuria) † / •ABUTI (Asymptomatic bacteremic UTI) ‡ • OUTI (Other infections of the urinary tract) †/‡	• UTI-A (Symptomatic, microbiologically confirmed) • UTI-B (Symptomatic , not microbiologically confirmed) • UTI-C (Asymptomatic bacteriuria)
ICU-acquired HAI	• No evidence that the infection was present or incubating at the time of admission to the ICU	• Infection occurred later than 48 hours after admission in the ICU
Ventilator-associated	• A device to assist or control respiration continuously through a tracheostomy or by endotracheal intubation was present within the 48-hour period before the onset of infection, inclusive of the weaning period	• An invasive respiratory device was present (even intermittently) in the 48 hours preceding the onset of infection

*, not applicable.

†, until December 2008.

‡, since January 2009.

Since US and European definitions of UTI showed major differences because of recent modifications, UTI definitions were excluded from the study.

Participating ICUs

Surveillance was performed in 47 ICUs in 28 hospitals across 7 EU countries. The majority of participating ICUs were mixed ICUs, followed by medical and surgical ICUs. Three countries also surveyed paediatric patients in 9% of their participating ICUs. The characteristics of participating ICUs are presented in Table 2.

Agreement of definitions

For the study, 6,506 patients were assessed. The incidence of PN and of BSI were 2.8 and 1.9 per 100 patients, respectively. Overall, 180 PN and 123 BSI cases were identified by either the US definitions or the European definitions (Figures 1 and 2). Of all 180 PN cases, 178 were identified with the European definitions and 179 with the US definitions. Two PN cases were only identified with the US definitions due to age-dependent criteria that are not included in the European definitions. The third discordant case was a patient with microbiological findings that fulfilled a criterion for "PN 2" of the European definitions, but without sufficient criteria for PN according to the US definitions. These findings led to a kappa value of 0.99 for PN. Kappa values were lower when PN cases were subdivided into clinically defined PN ($\kappa = 0.90$) and microbiologically defined PN ($\kappa = 0.72$).

Since this subdivision did not take into account US-defined PNU3 cases (PN in immunocompromised patients), those cases were reclassified into US-defined PNU1 and PNU2. A repeated analysis of agreement within the new clinically and microbiologically defined PN groups resulted in equal agreement for clinically defined PN ($\kappa = 0.90$) and higher agreement for microbiologically defined PN ($\kappa = 0.84$).

Agreement of definitions for BSI showed a kappa value of 0.73. All 123 BSI cases were diagnosed by the European criteria. Forty-two percent of the BSI cases were missed when US definitions were used (Figure 2) because they were secondary to an infection at another site. In the remaining 72 cases, the BSI origin was either a catheter (central venous, peripheral or arterial) (30%) or unknown (29%). BSI concordance was perfect ($\kappa = 1.00$) when only primary BSI cases, i.e. Europe-defined BSI with either "catheter" or "unknown" origin and US-defined "LCBI", were analyzed.

For 245 (81%) of all cases the concordance of the key term "ICU-acquired" was analyzed. A few more HAI were classified as "ICU-acquired" according to the US definitions than to the European definitions (245 vs. 240); agreement was equal for ICU-acquired PN and for ICU-acquired BSI ($\kappa = 0.94$) (Table 3).

Discussion

HAI surveillance methods vary across Europe. Some countries use European definitions while other countries use US definitions. As a contribution to further harmonization of Europe-wide surveillance of HAI, this study assessed the concordance between US and European definitions of BSI and of PN, two major types of HAI that are partly preventable [27] and are under surveillance in most European countries. The recommendations of Landis and Koch for evaluating the strength of an agreement were used [28]. Overall, an "almost perfect" agreement was found for PN ($\kappa = 0.99$). This was different when PN cases were subdivided into clinically and microbiologically defined PN. More PN cases were classified as microbiologically-defined PN following the European definitions than the US definitions. This was still the case when Europe-defined PN2 cases which are based on the criteria "non-protective sample and quantitative culture" were considered as clinically defined PN. This difference was no longer evident when all

Table 2 Participating intensive care units (ICUs)

| Country | Number of ICUs / Number of hospitals | Number of ICUs per specialty* | | | | | Median number of beds per hospital | Median number of beds per ICU | Median number of beds with a ventilator per ICU (n) | Number of included patients |
		Mixed	Internal medicine	Surgery	Cardiac surgery	Other†				
Austria	7 / 1	3	3	0	0	1	2,137	8	8	132
Belgium	5 / 4	3	1	1	0	0	854	18	18	1,318
France	4 / 4	2	0	2	0	0	504	11	11	323
Germany	5 / 1	2	0	0	1	2	3,200	11	11	689
Hungary	15 / 10	7	1	2	2	3	1,163	10	10	2,311
Italy	7 / 4	2	1	2	0	2	474	8	8	1,031
Spain	4 / 4	3	0	0	0	1	600	19	16	702
All	**47 / 28**	**22**	**6**	**7**	**3**	**9**	**854**	**11**	**11**	**6,506**

* An ICU was defined as belonging to a specialty if ≥ 80% of patients in this ICU belonged to this specialty.
† Other: Neurosurgery, Paediatrics, Transplant surgery, Burn, Neurology.

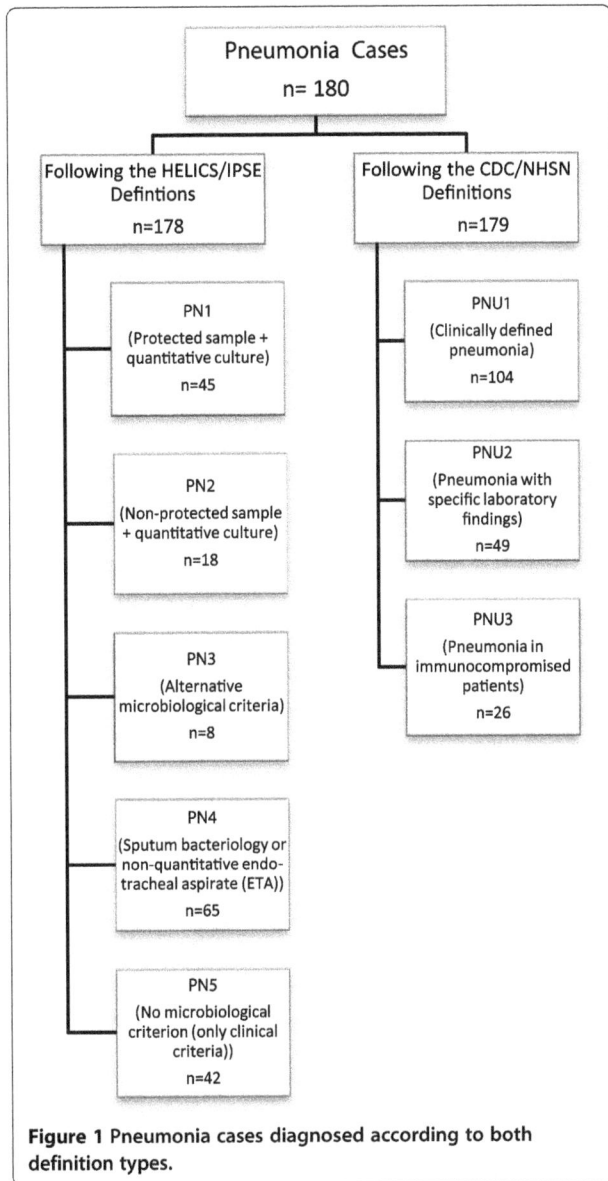

Figure 1 Pneumonia cases diagnosed according to both definition types.

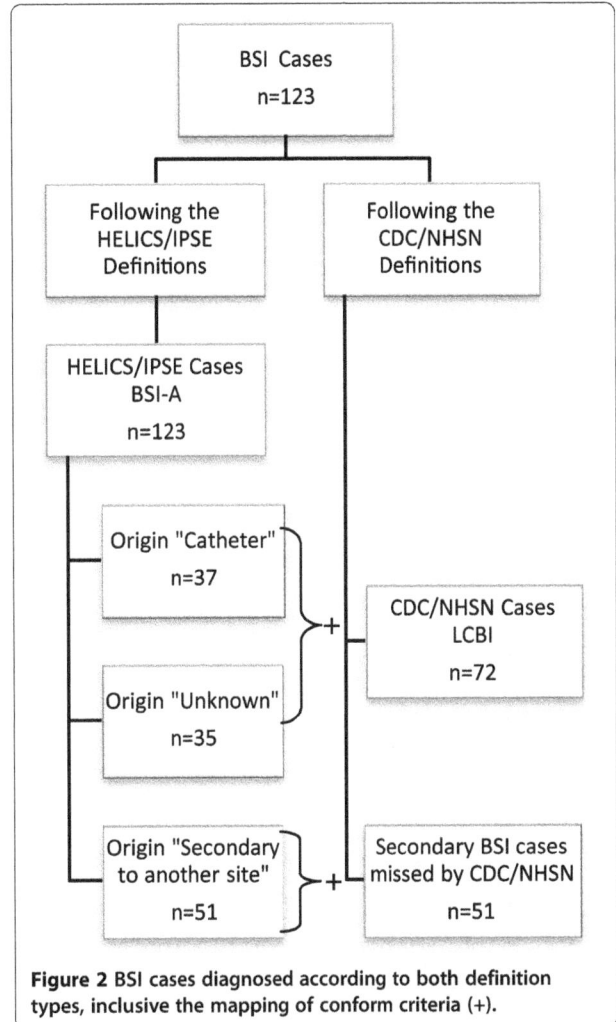

Figure 2 BSI cases diagnosed according to both definition types, inclusive the mapping of conform criteria (+).

US-defined PNU3 ("PN in immunocompromised patients") cases were reclassified into the US-defined categories PNU1 or PNU2. Since all 26 PNU3 cases could be classified as either PNU1 cases (n = 2) or PNU2 cases (n = 24), the results of this study suggest that the PNU3 subcategory may not be essential when performing surveillance of PN in immunocompromised patients.

As expected, concordance of BSI definitions was only "substantial" according to Landis and Koch [28]. Since one major criterion of US definitions, i.e. signs and symptoms of BSI must not be related to an infection at another site, is not included in the European definitions, 51 (42%) BSI cases were not identified with the US definition. With the European BSI definition, which includes the specification of the origin of the BSI, these

51 BSI cases were reported as "secondary to another infection site".

European definitions provide two more categories, i.e. "catheter" and "unknown", for origin of BSI [18]. The origin "catheter" was reported in 37 (30%) BSI cases and the origin "unknown" was reported in 35 (29%) BSI cases, which correspond to the "primary BSI" of the US definitions. All 72 of these BSI cases were also defined as LCBI cases with the US definitions. Thus for a potential comparison, US-defined LCBI cases should only be related to Europe-defined BSI cases with either "catheter" or "unknown" origin.

Definitions of the key term "ICU-acquired HAI" varied between the U.S. and Europe. According to European definitions 97% of HAI cases were defined as ICU-acquired (i.e. HAI occurring later than 48 hours after admission in the ICU). By contrast, according to the US definitions, all HAI cases were defined as ICU-acquired (i.e., no evidence that the infection was present or incubating at the time of admission to the ICU). Since US

Table 3 Concordance of HAI definitions, determined by Cohen's kappa statistic

Type of HAI or key term	Included cases based on:		Incidence of HAI (no. cases per 100 patients)	No. cases of HAI				No. patients without HAI	Cohen's kappa [95% confidence interval]
	US definitions	European definitions		According to either the European or the US definition	According to both the European and the US definitions	According to the European definition but not the US definition	According to the US definition but not the European definition		
Pneumonia	PNU1 + PNU2 + PNU3	PN1 + PN2 + PN3 + PN4 + PN5	2.8	180	177	1	2	6,326	0.99 [0.98 ; 1.00]
Clinically defined pneumonia	PNU1	PN2 + PN4 + PN5	2.0	127	102	23	2	6,379	0.89 [0.85 ; 0.93]
	PNU1	PN4 + PN5	1.8	119	92	15	12	6,387	0.87 [0.82 ; 0.92]
	PNU1*	PN2 + PN4 + PN5	2.0	127	104	21	2	6,379	0.90 [0.86 ; 0.94]
	PNU1*	PN4 + PN5	1.8	119	94	13	12	6,387	0.88 [0.83 ; 0.93]
Microbiologically defined pneumonia	PNU2	PN1 + PN3	1.0	65	37	16	12	6,441	0.72 [0.63 ; 0.82]
	PNU2	PN1 + PN2 + PN3	1.2	78	42	29	7	6,428	0.70 [0.60 ; 0.79]
	PNU2†	PN1 + PN3	1.1	73	53	0	20	6,433	0.84 [0.77 ; 0.91]
	PNU2†	PN1 + PN2 + PN3	1.3	84	60	11	13	6,422	0.83 [0.77 ; 0.90]
ICU-acquired pneumonia	Pneumonia not present or in incubation at admission	Pneumonia occurring >48 h after admission	2.3	147	144	0	3	28	0.94 [0.87 ; 1.00]
Mechanical ventilation	Continuous presence of device within 48 hours preceding pneumonia onset	Presence of device (even intermittently) within 48 hours preceding pneumonia onset	2.1	136	134	2	0	42	0.97 [0.93 ; 1.00]
Bloodstream infection (BSI)	Microorganism is not related to infection at another site	Origin of BSI is "catheter", "secondary to another site" or "unknown"	1.9	123	72	51	0	6,383	0.73 [0.66 ; 0.80]
Primary BSI	Microorganism is not related to infection at another site	Origin of BSI is "catheter" or "unknown"	1.1	72	72	0	0	51	1.00
ICU-acquired BSI	BSI not present or in incubation at admission	BSI occurring >48 h after admission	1.5	98	96	0	2	22	0.94 [0.87 ; 1.00]

*Including PNU3 cases (pneumonia in the immunocompromised patient) qualified as PNU1 after redistribution of PNU3 cases into PNU1 or PNU2.
† Including PNU3 cases (pneumonia in the immunocompromised patient) qualified as PNU2 after redistribution of PNU3 cases into PNU1 or PNU2.

definitions do not specify a time period between admission to the ICU and onset of symptoms, it is easy to explain why a few more HAI were recorded as ICU-acquired according to the US definitions. Nevertheless, agreement for the key term "ICU-acquired HAI" was still "almost perfect" according to Landis and Koch [28].

A strength of our study is that it was performed in seven European countries with different diagnostic methods and habits reflecting the variety of diagnostic practices in Europe. A limitation of the study is that the time of admission to the ICU and the time of onset of the HAI were recorded less precisely (in "days" instead of "hours") than in the original definition because the findings of the study pre-test revealed major difficulties in collecting time of onset data in "hours". As a consequence, all HAI occurring on or after the third day of ICU stay (rather than after 48 hours according to the European definitions), were defined as ICU-acquired. A further limitation was that specific patient groups, such as paediatric and immunocompromised patients, were likely to be underrepresented in the study.

In conclusion, countries using either US or European definitions for HAI surveillance can compare PN and primary BSI rates as long as the following points are taken into account. First, data should of course be valid and be collected following the original US and European definitions since country-specific modification of definitions may result in additional differences [29]. Second, PN data should always be compared in total, but not as subcategories of clinically defined and microbiologically defined PN. Third, for BSI the source should always be reported since all BSI cases with the origin "secondary to another site" according to European definitions should be excluded when making comparisons with US-defined BSI. Fourth, only Europe-defined BSI cases with either "catheter" or "unknown" origin should be compared to US-defined LCBI cases. Fifth, there are differences between US and European surveillance protocols, other than just case definitions of HAI, and these differences should be taken into account before performing comparison of HAI rates. Finally, comparisons are valid as long as US and European definitions do not change. Indeed, changing US definitions for PN to ventilator-associated complications under the influence of public reporting [30,31] would certainly affect the current good concordance between US and European definitions of PN.

Abbreviations
BSI: Bloodstream infection; CDC: Centers for disease control and prevention; ECDC: European Centre For Disease Prevention And Control; HAI: Healthcare-associated infection; HELICS: Hospitals in Europe Link for Infection Control through Surveillance; ICU: Intensive care unit; IPSE: Improving patient safety in Europe; k: Kappa; LCBI: Laboratory-confirmed bloodstream infection; NHSN: National Healthcare Safety Network; NNIS: System National Nosocomial Infection Surveillance System; PN: Pneumonia; PN1-5: Pneumonia case definitions (according to HELICS/IPSE); PNU1: Clinically defined pneumonia (according to CDC/NHSN); PNU2: Pneumonia with specific laboratory findings (according to CDC/NHSN); PNU3: Pneumonia in immunocompromised patients (according to CDC/NHSN); SSI: Surgical site infection; UTI: Urinary tract infection.

Competing interests
The study was supported by the European Centre for Disease Prevention and Control (ECDC) through a specific service contract (ECD.1781). The authors declare that they have no competing interests.

Authors' contributions
The study was designed by all members of the working group (PA, AB, PG, SH, WK, IM, MLM, MP, ES, CS) and by CG and DS. PG was the investigator of the study. SH coordinated the study. PA, AB, SH, IM, MLM, MP, ES performed the study in their respective countries. DS performed the statistical analysis. SH drafted the manuscript. All authors critically revised the manuscript and contributed substantially to the submitted version. All authors have read and approved the final manuscript.

Acknowledgements
The authors would like thank Michael Behnke and Florian Schmid, Charité – University Medicine Berlin, Germany, for support with data management and the following colleagues for making the surveillance data available:
Belgium: Karl Mertens, Scientific Institute of Public Health, Brussels; Pieter Depuydt, Ghent University Hospital, Gent; Pierre Damas, University Hospital Liège, Liège; Jacques Devriendt, Brugmann University Hospital, Brussels; Claire Boland, Clinique Saint-Jean, Brussels.
France: Jean-Winoc Decousser, Antoine Béclère Hospital, Clamart; Xavier Becanne, Hôtel Dieu Hospital, Paris; Anne Casetta, Hôtel Dieu Hospital, Paris; Alain Combès, General Hospital, Meaux; Jacques Merrer, Gilles Troché, General Hospital, Versailles.
Germany: Nadine Mönch, Andrea Landskron, Vivien Luchtenberg, Carola Schönborn, Charité – University Medicine, Berlin.
Hungary: Márta Patyi, Bács-Kiskun County Teaching Hospital, Kecskemét; Erika Rauth, University of Pecs Clinical Center; Sára Uray, Gabriella Csók, Gyula Prinz, Hungarian Institute of Cardiology, Budapest; Irén Németh, Military Hospital, Budapest; Erzsébet Rákay, Irén Heid, Tünde Aszalay, Szent János Hospital, Budapest; Erika Hemző, Szent Imre Hospital, Budapest; Kamilla Nagy, Renata Süli, University of Szeged, Albert Szent-Györgyi Clinical Center; Piroska Orosi, University of Debrecen; Zsuzsanna Fekete, Irén Kapus, Szent Lukács Hospital, Dombóvár; Zsófia Ozsvár, Szent György Hospital, Székesfehérvár.
Italy: Stefano Giordani, Massimo Girardis, Lucia Serio AUSL Modena; Maria Rita Melotti, Marco Adversi, Simonetta Baroncini AOU Bologna; Francesca Faccondini, Grazia Tura, AUSL Rimini; Veronica Cappelli, Davide Resi ASSR Emilia-Romagna.
Spain: MJ Lopez-Pueyo, Hospital Gral Yagüe, Burgos; Magda Campins, Hospital Vall Hebron, Barcelona; Josu Insausti, Hospital Provincial, Pamplona.

Author details
[1]Institute for Hygiene and Environmental Medicine, Charité – University Medicine Berlin, Campus Benjamin Franklin, Hindenburgdamm 27, D-12203, Berlin, Germany. [2]C-CLIN Nord - Département de santé publique, Université Pierre & Marie Curie, Paris, France. [3]Clinical Institute for Hygiene and Medical Microbiology, Medical University of Vienna, Vienna, Austria. [4]National Surveillance of Infections in Hospitals - NSIH, Operational Direction Public Health and Surveillance, Scientific Institute of Public Health, Brussels, Belgium. [5]Agenzia Sanitaria e Sociale Regione Emilia Romagna, Area di Programma Rischio Infettivo, Bologna, Italy. [6]Department of Intensive Care, Hospital Vall d'Hebron, Barcelona, Spain. [7]National Centre for Epidemiology, Department of Hospital Epidemiology, Budapest, Hungary. [8]European Centre for Disease Prevention and Control, Stockholm, Sweden.

References
1. Haley RW, Culver DH, White JW, Morgan WM, Emori TG, Munn VP, Hooton TM: The efficacy of infection surveillance and control programs in preventing nosocomial infections in US hospitals. Am J Epidemiol 1985, 121:182–205.
2. Geubbels E, Bakker HG, Houtman P, Van Noort-Klaassen MA, Pelk MS, Sassen TM, Wille JC: Promoting quality through surveillance of surgical site

infections: five prevention success stories. *Am J Infect Control* 2004, **32**:424–430.

3. Gastmeier P, Schwab F, Sohr D, Behnke M, Geffers C: **Reproducibility of the surveillance effect to decrease nosocomial infection rates.** *Infect Control Hosp Epidemiol* 2009, **30**:993–999.

4. Astagneau P, L'Hériteau F: **Surveillance of surgical-site infections: impact on quality of care and reporting dilemmas.** *Curr Opin Infect Dis* 2010, **23**:306–310.

5. Gastmeier P, Sohr D, Schwab F, Behnke M, Zuschneid I, Brandt C, Dettenkofer M, Chaberny IF, Rüden H, Geffers C: **Ten years of KISS: the most important requirements for success.** *J Hosp Infect* 2008, **70**(Suppl 1):11–16.

6. Gaynes R, Richards C, Edwards J, Emori TG, Horan T, Alonso-Echanove J, Fridkin S, Lawton R, Peavy G, Tolson J: **Feeding back surveillance data to prevent hospital-acquired infections.** *Emerg Infect Dis* 2001, **7**:295–298.

7. Horan TC, White JW, Jarvis WR, Emori TG, Culver DH, Munn VP, Thornsberry C, Olson DR, Hughes JM: **Nosocomial infection surveillance, 1984.** *MMWR CDC Surveill Summ* 1986, **35**:17–29.

8. Hughes JM: **Nosocomial infection surveillance in the United States: historical perspective.** *Infect Control* 1987, **8**:450–453.

9. Garner JS, Jarvis WR, Emori TG, Horan TC, Hughes JM: **CDC definitions for nosocomial infections, 1988.** *Am J Infect Control* 1988, **16**:128–140.

10. Horan TC, Gaynes RP, Martone WJ, Jarvis WR, Emori TG: **CDC definitions of nosocomial surgical site infections, 1992: a modification of CDC definitions of surgical wound infections.** *Infect Control Hosp Epidemiol* 1992, **13**:606–608.

11. Horan T, Gaynes R: **Surveillance of nosocomial infections.** In *Hospital Epidemiology and Infection Control.* 3rd edition. Edited by Mayhall CG. Philadelphia: Lippincott Williams &Wilkins; 2004:1659–1689.

12. Horan TC, Andrus M, Dudeck MA: **CDC/NHSN surveillance definition of health care-associated infection and criteria for specific types of infections in the acute care setting.** *Am J Infect Control* 2008, **36**:309–332.

13. Gould C, Allen-Bridson K, Horan T: **Surveillance definitions for urinary tract infections.** *Clin Infect Dis* 2009, **49**:1288–1289.

14. Horan TC, Emori TG: **Definitions of key terms used in the NNIS System.** *Am J Infect Control* 1997, **25**:112–116.

15. Gastmeier P, Kampf G, Wischnewski N, Schumacher M, Daschner F, Rüden H: **Importance of the surveillance method: national prevalence studies on nosocomial infections and the limits of comparison.** *Infect Control Hosp Epidemiol* 1998, **19**:661–667.

16. *Decision No 2119/98/EC of the European Parliament and of the Council of 24 September 1998 setting up a network for the epidemiological surveillance and control of communicable diseases in the Community;* http://ec.europa.eu/health/communicable_diseases/early_warning/comm_legislation_en.htm *(accessed on 2012-03-12).*

17. Suetens C, Savey A, Labeeuw J, Morales I: **The ICU-HELICS programme: towards European surveillance of hospital-acquired infections in intensive care units.** *Euro Surveill* 2002, **7**:127–128.

18. Suetens C, Morales I, Savey A, Palomar M, Hiesmayr M, Lepape A, Gastmeier P, Schmit JC, Valinteliene R, Fabry J: **European surveillance of ICU-acquired infections (HELICS-ICU): methods and main results.** *J Hosp Infect* 2007, **65**(Suppl 2):171–173.

19. European Centre for Disease Prevention and Control (ECDC): *Annual Epidemiological Report on Communicable Diseases in Europe 2008.* Stockholm: ECDC; 2008:16–38.

20. European Centre for Disease Prevention and Control (ECDC): **Epidemiology of communicable diseases in Europe, 2006.** In *Annual Epidemiological Report on Communicable Diseases in Europe 2008.* Stockholm: ECDC; 2008:289–295.

21. Cohen J: **A coefficient of agreement for nominal scales.** *Educ Psychol Meas* 1960, **20**:37–46.

22. Cohen J: **Weighted kappa: Nominal scale agreement with provision for scaled disagreement or partial credit.** *Psych Bull* 1968, **70**:213–220.

23. Minei JP, Hawkins K, Moody B, Uchal LB, Joy K, Christensen LL, Haley RW: **Alternative case definitions of ventilator associated pneumonia identify different patients in a surgical intensive care unit.** *Shock* 2000, **14**:331–337.

24. Wilson A, Gibbons C, Reeves B, Hiodgson B, Liu M, Plummer D, Krukowski ZH, Bruce J, Wilson J, Pearson A: **Surgical wound infection as a performance indicator: agreement of common definitions of wound infection in 4773 patients.** *BMJ* 2004, **329**:720.

25. Gastmeier P, Hentschel J, De Veer I, Obladen M, Rüden H: **Device-associated nosocomial infection surveillance in neonatal intensive care using specified criteria for neonates.** *J Hosp Infect* 1998, **38**:51–60.

26. Beck K, Gastmeier P: **Clinical or epidemiologic diagnosis of nosocomial pneumonia: Is there any difference?** *Am J Infect Control* 2003, **31**:331–335.

27. Harbarth S, Sax H, Gastmeier P: **The preventable proportion of nosocomial infections: an overview of published reports.** *J Hosp Infect* 2003, **54**:258–266.

28. Landis JR, Koch GG: **The measurement of observer agreement for categorical data.** *Biometrics* 1977, **33**:159–174.

29. Hansen S, Schwab F, Behnke M, Carsauw H, Heczko P, Klavs I, Lyytikäinen O, Palomar M, Riesenfeld Orn I, Savey A, Szilagyi E, Valinteliene R, Fabry J, Gastmeier P: **National influences on catheter-associated bloodstream infection rates: practices among national surveillance networks participating in the European HELICS project.** *J Hosp Infect* 2009, **71**:66–73.

30. Klompas M, Kleinman K, Khan Y, Evans RS, Lloyd JF, Stevenson K, Samore M, Platt R: **CDC Prevention Epicenters Program. Rapid and reproducible surveillance for ventilator-associated pneumonia.** *Clin Infect Dis* 2012, **54**:370–377.

31. Magill SS, Fridkin SK: **Improving surveillance definitions for ventilator-associated pneumonia in an era of public reporting and performance measurement.** *Clin Infect Dis* 2012, **54**:378–80.

Implementation of an antimicrobial stewardship program targeting residents with urinary tract infections in three community long-term care facilities: a quasi-experimental study using time-series analysis

Sarah B. Doernberg[1*], Victoria Dudas[2] and Kavita K. Trivedi[3]

Abstract

Background: Asymptomatic bacteriuria in the elderly commonly results in antibiotic administration and, in turn, contributes to antimicrobial resistance, adverse drug events, and increased costs. This is a major problem in the long-term care facility (LTCF) setting, where residents frequently transition to and from the acute-care setting, often transporting drug-resistant organisms across the continuum of care. The goal of this study was to assess the feasibility and efficacy of antimicrobial stewardship programs (ASPs) targeting urinary tract infections (UTIs) at community LTCFs.

Methods: This was a quasi-experimental study targeting antibiotic prescriptions for UTI using time-series analysis with 6-month retrospective pre-intervention and 6-month intervention period at three community LTCFs. The ASP team (infectious diseases (ID) pharmacist and ID physician) performed weekly prospective audit and feedback of consecutive prescriptions for UTI. Loeb clinical consensus criteria were used to assess appropriateness of antibiotics; recommendations were communicated to the primary treating provider by the ID pharmacist. Resident outcomes were recorded at subsequent visits. Generalized estimating equations using segmented regression were used to evaluate the impact of the ASP intervention on rates of antibiotic prescribing and antibiotic resistance.

Results: One-hundred and four antibiotic prescriptions for UTI were evaluated during the intervention, and recommendations were made for change in therapy in 40 (38 %), out of which 10 (25 %) were implemented. Only eight (8 %) residents started on antibiotics for UTI met clinical criteria for antibiotic initiation. An immediate 26 % decrease in antibiotic prescriptions for UTI during the ASP was identified with a 6 % reduction continuing through the intervention period (95 % Confidence Interval ([CI)] for the difference: −8 to −3 %). Similarly, a 25 % immediate decrease in all antibiotic prescriptions was noted after introduction of the ASP with a 5 % reduction continuing throughout the intervention period (95 % CI: −8 to −2 %). No significant effect was noted on resistant organisms or *Clostridium difficile*.

(Continued on next page)

* Correspondence: sarah.doernberg@ucsf.edu
[1]Department of Internal Medicine, Division of Infectious Diseases, University of California, San Francisco, 513 Parnassus Avenue, room S-380, Box 0645, San Francisco, CA 94143, USA
Full list of author information is available at the end of the article

(Continued from previous page)

Conclusion: Weekly prospective audit and feedback ASP in three community LTCFs over 6 months resulted in antibiotic utilization decreases but many lost opportunities for intervention.

Keywords: Urinary tract infection, Antimicrobial stewardship, Long-term care, Antimicrobial resistance

Background

Asymptomatic bacteriuria in the elderly commonly results in antibiotic administration despite evidence showing no clinical benefit [1–6]. In turn, antibiotic overuse contributes to antimicrobial resistance, adverse drug events, and increased costs in the long-term care facility (LTCF) population [7–17]. As the elderly population grows, these consequences become more problematic.

Currently, over 3 million individuals reside in LTCFs in the United States, and the complexity of underlying conditions is increasing [18]. Correspondingly, these residents frequently transition to and from the acute-care setting, often transporting drug-resistant organisms across the continuum of care [19, 20]. Recently published work assessing prevalence of drug-resistant organisms in LTCFs indicates that antimicrobial stewardship efforts are necessary [21, 22].

Antimicrobial stewardship programs (ASP) are viewed as resident safety initiatives designed to improve clinical outcomes while reducing adverse effects [23]. These types of programs have proven to be effective in acute care hospitals and LTCFs affiliated with tertiary care centers but have not been as well-studied in community LTCFs [24–34]. Because staffing levels, patient care models, and overall goals differ between the LTCF and the acute care settings, the ideal design and execution of an ASP in the LTCF setting will likely diverge. In addition, since September 2009 when the Interpretative Guidelines for Long-Term Care Facilities was issued, the Centers for Medicare and Medicaid Services (CMS) have stated that it is the LTCF physician's responsibility to prescribe appropriate antibiotics and to establish the indication for use of these medications; furthermore, consultant pharmacists are encouraged to review indications for antibiotic use and report findings to the physician [35]. Despite this regulatory backbone, it remains unclear how best to implement ASPs in the LTCF setting.

The objectives of this study were to assess the feasibility and efficacy of implementing an ASP utilizing a syndromic approach targeting urinary tract infections (UTIs) at community, stand-alone LTCFs.

Methods
Study design

A prospective quasi-experimental study was performed to implement an ASP targeted at UTIs diagnosed and treated at three community LTCFs in Northern California between September 2011 and May 2012. The ASP team consisted of an Infectious Diseases (ID)-trained clinical pharmacist and an ID physician, who worked closely with the infection control practitioners at each of the respective LTCFs.

The study period was divided into two phases: pre-intervention (7 months) and intervention (7 months). During the pre-intervention phase, baseline information on facility-level antimicrobial susceptibility patterns and antimicrobial utilization were collected from each LTCF. During the intervention phase, the ID pharmacist made weekly site visits to each LTCF to identify residents receiving antibiotics for UTIs which was determined by infection control and nursing administration records at each site. Individual variables, including resident demographics, comorbidities, vital signs, documented exam findings, laboratory results, and additional antibiotics for each resident on antibiotics for UTI, were collected weekly by the ID pharmacist by review of the medical record. The ID pharmacist and ID physician then consulted, and recommendations were formulated utilizing the Loeb clinical consensus criteria for initiation of antibiotics in the LTCF setting as a guideline [36]. For residents not meeting clinical consensus criteria, the ASP team used clinical judgement including input from subspecialists and the resident's predisposition for other infections, to determine if antibiotics were indicated and to help formulate recommendations. The ID pharmacist subsequently conveyed the ASP recommendations to the primary treating provider via telephone or fax. Fax was utilized a minority of the time with one specific provider who expressed a preference for this form of communication. Implementation of recommendations and clinical course of each resident was recorded at subsequent visits, including vital sign abnormalities, white blood cell count, change in antibiotics, need to transfer to acute care, or death. Data on facility-level antibiotic susceptibility patterns and antibiotic utilization was collected, in a similar manner to the pre-intervention phase, for the intervention phase.

Ethics, consent, and permissions

This study was reviewed by the Committee for the Protection of Human Subjects of the California Health and Human Services Agency and was deemed not to be research and therefore exempt from approval. As a result and because implementation of this study was evaluated as a quality improvement initiative, consent was not obtained from residents in the participating facilities.

Setting and population

This intervention took place at three community, stand-alone LTCFs in Northern California: facility A is licensed for 77 subacute beds and 82 skilled nursing beds with 3 physicians; facility B has 478 licensed skilled nursing beds with 5 physicians and 1 nurse practitioner; facility C is comprised of two sister facilities located blocks away from each other and licensed for 60 and 65 skilled nursing beds respectively with 2 physicians and 1 nurse practitioner. Because the medical staff and population of these latter two facilities overlap significantly, facility C was analyzed as one LTCF. Subjects included any resident of the skilled nursing or subacute sections of these LTCFs being treated for UTI with an antibiotic at the time of the ID pharmacist visit each week. Subjects were excluded if they resided in the psychiatric or acute rehabilitation units at each facility or if antibiotic initiation for UTI occurred at an acute care facility.

Process and outcome measurements

Outcome of recommendations and clinical course for residents experiencing ASP interventions were recorded at subsequent visits through chart review. Recommendations were considered "accepted" if the suggested change (or discontinuation) of antimicrobials was made within 24 h of the ASP recommendation being communicated. Resident-days were collected from each facility. Antibiotic use was measured as antibiotic starts per 1000 resident-days. Data on antibiotic starts were obtained from the infection control practitioner at each facility. All LTCFs utilized a maintenance log of all antibiotic starts, which included indication for the antibiotic, allowing for determination of both a UTI and overall rate of antibiotic use.

Culture data, including information on susceptibility, was obtained from the diagnostic laboratories utilized by each of the facilities. As a marker for potential downstream consequence of antibiotic pressure, we collected information on rates of *Clostridium difficile*, ceftriaxone-resistant *Enterobacteriaceae* (including extended-spectrum β-lactamase (ESBL) producing organisms), fluoroquinolone-resistant *Pseudomonas aeruginosa*, and vancomycin-resistant Enterococci isolated from any site for each facility. Rates of these organisms were calculated from cultures that were collected as a part of routine clinical care. An individual resident could contribute more than one clinical culture since the unit of measurement was the culture. Rates were calculated based on number of cases of each resistant organism normalized to resident-days.

Analysis

Generalized estimating equations using segmented regression and a Poisson distribution accounting for clustering by facility were used to evaluate the impact of the ASP intervention on rates of antibiotic prescribing and antibiotic resistance. This model generated four important estimates: 1. The pre-intervention trend in incidence ($\beta 1$); 2. The immediate change upon initiation of the ASP ($\beta 2$); 3. The difference between the pre- and intervention trend ($\beta 3$); and 4. The intervention period rate change ($\beta 1 + \beta 3$) [37]. The combination of $\beta 1$ and $\beta 3$ prevented the attribution of changes preceding the intervention from being attributed to the effects of the intervention. Because of the concern for autocorrelation between observations over the time of this study given the time-series design, first order positive and negative autocorrelation was assessed using the Durbin-Watson statistic, which did not suggest evidence of autocorrelation in these models. Robust standard errors were used to estimate variance. Significance was defined as $P \le 0.05$. STATA software (ver 11, StataCorp 2009) was used for all statistical analyses except the Durbin-Watson statistic, which were performed with SAS version 9.3 (SAS Institute Inc., Cary, NC).

Results

Resident characteristics

During the historical pre-intervention phase (April 2011–October 2012), there were combined 118,070 resident-days from the participating LTCFs. During the intervention phase (November 2012–May 2012), there were combined 113,220 resident-days from the LTCFs. Table 1 demonstrates the baseline characteristics of the 104 reviewed prescriptions during the intervention. The average temperature and white blood cell counts for residents were within the normal range. Most residents had pyuria and positive markers of urinary tract inflammation on urinalysis. Despite these findings, only 8 % of residents started on antibiotics for UTI who were evaluated during the intervention met the Loeb minimum criteria for antibiotic initiation [36]. Of those meeting Loeb criteria, 6 % were not catheterized and 2 % catheterized. Both of the catheterized residents met Loeb criteria on fever alone. In those non-catheterized residents meeting criteria, 33 % had dysuria plus urinary frequency, 33 % had dysuria plus incontinence, 17 % had fever plus hematuria, and 17 % had fever plus incontinence.

Escherichia coli was the most common urinary organism treated (in 70 % of residents), and gram-negative rods predominated the positive urine cultures (accounting for 95 % of treated urine cultures). Of the prescriptions that were reviewed, fluoroquinolones were the most commonly prescribed antibiotics (9 prescriptions, 39 %), followed by

Table 1 Characteristics of residents started on antibiotics for urinary tract infection who were reviewed during the intervention

Baseline characteristic	Intervention (n = 104)
Age, mean, years (Standard Deviation (SD))	80.8 (14.4)
Male gender, number (%)	70 (67)
Facility, number (%)	–
A	22 (21)
B	63 (61)
C	19 (18)
Charlson comorbidity index, median (IQR)	2 (1–3)
Temperature, mean, F (SD)	98.2 (1.1)
Indwelling catheter in prior 48 h, number (%)	7 (7)
WBC $\times 10^9$/L, mean (range)	9.9 (4.1–21.3)
Urine WBCs/hpf >10, n (%)	89 (86)
Urine leukocyte esterase, number/total sent (%)	89/91 (98)
Urine nitrites, number/total sent (%)	51/91 (56)
Meets criteria for UTI, n (%)	8 (8)
No catheter	6 (75)
Catheter	2 (25)

IQR interquartile range, *WBC* white blood cell count, *hpf* high-powered field, *SD* standard deviation, *UTI* urinary tract infection

nitrofurantoin (5 prescriptions, 22 %), trimethoprim-sulfamethoxazole (4 prescriptions, 17 %), cephalexin (3 prescriptions, 13 %), and amoxicillin +/– clavulanate (2 prescriptions, 9 %). Intravenous therapy was infrequently prescribed.

Process measures

There were 292 prescriptions for UTI during the pre-intervention phase and 183 during the intervention. Of the 183 prescriptions for UTI, 104 were able to be reviewed by the Pharmacist. Of these, recommendations for change in therapy were made in 38 %, and 10 (25 %) were accepted. Twenty-four percent of the recommendations were to discontinue antibiotics; 2 % to streamline antibiotics; and 11 % to shorten the course of antibiotics. No recommendations were made to broaden antibiotics, lengthen course, or change route. The majority of recommendations were made by phone. A small minority (<5 %) were made by fax.

Of the 59 % of antibiotic prescriptions for UTI where recommendations were not communicated to the primary provider, there was either agreement with current management (12 residents, 19 %) or completion of the antibiotic course within 2 days from the time of review (52 residents, 81 %). Because the antimicrobial course was due to end concurrently with review, interventions were not made in the latter group. Of this group of 52 residents, antibiotics were not felt to be indicated in 44 (85 %). Of note, the percentage of residents where there

was concordance with antibiotic management exceeded the percentage meeting Loeb criteria for UTI. In the cases where there was a discrepancy, the ASP team considered extenuating circumstances, including recommendations for antibiotics from other subspecialists, family dynamics, and concurrent treatment for other infections. The remainder of antibiotic prescriptions was not reviewed due to an inability to determine if the prescription was for UTI, the entire antibiotic course was completed in between weekly ID Pharmacist visits, or the antibiotic was initiated in an acute care setting.

Outcome measures

Crude incidence rates for antibiotic prescriptions and resistant organisms are shown in Table 2. Incidence rate ratios for the segmented regression for antibiotic utilization are shown in Table 3. Monthly rates, both measured and predicted by our statistical model, for antibiotic starts are shown in Fig. 1. During the pre-intervention phase, there was a trend towards a significant increase in antibiotic starts for UTI (4 % increase, $P = 0.06$). Upon initiation of the ASP intervention, a 26 % immediate decrease in antibiotic prescriptions for UTI was observed, and there was a 9 % change in the trend from the pre-intervention phase to the intervention phase. After the initial intervention effect, there was a 6 % decrease in the rate of antibiotic prescriptions for UTI per month continuing throughout the intervention period (95 % Confidence Interval [CI]: –8 to –3 %). There was no change in antibiotic prescription rates for all indications during the pre-intervention phase. With the introduction of the intervention, there was a 25 % decrease in all antibiotic

Table 2 Crude incidence rates for antibiotic starts

Month	Antibiotic starts, UTI[a]	Antibiotic starts, all indications
1	1.8	4.8
2	2.4	5.1
3	2.1	4.6
4	3.5	6.5
5	2.7	5.8
6	2.4	5.6
7	2.4	6.2
Intervention began		
8	2.6	4.4
9	1.5	4.2
10	1.3	3.8
11	1.2	3.6
12	1.5	4.3
13	1.2	2.8
14	1.9	3.4

UTI urinary tract infection
[a]N/1000 resident-days for antibiotic measurements

Table 3 Incidence rate-ratios for an interrupted time-series model of antibiotic prescriptions

Parameter	Co-efficient	Incidence rate ratio (95 % confidence interval)	P-value
		Antibiotic starts, UTI	
Pre-intervention trend	β1	1.04 (1.00–1.07)	0.06
Immediate intervention change	β2	0.74 (0.64–0.84)	<0.001
Change in trend after intervention	β3	0.91 (0.89–0.93)	<0.001
Intervention trend	β1 + β3	0.94 (0.92–0.97)	<0.001
		All antibiotic starts	
Pre-intervention trend	β1	1.04 (0.96–1.13)	0.30
Immediate intervention change	β2	0.75 (0.67–0.84)	<0.001
Change in trend after intervention	β3	0.91 (0.81–1.02)	0.09
Intervention trend	β1 + β3	0.95 (0.92–0.98)	0.001

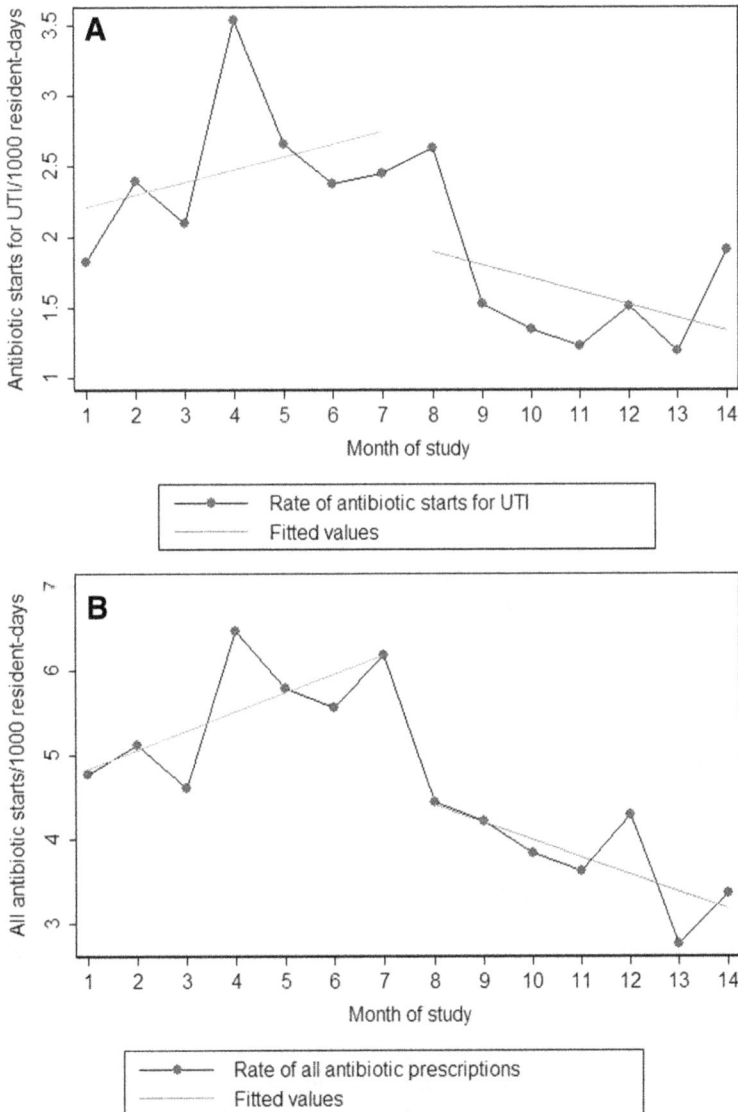

Fig. 1 a Predicted and actual rates for antibiotic starts for UTI per 1000 resident-days; (**b**) Predicted and actual rates for antibiotic starts for all indications per 1000 resident-days. Predicted rates are based on the intervention trend calculated from the time-series model. The intervention started in month 8

prescriptions. After this initial decrease, there was a non-significant trend toward decreasing antibiotic prescriptions compared to the pre-intervention phase (95 % CI: −19 to 2 %). During the entire intervention phase, there was a 5 % decrease in all antibiotic starts.

To evaluate the consequence of antibiotic pressure on clinical cultures for common resistant organisms, rates of *Clostridium difficile*, ceftriaxone-resistant *Enterobacteriaceae*, fluoroquinolone-resistant *Pseudomonas aeruoginosa*, and vancomycin-resistant *Enterococci* were examined. There were no significant changes in rates of any of these organisms throughout the study period (data not shown).

Discussion

Introduction of a weekly prospective audit and feedback ASP in three community LTCFs resulted in modest decreases in antibiotic utilization but encountered several barriers to effective ASP implementation. Despite having a dedicated ID pharmacist and physician available once weekly for reviews, there were many missed opportunities for intervention and low acceptance rates when recommendations were made.

Given the modest effect observed with implementation of our ASP in this study, we have identified several areas for improvement in future interventions. First, given that 85 % of the prescriptions that were not reviewed were deemed unnecessary, an ASP with more frequent review of residents on antibiotics might be more useful, though it may not be feasible with resource limitations and the general unavailability of ID physicians and pharmacists in the LTCF setting. More education and training of non-Infectious Diseases specialized providers may help to bolster a more robust ASP at these facilities.

Second, there were many missed opportunities for intervention to improve or to identify prescribing habits associated with good antimicrobial stewardship, even if the recommendation would not affect that particular course of antimicrobials (e.g. in the case of a resident whose course was scheduled to end the day of review). In future studies, educational feedback with the goal of broadly changing antimicrobial prescribing habits may be more successful. The large initial decrease in antimicrobial prescriptions suggests that knowledge of program implementation itself may have affected prescribing practice; whether this decrease would have been sustained longer than 6 months warrants further investigation.

In addition, our largest barrier was establishing relationships with prescribers in this setting as compared with acute care. Because much of the medical care occurs remotely in the LTCF population, establishing interpersonal relationships between the ASP and the primary treating providers proved challenging due to lack of face-to-face interaction and lack of a prior provider-to-provider relationship. This barrier limited physician and

advanced care practitioner buy-in and implementation of recommendations. In future interventions, it may be helpful if the ASP champion was identified from within the institution, though this may be problematic if sufficient knowledge of antimicrobial stewardship principles is lacking at the local level. If stewardship is to be initiated by an outside consultant, concerted efforts to establish a relationship with providers should be pursued, such as educational seminars, face-to-face meetings, and collaboration in design of the program.

Lastly, primary treating providers reported feeling pressured by nursing staff and, to some extent, resident families to send urinalyses and urine cultures for indications such as cloudy urine, foul-smelling urine, or temporary behavior changes. When these cultures tested positive, regardless of whether the symptoms had disappeared prior to therapy, the residents were often treated. Front-line staff education must remain a specific focus of future ASP interventions in the LTCF setting since this group plays a vital role in establishing the prescribing culture of an institution. A recent study at the VA Healthcare System, which included an associated long-term care facility, found that an educational campaign aimed to improve treatment for catheter-associated UTI decreased the number of urine cultures sent by 71 %, which corresponded to a 76 % decrease in overtreatment for asymptomatic bacteruria [38]. The decreases were most pronounced in the LTCF portion of the study. Stewardship of urinalysis and urine culture, including among nursing staff and families, may be an effective upstream method for decreasing inappropriate antibiotic use for UTI in the LTCF setting. In fact, in the acute care setting, a recent pilot study demonstrated that suppressing urine culture results in noncatheterized patients resulted in decreased treatment of asymptomatic bacteriuria without any untoward consequences [39]. Though this degree of intervention may be risky and require more resources, it does support the notion that limiting cultures may limit overtreatment of asymptomatic bacteriuria.

Our study has several additional important limitations aside from the barriers to success. Because it took place over a 14-month period, the pre-intervention and intervention phases occurred during different seasons, so temporal trends could not be eliminated. We attempted to adjust for this with our statistical analyses by using a time-series analysis approach. In addition, the 2011–2012 influenza season was accounted for mainly during the intervention phase, so antibiotic prescriptions would be expected to increase during the intervention, which is the opposite of what was observed. We only identified 104 cases of treated UTI in three nursing homes in 6 months of our study intervention so our study power was lower than expected but sometimes unavoidable in real-life research. In order to identify cases we relied on Infection

Control reports of antimicrobial prescriptions, which may have been limited by recall bias. Obtaining prescription data would have allowed for a more objective measurement of prescriptions during the pre- and post-intervention periods. It would also have allowed for more information regarding days of therapy and length of therapy. Unfortunately, we did not have access to pharmacy records at two of the sites due to pharmacies being located off-site and operated by third-party vendors.

Several other groups have implemented stewardship initiatives in the LTCF setting with varied success. Jump and colleagues found an even larger decrease in antimicrobial utilization with initiation of an ID service at a LTCF associated with a Veterans Affairs Hospital [40]. That study included a more resource-intensive and comprehensive approach to antimicrobial stewardship with a team that physically staffed consults during weekly visits and took additional calls throughout the week, a model that is unlikely to be feasible, especially at LTCFs that are not academically affiliated. Several other studies have explored less resource-intensive approaches, such as educational interventions. Two studies have demonstrated approximately 30 % decrease in antimicrobial prescribing for UTI after educational interventions aimed at appropriate evaluation and treatment of UTI versus asymptomatic bacteriuria [29, 33]. Additional studies have demonstrated 12–30 % decreases in antibiotic use with educational interventions focused on appropriate diagnosis and treatment of common infectious syndromes [31, 32]. The decrease in antibiotic use in our study was lower than that seen with the educational interventions alone. However, the most effective published strategy is an educational intervention consisting of mailing an antibiotic prescribing guide combined with physician-specific antibiotic prescribing profiles (physicians in the experimental group were 64 % less likely to prescribe non-adherent antibiotics than those in the control group (Odds Ratio = 0.36, 95 % CI = 0.18–0.73), suggesting that physician feedback is an essential component [30]. Provider characteristics have been demonstrated to play an important role in duration of antibiotic prescriptions independent of severity of underlying disease, suggesting that high-prescribing physicians may be good targets for these types of ASP interventions [41]. Combining education with an audit and feedback ASP would allow for targeted physician feedback and therefore even more benefit on improving prescribing habits.

Conclusion

Our findings suggest that an ASP with a syndromic approach has the potential to be effective in the LTCF setting but further studies are needed to determine the most robust and efficient design for such an intervention. The addition of an educational program with prescriber

feedback, which has proven beneficial in prior studies, might strengthen the benefits of an audit and feedback ASP alone. Our ASP was not able to provide as much educational support given that the ASP team and primary treating providers were not often at the LTCF at the same time. A dedicated educational aspect to the ASP would also allow for institutional changes such as educating the nursing staff in identifying residents at risk and diagnosing bacteriuria as well as the conviction from providers that positive cultures mandate therapy. Moving forward, qualitative analyses may be important to identify key stakeholders in the antibiotic prescribing process in LTCFs. Design of future interventions should incorporate education targeting these stakeholders as well as focused audit and feedback of prescriptions for specific common infectious syndromes.

Competing interests
All authors report no competing interests relevant to this article.

Authors' contributions
Study design: SD, VD, KT. Data collection: SD, VD. Data analysis: SD, KT. Drafting manuscript: SD, KT. All authors read and approved the final manuscript.

Acknowledgements
Financial support: Supported in part by a research grant from the Investigator Initiated Studies Program of Merck Sharp & Dohme Corp to the National Foundation for the Centers for Disease Control and Prevention Inc.The opinions expressed in this paper are those of the authors and do not necessarily represent those of Merck Sharp & Dohme Corp. SD received salary support from the National Institutes of Health (T32 GM007546-34). *Thank yous*: We are grateful to Drs. Sarah Yi, Jonathan Edwards, and Alexander Kallen of the Centers for Disease Control for their assistance with statistical analysis. We are also grateful to Diagnostic Laboratories and Radiology for assistance with recruiting facilities and laboratory data. These studies were carried out in part with resources of the Jewish Home, San Francisco. We appreciate the assistance of the infection control practitioners and additional staff at all the involved facilities.

Author details
¹Department of Internal Medicine, Division of Infectious Diseases, University of California, San Francisco, 513 Parnassus Avenue, room S-380, Box 0645, San Francisco, CA 94143, USA. ²UCSF Medical Center, 505 Parnassus Avenue, San Francisco, CA 94143, USA. ³Trivedi Consultants, 1563 Solano Avenue, #443, Berkeley, CA 94707, USA.

References
1. Abrutyn E, Mossey J, Berlin JA, Boscia J, Levison M, Pitsakis P, et al. Does asymptomatic bacteriuria predict mortality and does antimicrobial treatment reduce mortality in elderly ambulatory women? Ann Intern Med. 1994;120(10): 827–33.
2. Nicolle LE, Bjornson J, Harding GKM, MacDonell JA. Bacteriuria in elderly institutionalized men. N Engl J Med. 1983;309(23):1420–5.
3. Nicolle LE, Mayhew WJ, Bryan L. Prospective randomized comparison of therapy and no therapy for asymptomatic bacteriuria in institutionalized elderly women. Am J Med. 1987;83(1):27–33.
4. Ouslander JG, Schapira M, Schnelle JF, Uman G, Fingold S, Tuico E, et al. Does eradicating bacteriuria affect the severity of chronic urinary incontinence in nursing home residents? Ann Intern Med. 1995;122(10):749–54.
5. Rotjanapan P, Dosa D, Thomas KS. Potentially inappropriate treatment of urinary tract infections in two Rhode Island nursing homes. Arch Intern Med. 2011;171(5):438–43.

6.   Rummukainen M, Jakobsson A, Matsinen M, Järvenpää S, Nissinen A, Karppi P, et al. Reduction in inappropriate prevention of urinary tract infections in long-term care facilities. Am J Infect Control. 2012;40(8):711–4.

7.   D'Agata E, Mitchell SL. Patterns of antimicrobial use among nursing home residents with advanced dementia. Arch Intern Med. 2008;168(4):357–62.

8.   Daneman N, Gruneir A, Newman A, Fischer HD, Bronskill SE, Rochon PA, et al. Antibiotic use in long-term care facilities. J Antimicrob Chemother. 2011;66(12):2856–63.

9.   Katz PR, Beam Jr TR, Brand F, Boyce K. Antibiotic use in the nursing home: physician practice patterns. Arch Intern Med. 1990;150(7):1465–8.

10. Koch AM, Eriksen HM, Elstrøm P, Aavitsland P, Harthug S. Severe consequences of healthcare-associated infections among residents of nursing homes: a cohort study. J Hosp Infect. 2009;71(3):269–74.

11. Loeb M, Simor AE, Landry L, Walter S, McArthur M, Duffy J, et al. Antibiotic use in Ontario facilities that provide chronic care. J Gen Intern Med. 2001; 16(6):376–83.

12. Loeb MB, Craven S, McGeer AJ, Simor AE, Bradley SF, Low DE, et al. Risk factors for resistance to antimicrobial agents among nursing home residents. Am J Epidemiol. 2003;157(1):40–7.

13. March A, Aschbacher R, Dhanji H, Livermore DM, Böttcher A, Sleghel F, et al. Colonization of residents and staff of a long-term-care facility and adjacent acute-care hospital geriatric unit by multiresistant bacteria. Clin Microbiol Infect. 2010;16(7):934–44.

14. Muder RR, Brennen C, Goetz AM, Wagener MM, Rihs JD. Association with prior fluoroquinolone therapy of widespread ciprofloxacin resistance among gram-negative isolates in a Veterans Affairs medical center. Antimicrob Agents Chemother. 1991;35(2):256–8.

15. Pakyz A, Dwyer L. Prevalence of antimicrobial use among United States nursing home residents: results from a national survey. Infect Control Hosp Epidemiol. 2010;31(6):661–2.

16. Pop-Vicas A, Mitchell SL, Kandel R, Schreiber R, D'Agata EM. Multidrug-resistant gram-negative bacteria in a long-term care facility: prevalence and risk factors. J Am Geriatr Soc. 2008;56(7):1276–80.

17. Wiener J, Quinn JP, Bradford PA, Goering RV, Nathan C, Bush K, et al. Multiple antibiotic–resistant Klebsiella and Escherichia coli in nursing homes. JAMA. 1999;281(6):517–23.

18. Centers for Medicare and Medicaid Services Nursing Home Data Compendium, 2013 Edition. https://www.cms.gov/Medicare/Provider-Enrollment-and-Certification/CertificationandComplianc/downloads/nursinghomedatacompendium_508.pdf. Updated 2013. Accessed 14 September 2014.

19. Burke L, Humphreys H, Fitzgerald-Hughes D. The revolving door between hospital and community: extended-spectrum beta-lactamase-producing Escherichia coli in Dublin. J Hosp Infect. 2012;81(3):192–8.

20. Elizaga ML, Weinstein RA, Hayden MK. Patients in long-term care facilities: a reservoir for vancomycin-resistant enterococci. Clin Infect Dis. 2002;34(4):441–6.

21. Rhee SM, Stone ND. Antimicrobial stewardship in long-term care facilities. Infect Dis Clin North Am. 2014;28(2):237–46.

22. Mortensen E, Trivedi KK, Rosenberg J, Cody SH, Long J, Jensen BJ, et al. Multidrug-resistant Acinetobacter baumannii infection, colonization, and transmission related to a long-term care facility providing subacute care. Infect Control Hosp Epidemiol. 2014;35(4):406–11. Special Topic Issue: Carbapenem-Resistant Enterobacteriaceae and Multidrug-Resistant Organisms.

23. Dellit TH, Owens RC, McGowan JE, Gerding DN, Weinstein RA, Burke JP, et al. Infectious Diseases Society of America and the Society for Healthcare Epidemiology of America guidelines for developing an institutional program to enhance antimicrobial stewardship. Clin Infect Dis. 2007;44(2):159–77.

24. Camins B, King M, Wells J, Googe HL, Patel M, Kourbatova EV, et al. Impact of an antimicrobial utilization program on antimicrobial use at a large teaching hospital: a randomized controlled trial. Infect Control Hosp Epidemiol. 2009;30(10):931–8.

25. Evans RS, Classen DC, Pestotnik SL, Lundsgaarde HP, Burke JP. Improving empiric antibiotic selection using computer decision support. Arch Intern Med. 1994;154(8):878–84.

26. Evans RS, Pestotnik SL, Classen DC, Clemmer TP, Weaver LK, Orme Jr JF, et al. A computer-assisted management program for antibiotics and other antiinfective agents. N Engl J Med. 1998;338(4):232–8.

27. Linares LA, Thornton DJ, Strymish J, Baker E, Gupta K. Electronic memorandum decreases unnecessary antimicrobial use for asymptomatic bacteriuria and culture-negative pyuria. Infect Control Hosp Epidemiol. 2011;32(7):644–8.

28. Lutters M, Harbarth S, Janssens J, Freudiger H, Herrmann F, Michel JP, et al. Effect of a comprehensive, multidisciplinary, educational program on the use of antibiotics in a geriatric university hospital. J Am Geriatr Soc. 2004; 52(1):112–6.

29. Loeb M, Brazil K, Lohfeld L, Simor A, Stevenson K, Zoutman D, et al. Effect of a multifaceted intervention on number of antimicrobial prescriptions for suspected urinary tract infections in residents of nursing homes: cluster randomised controlled trial. BMJ. 2005;331(7518):669.

30. Monette J, Miller MA, Monette M, Laurier C, Boivin JF, Sourial N, et al. Effect of an educational intervention on optimizing antibiotic prescribing in long-term care facilities. J Am Geriatr Soc. 2007;55(8):1231–5.

31. Pettersson E, Vernby Å, Mölstad S, Lundborg CS. Can a multifaceted educational intervention targeting both nurses and physicians change the prescribing of antibiotics to nursing home residents? A cluster randomized controlled trial. J Antimicrob Chemother. 2011;66(11):2659–66.

32. Schwartz DN, Abiad H, DeMarais PL, Armeanu E, Trick WE, Wang Y, et al. An educational intervention to improve antimicrobial use in a hospital-based long-term care facility. J Am Geriatr Soc. 2007;55(8):1236–42.

33. Zabarsky TF, Sethi AK, Donskey CJ. Sustained reduction in inappropriate treatment of asymptomatic bacteriuria in a long-term care facility through an educational intervention. Am J Infect Control. 2008;36(7):476–80.

34. Nicolle LE. Antimicrobial stewardship in long term care facilities: what is effective? Antimicrob Resist Infect Control. 2014;3(1):6. -2994-3-6.

35. Centers for Medicare and Medicaid Services (CMS) Interpretative Guidelines for Long-Term Care Facilities . http://www.cms.gov/Regulations-and-Guidance/Guidance/Manuals/downloads/som107ap_pp_guidelines_ltcf.pdf. Updated 2009. Accessed 14 September 2014.

36. Loeb M, Bentley DW, Bradley S, Crossley K, Garibaldi R, Gantz N, et al. Development of minimum criteria for the initiation of antibiotics in residents of long-term-care facilities: results of a consensus conference. Infect Control Hosp Epidemiol. 2001;22(2):120–4.

37. Wagner AK, Soumerai SB, Zhang F, Ross-Degnan D. Segmented regression analysis of interrupted time series studies in medication use research. J Clin Pharm Ther. 2002;27(4):299–309.

38. Trautner BW, Grigoryan L, Petersen NJ, Hysong S, Cadena J, Patterson JE, et al. Effectiveness of an antimicrobial stewardship approach for urinary catheter-associated asymptomatic bacteriuria. JAMA Intern Med. 2015; 175(7):1120–7.

39. Leis JA, Rebick GW, Daneman N, Gold WL, Poutanen SM, Lo P, et al. Reducing antimicrobial therapy for asymptomatic bacteriuria among noncatheterized inpatients: a proof-of-concept study. Clin Infect Dis. 2014; 58(7):980–3.

40. Jump RP, Olds DM, Seifi N, Kypriotakis G, Jury LA, Peron EP, et al. Effective antimicrobial stewardship in a long-term care facility through an infectious disease consultation service: keeping a lid on antibiotic use. Infect Control Hosp Epidemiol. 2012;33(12):1185–92.

41. Daneman N, Gruneir A, Bronskill SE, Newman A, Fischer HD, Rochon PA, et al. Prolonged antibiotic treatment in long-term care: role of the prescriber. JAMA Intern Med. 2013;173(8):673–82.

Correlation between biofilm formation and resistance toward different commonly used antibiotics along with extended spectrum beta lactamase production in uropathogenic *Escherichia coli* isolated from the patients suspected of urinary tract infections visiting Shree Birendra Hospital, Chhauni, Kathmandu, Nepal

Sanjeev Neupane[1], Narayan Dutt Pant[2]* (iD), Saroj Khatiwada[3], Raina Chaudhary[4] and Megha Raj Banjara[1]

Abstract

Background: *Escherichia coli* is the most predominant causative agent of urinary tract infection (UTI). Recently, increase in drug resistance among the uropathogenic bacteria has caused great problem in treatment of UTI. The main objective of this research is to determine the correlation between biofilm formation and resistance toward different commonly used antibiotics along with extended spectrum beta lactamase production in uropathogenic *Escherichia coli*.

Methods: The urine samples collected from the patients suspected of urinary tract infections (visiting Shree Birendra Hospital, Chhauni, Kathmandu, Nepal between July to December 2013) were cultured in cystine lactose electrolyte deficient (CLED) agar by using semi quantitative culture technique. Extended spectrum beta lactamase (ESBL) production was detected by combined disc diffusion technique and biofilm formation was detected by Congo red agar method. Chi-square test was applied and p-value < 0.05 was considered statistically significant.

Results: Out of 1480 urine samples, *E. Coli* was isolated from 208 (14.1 %) samples. Of total 69 (33.2 %) ESBL producing uropathogenic strains of *E. coli*, 20 (29 %) were strong biofilm producers, 22 (31.9 %) were moderate biofilm producers, 11 (15.9 %) were weak biofilm producers and 16 (23.2 %) were biofilm non producers. Whereas among 139 ESBL non producing *E. coli*, 22 (15.8 %) were strong biofilm producers, 20 (14.4 %) were moderate biofilm producers, 13 (9.4 %) were weak biofilm producers and 84 (60.4 %) were biofilm non producers. Among total 108 biofilm producing *E. coli*, maximum resistance was observed toward cephalexin followed by amoxicillin and highest susceptibility was seen toward amikacin.

(Continued on next page)

* Correspondence: ndpant1987@gmail.com
[2]Department of Microbiology, Grande International Hospital, Dhapasi, Kathmandu, Nepal
Full list of author information is available at the end of the article

(Continued from previous page)

Conclusion: The ability of biofilm formation was found to be significantly higher in ESBL producing strains of *E. coli* than that in ESBL non producing strains ($p < 0.05$). There was higher resistance rate to antimicrobial agents among biofilm producing strains of *E. coli* than that in biofilm non producing strains. According to our antimicrobial susceptibility pattern for *E. coli*, to start preliminary treatment for UTI in Nepal, we recommend to use amikacin or nitrofurantoin. Further, for the treatment of the UTI, the antibiotics should be selected on the basis of the urine culture and sensitivity report.

Keywords: *Escherichia coli*, Urinary tract infection, Extended spectrum beta lactamase, Biofilm, Nepal

Background

Urinary tract infection (UTI) is one of the most common bacterial infections acquired both in the community and hospital settings, affecting all age groups [1, 2]. Worldwide, around 150 million cases of UTI are diagnosed each year [3] and *Escherichia coli* is identified as the most common cause of UTI, accounting for 80 to 85 % of the cases [4–6].

Recently the haphazard uses of antibiotics have resulted in the worldwide spread of antibiotic resistance among the bacteria causing a major problem [7]. The emergence and worldwide rapid increase in prevalence of extended spectrum beta-lactamase (ESBL) producing bacteria that are multidrug resistant, pose treatment problem resulting in high morbidity, high mortality, and increased health care costs [8]. Biofilm production is a mechanism exhibited by several microbes to survive in unfavorable conditions. The bacterial biofilm is a structured community of bacterial cells enclosed in polymeric matrix and adherent to a surface [9]. Biofilm producing uropathogenic bacteria may be responsible for many recurrent UTIs [10]. The bacteria enclosed in the biofilm are highly resistant to antibiotic treatment [9].

In this study we are investigating the incidence of the ESBL producing *E. coli* in causing UTI. Further we are determining the correlation between biofilm formation and drug resistance with commonly used antibiotics (for treatment of UTI) along with ESBL production in *E. coli* isolated from the urine samples of the patients suspected of urinary tract infections. This is the first this type of study conducted in Nepal.

Methods

A cross sectional study was conducted among the patients suspected of urinary tract infections (having symptoms like burning micturation, frequent or intense urge to urinate, back pain or lower abdominal pain, fever or chills etc.) visiting Shree Birendra Hospital, Chhauni, Kathmandu, Nepal since May to October 2013.

Total 1480 mid stream urine samples collected from the patients (out patients and in patients) suspected of urinary tract infections were cultured by the semi-quantitative culture technique [11]. The patients having laboratory or radiological evidence of other infections as the cause of the symptoms, patients with urinary catheterization and those who already have received antibiotics were excluded from our study. The bacterial isolates from the urine samples were identified by using microbiological techniques as described in the Bergey's manual which include morphological appearance of the colonies, staining reactions and biochemical properties. The antimicrobial susceptibility testing was done by Kirby-Bauer disk diffusion technique as recommended by clinical and laboratory standards institute (CLSI) [12].

Detection of ESBL producers

Among the uropathogens isolated from suspected cases of UTI, only the strains of *E. coli* were subjected for detection of ESBL production. The phenotypic confirmation of the ESBL producing strains was done by combined disk method (Fig. 1) [12].

Detection of biofilm producers

Detection of biofilm production was done for both ESBL positive and ESBL negative strains of *E. coli* by Congo red agar method (CRA) (Fig. 2) [13].

On the basis of the intensity of color change of CRA medium after inoculation of the organisms, which is directly proportional to the amount of biofilm produced

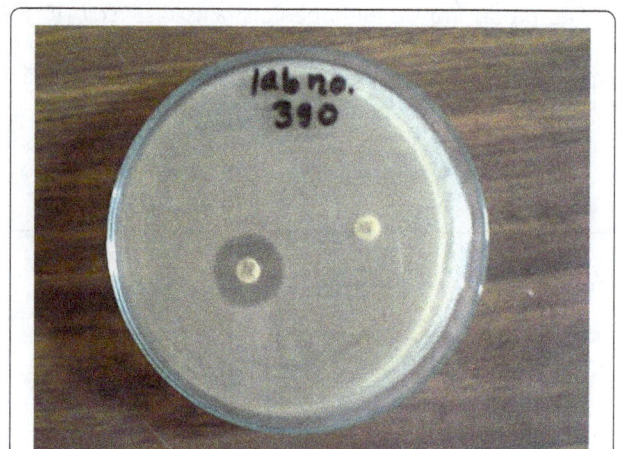

Fig. 1 Confirmation of ESBL producer *E. coli* by combined disk method

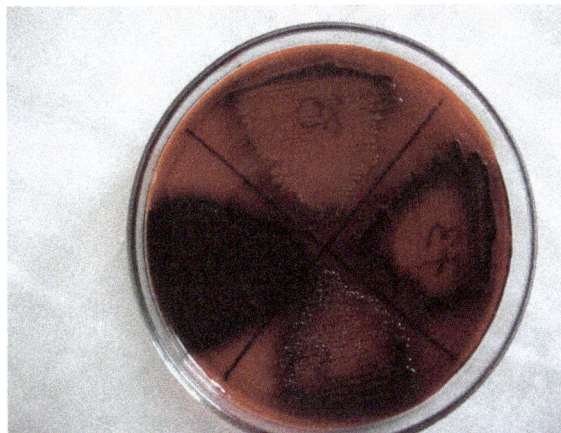
Fig. 2 Biofilm detection test for *Escherechia coli* showing positive result on Congo red agar medium

by the organisms, the biofilm producing organisms were classified into three categories as strong biofilm producers, moderate biofilm producers and weak biofilm producers [14, 15].

Data analysis
SPSS version 16.0 statistical software package was used for statistical analysis. Chi-square test was applied. P-value < 0.05 was considered statistically significant.

Results
Out of 1480 mid stream urine samples 278, (18.8 %) samples showed significant growth ($\geq 10^5$ cfu/ml). *E. coli* was isolated from 208 (74.82 %) samples. Out of 208 *E. coli* isolates 69 (33.2 %) were found to be ESBL producers and 139 (66.8 %) were ESBL non producers. Among 208 *E. coli* isolates 42 (20.192 %) were found to be strong biofilm producers, 42 (20.192 %) were moderate biofilm producers, 24 (11.538 %) were weak biofilm producers and 100 (48.076 %) were biofilm non producers.

Antibiotic resistance pattern of *E. coli* among biofilm producers and biofilm non producers
The antibiotic resistance among biofilm producing *E. coli* was found significantly higher than that of biofilm non producing *E. coli* ($p < 0.05$). The correlation between biofilm production and antibiotic resistance was found statistically significant ($p < 0.05$) in most of the antibiotics (ciprofloxacin, ofloxacin, norfloxacin, amikacin, gentamicin, cotrimoxazole, cephalexin, cefixime, ceftazidime, cefotaxime, ceftriaxone and cefepime) but the correlation was not found to be significant in case of amoxicillin and nitrofurantoin (Table 1).

Antibiotic susceptibility pattern of the uropathogenic *E. coli* isolated
Of total 208 *E. coli* isolates, the highest numbers of the strains were susceptible to amikacin followed by nitrofurantoin, gentamicin, ceftriaxone and cefepime. Similarly least numbers of the strains were susceptible to amoxicillin (Table 1).

Association of ESBL production and biofilm formation among *E. coli* isolates
Out of 69 ESBL producing uropathogenic strains of *E. coli*, 20 (29 %) were strong biofilm producers, 22 (31.9 %) were moderate biofilm producers, 11 (15.9 %) were weak biofilm producers and 16 (23.2 %) were biofilm non producers. Whereas among 139 ESBL non producing *E. coli*, 22 (15.8 %) were strong biofilm producers, 20 (14.4 %) were moderate biofilm producers, 13 (9.4 %) were weak biofilm producers and 84 (60.4 %) were biofilm non producers. The ability of biofilm formation was found to be significantly higher in ESBL producing strains of *E. coli* than that in ESBL non producing strains ($p < 0.05$).

Discussion
Among 208 *E. coli* isolates, 108 (51.92 %) were biofilm producers. This finding agrees with the findings of different authors from different parts of the world [16, 17]. Biofilm protects bacteria from host defense mechanisms, along with the antibiotics [18].

In this study, the antibiotic resistance of biofilm producing *E. coli* was found significantly higher than that of biofilm non producing *E. coli* ($p < 0.05$). Among biofilm producing *E. coli*, higher antibiotic resistance was observed in strong and moderate biofilm producers. The association between biofilm production and antibiotic resistance was found to be statistically significant ($p < 0.05$) except in case of amoxicillin and nitrofurantoin. Microorganisms growing in a biofilm are intrinsically resistant to many antibiotics increasing the antibiotic resistance up to 1000 folds and high antimicrobial concentrations are required to inactivate organisms growing in a biofilm [19, 20]. This may be because of the insufficient concentration of the antibiotics reaching some areas of the biofilms and metabolic inactiveness (along with the presence of active antibiotic degradation mechanisms contributing to halt the accumulation of the drugs up to an effective concentration) of the bacteria located at the base of the biofilms [9].

The biofilm forming ability was found to be significantly higher in ESBL positive strains of uropathogenic *E. coli* than that of ESBL negative strains [$p < 0.05$]. The study by Subramanian et al. in India also reported the higher ability of the ESBL producing organisms to form biofilm in comparison to that of ESBL non-producing isolates. It has been postulated that during occurrence of the large numbers of the chromosomal gene rearrangements upon

Table 1 Antibiotic resistance pattern of E. coli among biofilm producers and non producers along with the antibiotic susceptibility pattern of all the E. coli isolates

Antibiotics used	Resistance pattern of biofilm producers and biofilm non producers				Total Resistant	Total susceptible
	Strong producers N = 42	Moderate producers N = 42	Weak producers N = 24	Non producers N = 100		
	No (%)	No (%)	No (%)	No (%)	No (%)	No (%)
Ciprofloxacin	32 (76.2)	32 (76.2)	17 (70.8)	45 (45.0)	126 (60.6)	82 (39.4)
Ofloxacin	30 (71.4)	30 (71.4)	14 (58.3)	39 (39.0)	113 (54.3)	95 (45.7)
Norfloxacin	33 (78.6)	32 (76,2)	16 (66.7)	45 (45.5)	126 (60.6)	82 (39.4)
Gentamicin	24 (57.1)	26 (61.9)	6 (25.0)	26 (26.0)	82 (39.4)	126 (60.6)
Amikacin	7 (16.7)	11 (26.2)	3 (12.5)	5 (5.0)	26 (12.5)	182 (87.5)
Cotrimoxazole	27 (64.3)	29 (69,0)	17 (70.8)	42 (42.0)	115 (55.3)	93 (44.7)
Amoxicillin	40 (95.2)	37 (88.1)	22 (91.7)	87 (87.0)	186 (89.4)	22 (10.6)
Cephalexin	41 (97.6)	38 (90.5)	22 (91.7)	74 (74.0)	175 (84.1)	33 (15.9)
Cefixime	37 (88.1)	41 (97.6)	20 (83.3)	59 (59.0)	157 (75.5)	51 (24.5)
Ceftazidime	31 (73.8)	36 (85.7)	15 (62.7)	40 (40.0)	122 (58.7)	86 (41.3)
Cefotaxime	34 (81.1)	34 (81.0)	14 (58.3)	35 (35.0)	117 (56.2)	91 (43.8)
Ceftriaxone	29 (69.0)	28 (66.7)	15 (62.5)	28 (28.0)	100 (48.1)	108 (51.9)
Cefepime	31 (73.8)	27 (64.3)	12 (50.0)	33 (33.0)	103 (49.5)	105 (50.5)
Nitrofurantoin	12 (28.6)	11 (26.2)	6 (26.0)	28 (28.0)	57 (27.4)	151 (72.6)

acquisition of the ESBL plasmids the bacteria express several virulence genes [21].

ESBLs are enzymes that are responsible for resistance of bacteria toward third generation cephalosporins and monobactams [22]. Most of the plasmids responsible for ESBL production carry genes encoding resistance to other drugs also [23]. Due to frequent presence of cross-resistance to several other classes of antibiotics (like aminoglycosides and fluoroquinolones), in ESBL-producing organisms, the treatment of the infections by these bacteria are often present as the therapeutic challenges [22]. Further higher ability of the ESBL producing organisms to form biofilm makes the treatment even more difficult, increasing the mortality and severity of the infections [21]. Macrolides (erythromycin, clarithromycin, and azithromycin) are known to have antibiofilm activity against biofilm producing organisms by inhibiting a key component of the biofilm, alginate. And several studies have recommended, the combined therapy (being macrolides one of the first antibiotics chosen) as the treatment of choice in infections caused by biofilm producing organisms [9].

Increasing irrational and haphazard use of antibiotics, sales of substandard antibiotics and transmission of drug resistant bacteria among people may be responsible for the rise in antibiotic resistance among the bacteria [24]. Antimicrobial resistance has become a serious global public health issue. Infections caused by drug resistant bacteria are responsible for increased morbidity and mortality [25]. The selection of the antibiotics for treatment of the bacterial infections should be based on culture and sensitivity reports.

Conclusion

The ability of biofilm formation was found higher among ESBL producing strains of E. coli. There was higher resistance rate among biofilm producing E. coli isolates to almost all the antimicrobial agents except a few. According to our antimicrobial susceptibility pattern for E. coli, to start preliminary treatment for UTI in Nepal, we recommend to use amikacin or nitrofurantoin. Further, for the treatment of the UTI, the antibiotics should be selected on the basis of the urine culture and sensitivity report.

Limitations of the study

Due to lack of easy availability of the advanced laboratory in Nepal and due to lack of the fund we could not confirm the ESBL producing and biofilm producing organisms by using molecular technology.

Abbreviations
ATCC: American type culture collection; CLED: Cystine lactose electrolyte deficient agar; CLSI: Clinical and laboratory standards institute; CRA: Congo red agar; ESBL: Extended spectrum beta lactamase; MHA: Mueller Hinton agar; SPSS: Statistical package for the social sciences; UTI: Urinary tract infection.

Competing interests
The authors declare that they have no competing interests.

Authors' contributions
SN designed the study, collected and processed the samples and analysed the data, NDP designed the study, analysed the data and prepared the manuscript, SK analysed the data, RC and MRB monitored the study. All authors read and approved the final manuscript.

Acknowledgements
The authors would like to thank all who contributed directly or indirectly in conduction of this research.

Author details
[1]Central Department of Microbiology, Tribhuvan University, Kirtipur, Kathmandu, Nepal. [2]Department of Microbiology, Grande International Hospital, Dhapasi, Kathmandu, Nepal. [3]Department of biochemistry, CIST College, Kathmandu, Nepal. [4]Shree Birendra Hospital, Chhauni, Kathmandu, Nepal.

References
1. Ramesh N, Sumathi CS, Balasubramanian V, Palaniappan KR, Kannan VR. Urinary tract infection and antimicrobial susceptibility pattern of extended spectrum beta lactamase producing clinical isolates. Adv Biol Res. 2008;2:78–82.
2. Dromigny JA, Nabeth P, Perrier Gros Claude JD. Distribution and susceptibility of bacterial urinary tract infection in Dakar, Senegal. Int J Antimicrob Agents. 2002;20:339–47.
3. Gupta K. Increasing antimicrobial resistance and the management of uncomplicated community acquired urinary tract infections. Int J Antimicrob. 2001;135:41–50.
4. Nicolle LE. Uncomplicated urinary tract infection in adults including uncomplicated pyelonephritis. Urol Clin North Am. 2008;35:1–12.
5. Bhatta CP, Shrestha B, Khadka S, Swar S, Shah B, Pun K. Etiology of urinary tract infection and drug resistance cases of uropathogens. J Kath Med coll. 2012;2:114–20.
6. Sahm DF, Thornsberry C, Mayfield DC, Jones ME, Karlowsky JA. Multidrug-resistant urinary tract isolates of E. coli: prevalence and patient demographics in the United States. J Antimicrob Chemother. 2001;45:1402–6.
7. Goldstein FW. Antibiotic susceptibility of bacterial strains isolated from patients with community-acquired urinary tract infections in France. Multicentre Study Group. Eur J Clin Microbiol Infect Dis. 2000;19:112–7.
8. Schwaber MJ, Carmeli Y. Mortality and delay in effective therapy associated with extended-spectrum -lactamase production in Enterobacteriaceae bacteraemia: a systemic review and meta-analysis. J Antimicrob Chemother. 2007;60:913–20.
9. Soto SM. Importance of biofilms in urinary tract infections: new therapeutic approaches. Adv Biol. 2014;2014(2014):543974.
10. Rijavec M, Muller-Premru M, Zakotnik B, Bertok DZ. Virulence factors and biofilm production among Escherichia coli strains causing bacteraemia of urinary tract origin. J Med Microbio. 2008;57:1329–34.
11. Cheesbrough M. District laboratory practice in tropical countries, part II. 2nd ed. New York: Cambridge university press; 2006. p. 112–3.
12. Clinical Laboratory Standards Institute. (CLSI) CLSI document M100S-S22. Performance standards for antimicrobial susceptibility testing: Twenty second informational supplement ed. Wayne: CLSI; 2012.
13. Mathur T, Singhal S, Khan S, Upadhyay DJ, Fatma T, Rattan A. Detection of biofilm formation among the clinical isolates of staphylococci: an evaluation of three different screening methods. Indian J Med Microbiol. 2006;24:25–9.
14. Poovendran P, Vidhya N, Murugan S. Antimicrobial susceptibility pattern of ESBL and non-ESBL producing uropathogenic Escherichia coli (UPEC) and their correlation with biofilm formation. Intl J Microbiol Res. 2013;4:56–63.
15. Christensen GD, Simpson WA, Bisno AL, Beachey EH. Adherence of slime producing strains of Staphylococcus epidermidis to smooth surface. Infec Immun. 1982;37:318–26.
16. Anandkumar H, Soham G, Vinodkumar CS, Rao A, Srinivasa H. Detection of Cell Surface Hydrophobicity and Biofilm formation among ESBL and non-ESBL producing uropathogenic Escherichia coli. J Med Educ Res. 2012;2:12–20.
17. Nair BT, Bhat KG, Shantaram M. In vitro biofilm production and virulence factors of uropathogenic Escherichia coli. Int J Pharm Bio Sci. 2013;4:951–6.
18. Hanna A, Berg M, Stout V, Razatos A. Role of capsular colanic acid in adhesion of uropathogenic Escherichia coli. Appl Environ Microbiol. 2003;69:4474–81.
19. Thien-fah UK, George PA. Mechanism of biofilm resistance to antimicrobial agents. Trends Microbiol. 2001;9:34–9.
20. Stewart PS, Costerton JW. Antibiotic resistance of bacteria in biofilms. Lancet. 2001;358:135–8.
21. Subramanian P, Umadevi S, Kumar S, Stephen S. Determination of correlation between biofilm and extended spectrum β lactamases producers of Enterobacteriaceae. Scho Res J. 2012;2:2–6.
22. Black JA, Moland ES, Thomson KS. AmpC disk test for detection of plasmid-mediated AmpC-b lactamases in Enterobacteriaceae lacking chromosomal AmpC-b lactamases. J Clin Microbiol. 2005;43:3110–3.
23. Paterson DL, Bonomo RA. Extended-spectrum beta-lactamases: a clinical update. Clin Microbiol Rev. 2005;18:657–86.
24. Gautam R, Chapagain ML, Acharya A, Rayamajhi N, Shrestha S, Ansari S, et al. Antimicrobial susceptibility patterns of Escherichia coli from various clinical sources. JCMC. 2013;3:14–7.
25. Awasthi TR, Pant ND, Dahal PR. Prevalence of Multidrug Resistant Bacteria in Causing Community Acquired Urinary Tract Infection Among the Patients Attending Outpatient Department of Seti Zonal Hospital, Dhangadi, Nepal. Nepal J Biotechnol. 2015;3(1):55–9.

4

Regional variations in fluoroquinolone non-susceptibility among *Escherichia coli* bloodstream infections within the Veterans Healthcare Administration

Daniel J. Livorsi[1,2*], Michihiko Goto[1,2], Margaret Carrel[3], Makoto M. Jones[4,5], Jennifer McDanel[1,6], Rajeshwari Nair[1,7], Bruce Alexander[1], Brice Beck[1], Kelly K. Richardson[1] and Eli N. Perencevich[1,7]

Abstract

Objectives: We sought to define regional variations in fluoroquinolone non-susceptibility (FQ-NS) among bloodstream isolates of *Escherichia coli* across the Veterans Health Administration (VHA) in the United States.

Methods: We analyzed a retrospective cohort of patients managed at 136 VHA hospitals who had a blood culture positive for *E.coli* between 2003 and 2013. Hospitals were classified based on US Census Divisions, and regional variations in FQ-NS were analyzed.

Results: Twenty-four thousand five hundred twenty-three unique *E.coli* bloodstream infections (BSIs) were identified between 2003 and 2013. 53.9 % of these were community-acquired, 30.7 % were healthcare-associated, and 15.4 % were hospital-onset BSIs. The proportion of *E.coli* BSIs with FQ-NS significantly varied across US Census Divisions ($p < 0.001$). During 2003–2013, the proportion of *E.coli* BSIs with FQ-NS was highest in the West South-Central Division (32.7 %) and lowest in the Mountain Division (20.0 %). Multivariable analysis showed that there were universal secular trends towards higher FQ-NS rates ($p < 0.001$) with significant variability of slopes across US Census Divisions ($p < 0.001$).

Conclusion: There has been a universal increase in FQ-NS among *E.coli* BSIs within VHA, but the rate of increase has significantly varied across Census Divisions. The reasons for this variability are unclear. These findings reinforce the importance of using local data to develop and update local antibiograms and antibiotic-prescribing guidelines.

Keywords: Fluoroquinolones, Antimicrobial resistance, Epidemiology, *Escherichia coli*,

Introduction

Fluoroquinolones are a synthetic class of antibiotics that have been used in clinical medicine since the 1970s. Fluoroquinolones have excellent oral bioavailability, provide a broad-spectrum of antibacterial activity, and are highly efficacious in the treatment of a variety of infections. However, the overuse of these agents has led to rising rates of FQ non-susceptibility (FQ-NS) [1–3].

Historically, fluoroquinolones have been reliably active against *Escherichia coli*, a common cause of urinary tract infections, bloodstream infections, and intra-abdominal infections. National antibiotic-prescribing guidelines still recommend the empiric use of fluoroquinolones for infections that commonly involve *E.coli* [4, 5], but given the rising prevalence of FQ-NS, the empiric use of fluoroquinolones may no longer be appropriate in some geographic regions [1–3].

In this study, we sought to define regional variations in FQ-NS among bloodstream isolates of *E.coli* in the Veterans Health Administration (VHA) over an 11-year period. Identifying temporal and regional differences in

* Correspondence: daniel-livorsi@uiowa.edu
[1]Iowa City VA Health Care System, Iowa City, IA, USA
[2]Division of Infectious Diseases, Department of Internal Medicine, University of Iowa Carver College of Medicine, 200 Hawkins Drive, Iowa City, IA 52242, USA
Full list of author information is available at the end of the article

resistance patterns may inform development of national versus regional or local treatment guidelines.

Methods

We constructed a retrospective cohort of all patients within the VHA who had a blood culture positive for *E.coli* between January 1, 2003 and December 31, 2013. Data from 136 acute care hospitals in 48 US states contributed to the cohort. FQ-NS was defined as a non-susceptible result to at least one FQ: ciprofloxacin, levofloxacin, and/or moxifloxacin. In line with guidelines from the Clinical and Laboratory Standards Institute, only the first isolate was included when the patient had more than one blood culture positive for *E. coli* in the same calendar year [6].

Bloodstream infections (BSIs) were defined as hospital-onset, healthcare-associated, or community-acquired. Hospital-onset BSIs were defined as an *E.coli*-positive blood culture that was obtained after the patient had been hospitalized for ≥48 h. Healthcare-associated BSIs were defined as an *E.coli*-positive blood culture obtained at the time of admission or <48 h of admission if the patient met established criteria for healthcare exposure [7]. Community-acquired BSIs were defined as *E.coli*-positive blood cultures obtained at the time of admission or <48 h of admission in patients who did not meet criteria for healthcare-associated infections.

Hospitals were regionalized based on US Census Divisions (https://www.census.gov/geo/reference/gtc/gtc_census_divreg.html), and annual averages of FQ-NS were mapped. Monthly and annual counts of isolates with and without FQ-NS were measured as outcomes.

Poisson regression models were used to predict the number of isolates with FQ-NS while incorporating total number of isolates as an offset variable. The generalized estimating equations (GEE) method was used to account for grouping effect within Census Divisions. Residual plots were inspected to ensure the appropriateness of all models. An interaction term between time and region was included in the model, and region-specific incidence rate ratios (IRRs) by month and year were estimated to assess variability of slopes across divisions.

Results

Twenty-four thousand five hundred twenty-three unique *E.coli* (BSIs) were identified between 2003 and 2013 across 136 hospitals and 9 Census Divisions (Table 1). A majority of these BSIs were classified as community-acquired (53.9 %); 30.7 % were healthcare-associated and 15.4 % were hospital-onset BSIs.

The prevalence of FQ-NS increased with healthcare exposure. The frequency of FQ-NS was 20.2 % for community-acquired *E.coli*-BSIs, 37.0 % for healthcare-

Table 1 Number of VHA hospitals and *E.coli* bloodstream isolates (BSIs) from each census region, 2003–2013

Census region	Number of hospitals	Number of included E. coli BSIs (%)
East North Central	18	2799 (11.4 %)
East South Central	11	2146 (8.8 %)
Middle Atlantic	18	2544 (10.4 %)
Mountain	13	2010 (8.2 %)
New England	7	783 (3.2 %)
Pacific Central	13	3253 (13.3 %)
South Atlantic	26	5358 (21.8 %)
West North Central	16	1896 (7.7 %)
West South Central	14	3734 (15.2 %)

associated *E.coli*-BSIs, and 37.7 % for hospital-onset *E.coli*-BSIs.

Throughout the VHA, the percentage of *E.coli*-BSIs with FQ-NS increased from 13.9 % in 2003 to 31.3 % in 2008 and 32.6 % in 2013. Among *E.coli* strains demonstrating FQ-NS, the frequency of non-susceptibility to other antibiotic classes was as follows: 16.6 % extended-spectrum cephalosporins, 34.4 % aminoglycosides, and 0.3 % carbapenems.

The proportion of *E.coli*-BSIs with FQ-NS significantly varied across Census Divisions (range: 20.0–32.7 %; $p < 0.001$). During 2003–2013, the proportion of *E.coli* BSIs with FQ-NS was highest in the West South Central Division (32.7 %) and lowest in the Mountain Division (20.0 %, Fig. 1). In 2013 alone, the highest frequency of FQ-NS among *E.coli*-BSIs was seen in the East South Central Division (39.6 %) and the lowest frequency of FQ-NS was seen in the Pacific Central Division (25.4 %).

Regression analysis showed that there were universal temporal trends towards higher FQ-NS rates ($p < 0.001$) with significant variability of slopes across Census Divisions ($p < 0.001$, Fig. 2). The annual mean rate of increase in FQ-NS was as follows: East North Central 0.41 % /month; Mountain 0.86 % /month; South Atlantic 0.54 % /month; East South Central 0.51 % /month; New England 0.44 % /month; West North Central 0.89 % /month; Middle Atlantic 0.45 % /month; Pacific Central 0.19 % /month; West South Central 0.40 % /month.

Discussion

Our study has demonstrated a sustained increase in the frequency of FQ-NS among *E.coli* BSIs across VHA during 2003–2013. The rate of change has significantly varied across Census Divisions. The high prevalence of FQ-NS in some divisions could influence the empiric use of fluoroquinolones for infections thought to involve

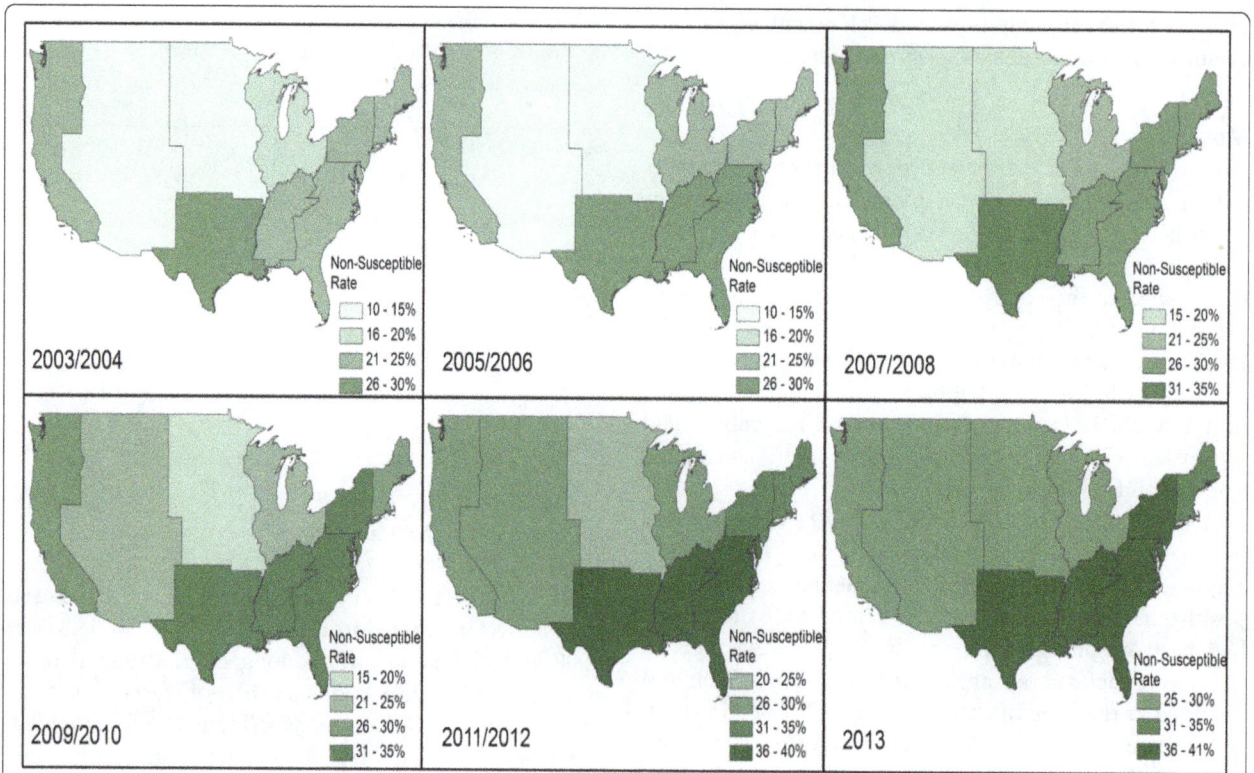

Fig. 1 Region-specific changes in FQ-NS among *E.coli* BSIs in the Veterans Health Administration, 2003–2013

E.coli and suggests that regional or even local guidelines might be preferred over national guidelines.

The clonal expansion of sequence type (ST) 131 *E.coli* is likely a major driver of this rising prevalence of fluoroquinolone resistance [8–11]. ST131 represents one of more than 1000 STs of *E.coli* defined by multilocus sequence typing (MLST). The clonal expansion of ST131 has been a global phenomenon that has not spared the VHA. In a 2011 analysis of *E.coli* clinical isolates from 24 VHA medical centers, ST131 accounted for 78 % of fluoroquinolone-resistant isolates and 28 % of all isolates [12]. The aminoglycoside and carbapenem susceptibility profiles of ST131 strains described in this 2011 study are similar to that of FQ-NS strains in our report. Studies outside of VHA have also found that ST131 accounts for 70–80 % of fluoroquinolone-resistant *E.coli* infections [12–14]. A specific subclone, which represents the vast majority of fluoroquinolone-resistant ST131 isolates, first emerged around 2000 and has since expanded rapidly around the world [15].

The global dissemination of ST131 and its subclones is not well understood. Possible microbiologic contributors include the clone's enhanced transmissibility, its increased virulence, its resistance to multiple antibiotics, and its success at colonizing the human body [8].

In certain healthcare settings, there is a high colonization pressure with ST131, and this likely facilitates

patient-to-patient transmission. Long-term care facilities may serve as reservoirs of this clone [16, 17]. At 2 long-term care facilities in Minnesota, 24 % of residents were colonized with ST131, and molecular analysis demonstrated evidence of intra-facility and inter-facility transmission [17]. Single-center studies at different acute care hospitals found that 50 % of inpatients are carriers [18] and that 13 % of stool samples sent to the microbiology laboratory grew *E.coli* ST131 [19].

Antibiotic-prescribing practices are probably also contributing to the spread of ST131. In a population-based cohort study, multivariable analysis showed that ST131 carriage was predicted by older age, healthcare exposure, and prior antibiotic use [13]. Specifically, prior use of fluoroquinolones, macrolides or extended-spectrum cephalosporins was predictive [13]. Other studies have found that prior fluoroquinolone-exposure is a risk factor for fluoroquinolone-resistant *E.coli*, but these studies did not describe the sequence type of the infecting strains of *E.coli* [2, 20, 21].

It's unclear why the frequency of FQ-NS significantly varied across Census Divisions within the VHA over time. These differences may reflect broad ecological trends beyond the VHA patient cohort. Alternately, specific infection control and antibiotic-prescribing practices within VHA may be influencing the spread of these strains of *E.coli*. Future research could examine

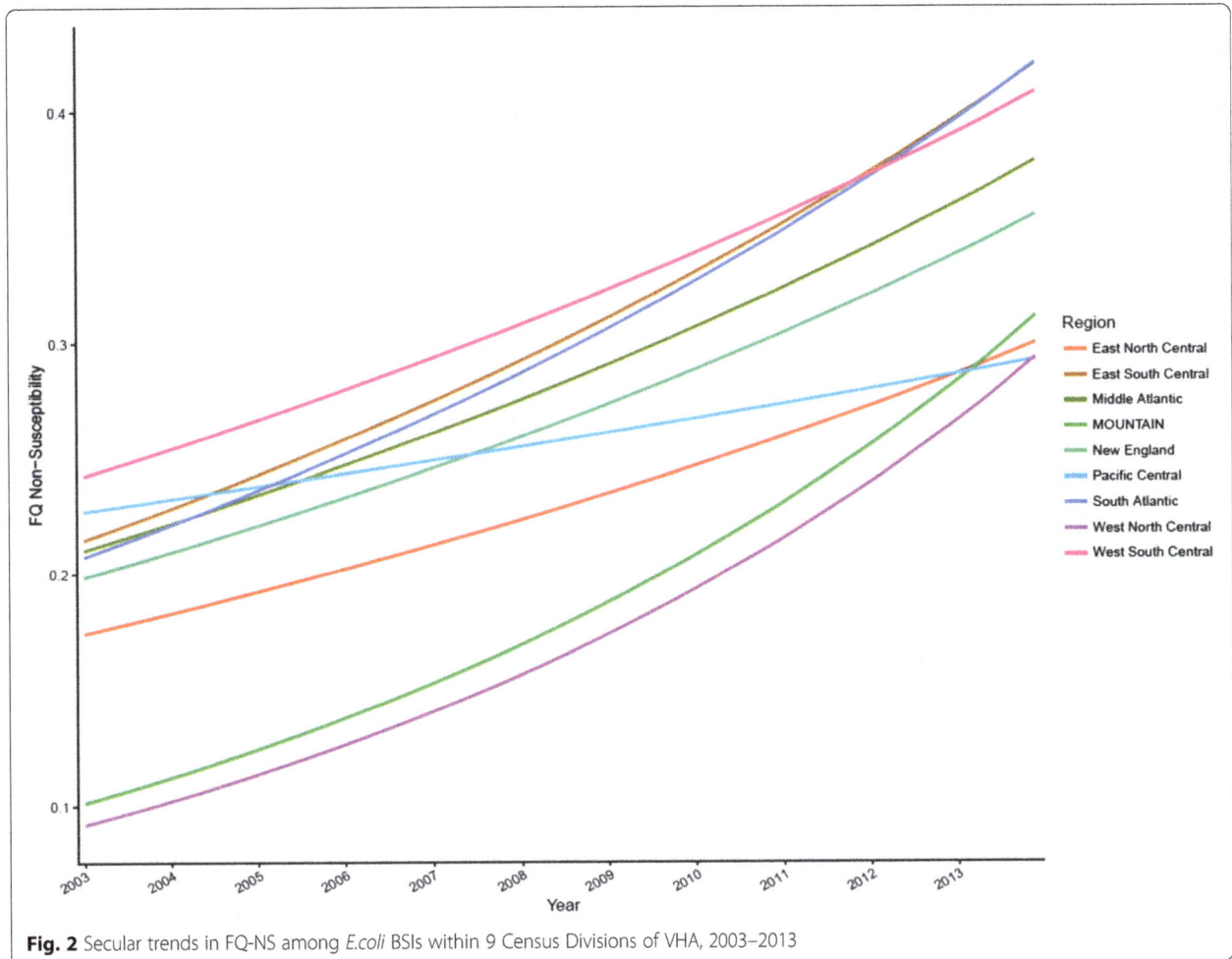

Fig. 2 Secular trends in FQ-NS among *E.coli* BSIs within 9 Census Divisions of VHA, 2003–2013

whether use of specific antibiotic agents varies across regions and, if so, whether the variations in antibiotic usage help explain the variability in FQ-NS.

There are several clinical implications to these changing resistance patterns among *E.coli*. Patients undergoing transrectal prostate biopsy typically receive fluoroquinolone prophylaxis. In one study, colonization with fluoroquinolone-resistant *E.coli* was the most important host characteristic associated with infection after transrectal prostate biopsy. Nearly two-thirds of these resistant strains were ST 131 [22]. A survey of Infectious Disease physicians found that there is a perceived increase in the incidence of infections after transrectal prostate biopsies [23]. Furthermore, rising rates of fluoroquinolone-resistant *E.coli* limit options for empiric antibiotic therapy. Among patients with *E.coli* bacteremia, inappropriate empiric antibiotic therapy was associated with worse outcomes in some [24, 25] but not all [26, 27] studies.

Our study has some limitations. First, the cohort included older patients who were predominantly male. As a result, the trends we observed may not be generalizable to other populations. Second, we have argued that ST131

is contributing to the changing epidemiology of *E.coli*, but we did not perform any microbiologic typing. A prior study, however, has demonstrated that ST 131 is prevalent within VHA [12].

Conclusion

In conclusion, there has been a universal increase in FQ-NS among *E.coli* BSIs within VHA, and the rate of increase has varied across Census Divisions. These findings reinforce the importance of using local data to develop and update local antibiograms and antibiotic-prescribing guidelines.

Abbreviations
BSI: Bloodstream infection; *E.coli*: *Escherichia coli*; FQ-NS: Fluoroquinolone non-susceptibility; GEE: Generalized estimating equations; VHA: Veterans Health Administration

Acknowledgements
Not applicable.

Funding
Not applicable.

Authors' contributions
Study design: DL. Data collection and analysis: MG, MJ, JM, RN, BA, BB, KR. Study supervision: EP. Manuscript writing: DL. Manuscript review: All authors. All authors read and approved the final manuscript.

Competing interests
The authors declare that they have no competing interests.

Author details
[1]Iowa City VA Health Care System, Iowa City, IA, USA. [2]Division of Infectious Diseases, Department of Internal Medicine, University of Iowa Carver College of Medicine, 200 Hawkins Drive, Iowa City, IA 52242, USA. [3]Department of Geographical and Sustainability Sciences, College of Liberal Arts and Sciences, University of Iowa, Iowa City, IA, USA. [4]Salt Lake City VA Health Care System, Salt Lake City, UT, USA. [5]University of Utah School of Medicine, Salt Lake City, UT, USA. [6]Department of Epidemiology, College of Public Health, University of Iowa, Iowa City, IA, USA. [7]Division of General Internal Medicine, Department of Internal Medicine, University of Iowa Carver College of Medicine, Iowa City, IA, USA.

References
1. Fasugba O, Gardner A, Mitchell BG, Mnatzaganian G. Ciprofloxacin resistance in community- and hospital-acquired Escherichia coli urinary tract infections: a systematic review and meta-analysis of observational studies. BMC Infect Dis. 2015;15:545.
2. Zervos MJ, Hershberger E, Nicolau DP, Ritchie DJ, Blackner LK, Coyle EA, Donnelly AJ, Eckel SF, Eng RH, Hiltz A, et al. Relationship between fluoroquinolone use and changes in susceptibility to fluoroquinolones of selected pathogens in 10 United States teaching hospitals, 1991–2000. Clin Infect Dis. 2003;37(12):1643–8.
3. Sanchez GV, Master RN, Karlowsky JA, Bordon JM. In vitro antimicrobial resistance of urinary Escherichia coli isolates among U.S. outpatients from 2000 to 2010. Antimicrob Agents Chemother. 2012;56(4):2181–3.
4. Solomkin JS, Mazuski JE, Bradley JS, Rodvold KA, Goldstein EJ, Baron EJ, O'Neill PJ, Chow AW, Dellinger EP, Eachempati SR, et al. Diagnosis and management of complicated intra-abdominal infection in adults and children: guidelines by the Surgical Infection Society and the Infectious Diseases Society of America. Clin Infect Dis. 2010;50(2):133–64.
5. Gupta K, Hooton TM, Naber KG, Wullt B, Colgan R, Miller LG, Moran GJ, Nicolle LE, Raz R, Schaeffer AJ, et al. International clinical practice guidelines for the treatment of acute uncomplicated cystitis and pyelonephritis in women: A 2010 update by the Infectious Diseases Society of America and the European Society for Microbiology and Infectious Diseases. Clin Infect Dis. 2011;52(5):e103–20.
6. CLSI. Analysis and presentation of cumulative antimicrobial susceptibility test data. Wayne: Clinical and Laboratory Standards Institute; 2014.
7. Friedman ND, Kaye KS, Stout JE, McGarry SA, Trivette SL, Briggs JP, Lamm W, Clark C, MacFarquhar J, Walton AL, et al. Health care–associated bloodstream infections in adults: a reason to change the accepted definition of community-acquired infections. Ann Intern Med. 2002;137(10):791–7.
8. Banerjee R, Johnson JR. A new clone sweeps clean: the enigmatic emergence of Escherichia coli sequence type 131. Antimicrob Agents Chemother. 2014;58(9):4997–5004.
9. Rogers BA, Sidjabat HE, Paterson DL. Escherichia coli O25b-ST131: a pandemic, multiresistant, community-associated strain. J Antimicrob Chemother. 2011;66(1):1–14.
10. Johnson JR, Johnston B, Clabots C, Kuskowski MA, Castanheira M. Escherichia coli sequence type ST131 as the major cause of serious multidrug-resistant E. coli infections in the United States. ClinInfect Dis. 2010;51(3):286–94.
11. Peirano G, Pitout JD. Molecular epidemiology of Escherichia coli producing CTX-M beta-lactamases: the worldwide emergence of clone ST131 O25:H4. Int J Antimicrob Agents. 2010;35(4):316–21.

12. Colpan A, Johnston B, Porter S, Clabots C, Anway R, Thao L, Kuskowski MA, Tchesnokova V, Sokurenko EV, Johnson JR, et al. Escherichia coli sequence type 131 (ST131) subclone H30 as an emergent multidrug-resistant pathogen among US veterans. Clin Infect Dis. 2013;57(9):1256–65.
13. Banerjee R, Johnston B, Lohse C, Porter SB, Clabots C, Johnson JR. Escherichia coli sequence type 131 is a dominant, antimicrobial-resistant clonal group associated with healthcare and elderly hosts. Infect Control Hosp Epidemiol. 2013;34(4):361–9.
14. Croxall G, Hale J, Weston V, Manning G, Cheetham P, Achtman M, McNally A. Molecular epidemiology of extraintestinal pathogenic Escherichia coli isolates from a regional cohort of elderly patients highlights the prevalence of ST131 strains with increased antimicrobial resistance in both community and hospital care settings. J Antimicrob Chemother. 2011;66(11):2501–8.
15. Johnson JR, Tchesnokova V, Johnston B, Clabots C, Roberts PL, Billig M, Riddell K, Rogers P, Qin X, Butler-Wu S, et al. Abrupt emergence of a single dominant multidrug-resistant strain of Escherichia coli. J Infect Dis. 2013;207(6):919–28.
16. Maslow JN, Lee B, Lautenbach E. Fluoroquinolone-resistant Escherichia coli carriage in long-term care facility. Emerg Infect Dis. 2005;11(6):889–94.
17. Burgess MJ, Johnson JR, Porter SB, Johnston B, Clabots C, Lahr BD, Uhl JR, Banerjee R. Long-Term Care Facilities Are Reservoirs for Antimicrobial-Resistant Sequence Type 131 Escherichia coli. Open Forum Infectious Diseases. 2015;2(1):ofv011.
18. Han JH, Johnston B, Nachamkin I, Tolomeo P, Bilker WB, Mao X, Clabots C, Lautenbach E, Johnson JR, Program CDCPE. Clinical and molecular epidemiology of Escherichia coli sequence type 131 among hospitalized patients colonized intestinally with fluoroquinolone-resistant E. coli. Antimicrob Agents Chemother. 2014;58(11):7003–6.
19. Mohamed M, Clabots C, Porter SB, Thuras P, Johnson JR. Isolation and Characterization of Escherichia coli Sequence Type 131 and Other Antimicrobial-Resistant Gram-Negative Bacilli from Clinical Stool Samples from Veterans. Antimicrob Agents Chemother. 2016;60(8):4638–45.
20. Loeb MB, Craven S, McGeer AJ, Simor AE, Bradley SF, Low DE, Armstrong-Evans M, Moss LA, Walter SD. Risk factors for resistance to antimicrobial agents among nursing home residents. Am J Epidemiol. 2003;157(1):40–7.
21. Carratala J, Fernandez-Sevilla A, Tubau F, Callis M, Gudiol F. Emergence of quinolone-resistant Escherichia coli bacteremia in neutropenic patients with cancer who have received prophylactic norfloxacin. Clin Infect Dis. 1995; 20(3):557–60.
22. Liss MA, Johnson JR, Porter SB, Johnston B, Clabots C, Gillis K, Nseyo U, Holden M, Sakamoto K, Fierer J. Clinical and microbiological determinants of infection after transrectal prostate biopsy. Clin Infect Dis. 2015;60(7):979–87.
23. Johnson JR, Polgreen PM, Beekmann SE. Transrectal prostate biopsy-associated prophylaxis and infectious complications: report of a query to the emerging infections network of the infectious diseases society of America. Open Forum Infectious Diseases. 2015;2(1):ofv002.
24. Peralta G, Sanchez MB, Garrido JC, De Benito I, Cano ME, Martinez-Martinez L, Roiz MP. Impact of antibiotic resistance and of adequate empirical antibiotic treatment in the prognosis of patients with Escherichia coli bacteraemia. J Antimicrob Chemother. 2007;60(4):855–63.
25. Kuikka A, Sivonen A, Emelianova A, Valtonen VV. Prognostic factors associated with improved outcome of Escherichia coli bacteremia in a Finnish university hospital. Eur J Clin Microbiol Infect Dis. 1997;16(2):125–34.
26. Thom KA, Schweizer ML, Osih RB, McGregor JC, Furuno JP, Perencevich EN, Harris AD. Impact of empiric antimicrobial therapy on outcomes in patients with Escherichia coli and Klebsiella pneumoniae bacteremia: a cohort study. BMC Infect Dis. 2008;8:116.
27. Kang CI, Kim SH, Park WB, Lee KD, Kim HB, Kim EC, Oh MD, Choe KW. Bloodstream infections due to extended-spectrum beta-lactamase-producing Escherichia coli and Klebsiella pneumoniae: risk factors for mortality and treatment outcome, with special emphasis on antimicrobial therapy. Antimicrob Agents Chemother. 2004;48(12):4574–81.

5

Assessment of extended-spectrum β-lactamases and integrons among *Enterobacteriaceae* in device-associated infections: multicenter study in north of Iran

Masoumeh Bagheri-Nesami[1], Alireza Rafiei[2], Gohar Eslami[3], Fatemeh Ahangarkani[4], Mohammad Sadegh Rezai[1*], Attieh Nikkhah[5] and Azin Hajalibeig[1]

Abstract

Background: Device-associated nosocomial infections (DA-NIs), due to MDR *Enterobacteriaceae*, are a major threat to patient safety in ICUs. We investigated on Extended-spectrum β-lactamases (ESBL) producing *Enterobacteriaceae* and incidence of integrons in these bacteria isolated from ventilator-associated pneumonia (VAP) and catheter-associated urinary tract infections (CAUTIs) in 18 governmental hospitals in the north of Iran.

Methods: In this cross-section study, the antibiotic susceptibility test was performed using the MIC method; also, phenotypically detection of ESBL-producing bacteria was carried out by the double-disk synergy (DDS) test. Presence of ESBL-related genes and integron Classes 1 and 2 was evaluated by the PCR method.

Results: Out of a total of 205 patients with DA-NIs, *Enterobacteriaceae* were responsible for (72.68%) of infections. The most common DA-NIs caused by *Enterobacteriaceae* were VAP (77.18%), CAUTI (19.46%), and sepsis due to VAP (3.35%). The most frequently *Enterobacteriaceae* were; *Klebsiella pneumoniae* 75 (24; 32% ESBL positive), *E. coli* 69 (6; 8.69% ESBL positive) and *Enterobacter spp.* 5 (5; 100% ESBL positive). Distribution of ESBL-related genes was as follows: bla-SHV (94.3%), bla-CTX (48.6%), bla-VEB (22.9%) and bla-GES (17.14%). The incidence rate of integron class 1 and class 2 was (82.92%) and (2.9%) respectively. Eight types of ESBL-producing bacteria were observed.

Conclusions: Due to the fact that the emergence rate of ESBL *Enterobacteriaceae* is increasing in DA-NIs, co-incidence of different types of ESBL genes with integrons in 75–100% of strains in our study is alarming for clinicians and healthcare safety managers. Therefore, regional and local molecular level estimations of ESBLs that are agents of DA-NIs are critical for better management of empiric therapy, especially for patients in ICUs.

Background

Device-associated nosocomial infections (DA-NIs), especially ventilator-associated pneumonia (VAP) and catheter-associated urinary tract infections (CAUTIs) pose the greatest threat to patient safety in the ICUs [1–3]. VAP is the most lethal among the two, however, CAUTIs are the most common *Enterobacteriaceae* that have been indicated as the most common cause of extended-spectrum β-lactamases (ESBL) producing bacteria in ICUs. These bacteria have a plethora of resistance mechanisms and often use multiple mechanisms against the same antibiotic or use a single mechanism to affect multiple antibiotics. Resistance to broad-spectrum cephalosporin is spreading quickly among *Enterobacteriaceae* and this is mostly related to acquisition of ESBL genes. Isolates that express ESBL phenotypes and hydrolize the beta lactam antibiotics are often multiple drug resistant (MDR) [4, 5]. The commonly genes related to the ESBL phenotype

* Correspondence: drmsrezaii49@gmail.com
[1]Infection Diseases Research Center with Focus on Nosocomial Infection, Mazandaran University of Medical Sciences, Sari, Iran
Full list of author information is available at the end of the article

are sulf-hydryl variable (SHV), cefotaxime-beta lactamases (CTX), Vietnam extended-spectrum β-lactamase (VEB) and Guyana Extended-Spectrum ß-lactamases (GES) genes. Integrons as mobile DNA elements, are capable of detention and excision of antibiotic-resistant genes. Integrons achieve this by site-specific recombination. The different combinations of gene cassettes can contribute to the diverse genetic organization of integrons. There are five different classes of integrons. Class 1 integrons are the most common type that are present in *Enterobacteriaceae*.

Class 2 integrons are associated with the Tn7 transposon, whose transposition activity is directed at specific attachment sites on chromosomes or plasmids. Many of the antibiotic-resistant genes found in clinical isolates of *Enterobacteriaceae* are part of a gene cassette inserted into an integron [6]. Due to the potential of integrons to capture and collect gene cassettes, it is likely that incidence of MDR bacteria such as ESBL-producing *Enterobacteriaceae*, will become more prevalent in the future and integrons will continue to threaten the usefulness of antibiotics as therapeutic agents [6–8]. ESBL genes can be located on integrons, which may facilitate the spread of such genetic elements. To the best of our knowledge, this study is the first of its kind on ESBL-producing *Enterobacteriaceae* and incidence of integrons in these bacteria isolated from VAP and CAUTI as a major threat to patient safety in ICU wards, which was conducted in 18 governmental hospitals of Mazandaran province (The largest province in the north of Iran in terms of area and population).

Methods
Study population and DA-NIs definitions
This cross-sectional study was conducted in 18 governmental hospitals that overall contained 1200 ward beds and 100 intensive care unit beds, in Mazandaran province, located in the north of Iran, during 2014 and 2015. This study was approved by the Ethics Committee of Mazandaran University of Medical Sciences (Code No: 879 Date: July 9, 2014).

DA-NIs were defined as: Catheter-Associated Urinary Tract Infection; patient with a urinary catheter that had fever, dysuria, frequency, flank pain, suprapubic pain, nausea and vomiting. In addition, the urine culture was positive for 10^5 colony forming units per mL or more, with no more than two microorganisms isolated or, must have had at least two symptoms such as fever, dysuria, frequency, flank pain, suprapubic pain, nausea and vomiting plus pyuria.

Ventilator-Associated Pneumonia; Ventilator-associated pneumonia was indicated in a mechanically ventilated patient with a chest radiograph that showed new or progressive infiltrates, cavitation, consolidation, or pleural effusion 48 h after hospitalization. The patient must have

had at least one of the following criteria: new onset of purulent sputum or change in character of sputum; organism cultured from blood or from a specimen obtained by tracheal aspirate, bronchoalveolar lavage or bronchial brushing, or biopsy.

Sepsis due to VAP; in patients ventilated more than 72 h, and bacteria separated from positive blood culture and tracheal tube aspirate positive culture were similar; while the patients had the symptoms of systemic inflammatory response syndrome (SIRS).

For all the patients whom were subject to ventilator and urinary catheter, certain prevention strategies were used against VAP and CAUTIs.

The prevention strategies for CAUTIs: insert catheters just for appropriate indications; leave catheters only as long as needed; only trained nurses insert and maintain catheters; hand hygiene; Insert catheters using aseptic technique and sterile equipment; aseptic insertion, maintain a closed drainage system; maintain unobstructed urine flow.

The prevention strategies for VAP are: elevation of the head of the bed; oral hygiene care; Prophylaxis interventions for peptic ulcer disease and deep vein thrombosis.

Sampling and microbiological methods
For VAP, a deep tracheal aspirate from the endotracheal tube was obtained, and for CAUTI, urine was aseptically aspirated from the sampling port of the urinary catheter for performing gram stain and culture on selective media. Sampling was done by the head nurses and the samples were immediately transported in a transport medium to the microbiology laboratory. All the samples were routinely cultured on MacConkey and blood agar plates. Blood samples were cultured in Blood culture bottles. Isolates were identified at the species level using standard biochemical tests and microbiological methods [9, 10].

Antibiotic susceptibility test
Susceptibility of the clinical isolates to routinely used antibiotics was determined by the standard broth dilution (micro dilution) technique. MIC was determined according to the recommendations of the standard protocol of CLSI 2010. The antibiotics were purchased from Sigma chemical company. Antibiotics used in this study were Amikacin, Ciprofloxacin, Imipenem, Gentamicin, Ceftazidime, Tobramycin, Piperacillin-Tazobactam, Cefepime, Colistin and Co-trimoxazole.

Phenotype detection of extended-spectrum beta-lactamase (ESBL) producing *enterobacteriaceae*
ESBL-producing *Enterobacteriaceae* was detected using the double-disk synergy (DDS) test [11, 12]. ESBL's presence was assayed using the following antibiotic

disks (MAST, UK): cefotaxime (30 μg), cefotaxime/clavulanic acid (30/10 μg), ceftazidime (30 μg), and ceftazidime/clavulanic acid (30/10 μg). *Escherichia coli* ATCC 25922 strain served as positive controls.

DNA extraction and detection of ESBL-related genes

Enterobacteriaceae that were phenotypically confirmed as ESBL, were evaluated for ESBL-related genes. DNA of ESBL-positive *Enterobacteriaceae* was extracted using a commercial gene extraction kit (DNA Zist, Iran) according to the company's instructions. ESBL-positive strains were screened by the PCR method for genes bla CTX, bla VEB, bla GES, bla SHV and also integrons class 1 and class 2. The set of primers and PCR amplification conditions are available in Additional file 1. After performing the PCR reaction, electrophoresis of PCR products was carried out in 2% agarose gel at 70 voltage for 50 min. Then, results were evaluated under UV light on the UV Trans illuminator. In all the experiments, the following reference strains were used as positive controls: *K. pneumoniae* 7881 (*CTXM*), *K. pneumoniae* 7881 strain (containing *SHV*), *P. aeruginosa* ATCC 27853 (VEB-1), and *K. pneumoniae* (GES). *E. coli* 96 K062 was used as a positive control for classes 1 and 2 integrons. A non-ESBL-producing strain (*E. coli* ATCC 25922) was used as negative control.

Statistical analysis

Data were analyzed using SPSS software version 16. Descriptive statistics, Chi- square and Fisher's exact tests were used for statistical analysis.

Results

Out of total of 205 hospitalized patients with DA-NIs in ICU wards of the mentioned hospitals during 2014–2015, *Enterobacteriaceae* were responsible of 149 (72.68%) of DA-NIs. The most frequently found *Enterobacteriaceae* were; *Klebsiella pneumoniae* 75 (24; 32% ESBL

positive & 51; 68% ESBL negative), *E. coli* 69 (6; 8.69% ESBL positive & 63; 91.30% ESBL negative) and *Enterobacter* spp. 5 (5; 100% ESBL positive). The most common DA-NIs caused by *Enterobacteriaceae* were VAP (77.18%), CAUTI (19.46%) and sepsis due to VAP (3.35%).

The demographic feature of patients with DA-NIs caused by ESBL *Enterobacteriaceae* was as follows; 27 VAP patients (15; 55.5% male and 12; 44.4% female) with average age of 66.5 ± 20.17 years and average duration of hospitalization in the ICU of 28.37 ± 20.03 days; three CAUTI patients (1; 33.3% male and 2; 66.6% female) with average age of 45.66 ± 21.93 years and average duration of hospitalization in the ICU of 19.33 ± 15.63 days; five patients of sepsis due to VAP (2;40% male and 3;60% female) with average age of 60.25 ± 14.79 years and average duration of hospitalization in the ICU of 10.75 ± 1.89 days.

In total, the distribution of ESBL-related genes was 33 (94.3%) bla-SHV, 17 (48.6%) bla-CTX, 8 (22.9%) bla-VEB and 6 (17.14%) bla-GES. Figure 1 that is the illustration of agarose gel, shows the strains containing VEB, SHV, int1 (integron class1), int2 (integron class 2), GES and CTX genes. The Antibiotic susceptibility pattern of *Enterobacteriaceae* containing ESBL-related genes is shown in detail in Table 1. The rate of antibiotic resistance among strains containing SHV gene was 27.3–78.8% whereas the rate of sensitivity was 6.1–48.5%. On the other hand, Gentamicin and Imipenem had the highest resistance and sensitivity rates respectively. The rate of antibiotic resistance among strains containing CTX gene was 41.2–88.2%, whereas the rate of sensitivity was 5.9–35%. In addition, Gentamicin and Ciprofloxacin had the highest resistance and sensitivity rates respectively. The rate of antibiotic resistance among strains containing VEB gene was 12.5–87%, whereas the rate of sensitivity was 12.5–75% and Ceftazidime and Ciprofloxacin had the highest resistance and sensitivity rates respectively. The rate of antibiotic resistance among strains containing

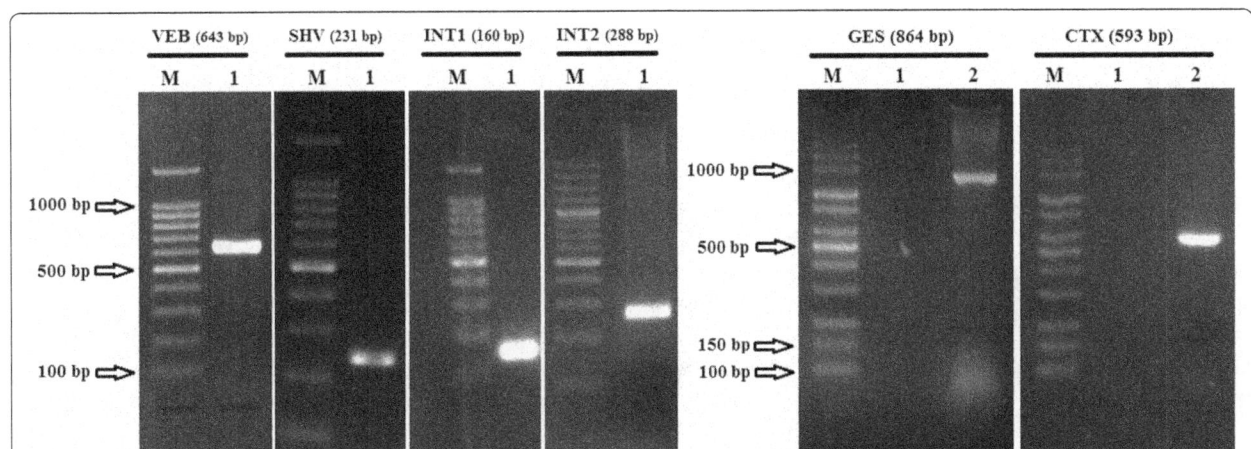

Fig. 1 Agarose gel showing the strains containing, VEB, SHV, int1 (integron class1), int2 (integron class 2), GES and CTX genes

Table 1 Antibiotic susceptibility pattern of *Enterobacteriaceae* containing ESBL related genes

		Klebsiella pneumoniae N=24 Positive ESBL related genes				Enterobacter .spp N=5				E.coli N=6			
		SHV N=22	CTX N=14	VEB N=4	GES N=4	SHV N=5	CTX N=2	VEB N=3	GES N=1	SHV N=6	CTX N=1	VEB N=1	GES N=1
Amikacin	R	50	50	25	25	60	100	33	0	66.6	100	100	100
	I	27.2	28.5	50	25	40	0	66	100	16.6	0	0	0
	S	22.7	21.5	25	50	0	0	0	0	16.6	0	0	0
Ciprofloxacin	R	40.9	50	0	25	0	0	0	0	33.3	0	0	100
	I	31.8	28.5	50	50	0	0	0	0	-	-	-	-
	S	27.2	21.5	50	25	100	100	100	100	66.6	100	100	0
Imipenem	R	36.3	50	25	50	0	0	0	0	16.6	0	0	0
	I	27.2	28.5	25	25	20	50	33	100	16.6	0	0	100
	S	36.3	21.5	50	25	80	50	66	0	66.6	100	100	0
Gentamicin	R	81.8	85.7	50	100	80	100	33	0	83.33	100	100	100
	I	4.54	0	0	0	20	0	33	100	16.6	0	0	0
	S	13.63	14.2	50	0	0	0	33	0	-	-	-	-
Ceftazidime	R	72.7	57.14	75	50	60	50	100	100	50	100	100	0
	I	27.2	35.7	25	25	40	50	0	0	33.3	0	0	100
	S	13.63	7.1	0	25	0	0	0	0	16.6	0	0	0
Tobramycin	R	59	64.28	50	25	60	100	33	0	33.3	0	0	100
	I	31.8	28.57	50	50	0	0	0	0	16.6	0	100	0
	S	9.1	7.1	0	25	40	0	66	100	50	100	0	0
Piperacillin-Tazobactam	R	63.6	64.28	50	75	60	0	33	100	16.6	0	0	0
	I	31.8	28.57	25	25	0	50	66	0	66.6	100	100	100
	S	4.54	7.1	25	0	40	50	0	0	16.6	0	0	0
Cefepime	R	72.7	85.71	25	100	60	100	66	100	33.3	0	100	0
	I	9.1	7.1	25	0	20	0	0	0	16.6	0	0	100
	S	18.18	7.1	50	0	20	0	33	0	50	100	0	0
Colistin	R	72.7	71.42	50	25	40	100	33	0	33.3	0	0	100
	I	27.2	14.2	25	25	20	0	0	0	16.6	100	0	0
	S	13.63	14.2	25	50	40	0	66	100	50	0	100	0
Co-trimoxazole	R	81.8	85.71	75	75	80	100	66	0	33.3	0	100	100
	I	-	-	-	-	0	0	0	0	-	-	-	-
	S	18.2	14.2	25	25	20	0	33	100	66.6	100	0	0

R resistant, *I* intermediate, *S* sensitive

GES gene was 16.7–83.3% whereas the rate of sensitivity was 16.7–66.7%. On the other hand, Cefepime and Imipenem had the highest resistance and sensitivity rates respectively. The incidence of integrons class 1 and class 2 was 29 (82.92%) and 1 (2.9%) respectively. Antibiotic susceptibility pattern of integron-positive *Enterobacteriaceae* is shown in Table 2.

The rate of antibiotic resistance among integron class 1 positive strain was 35–85%. The only integron class 2 positive strain was *Klebsiella pneumoniae* and this

isolate was resistant to all the antibiotics. Eight types of ESBL genes were seen among the isolates. Coincidence of each type of ESBL-producing bacteria and integron class 1 is shown in Table 3. Nine strains contained three ESBL genes (2 strains had GES, VEB, and SHV, 3 strains had GES, CTX, and SHV and 4 strains had VEB, CTX, and SHV). Fourteen strains contained 2 ESBL genes (10 strains had CTX and SHV, one strain had GES and SHV and three strains had VEB and SHV). Twelve strains had only one ESBL gene (11 strains contained

Table 2 Antibiotic susceptibility pattern of integron positive *Enterobacteriaceae*

		Klebsiella pneumoniae		Enterobacter .spp		E.coli	
		N = 24		N = 5		N = 6	
		Integron class 1	Integron class 2	Integron class 1	Integron class 2	Integron class 1	Integron class 2
		N = 20	N = 1	N = 4	N = 0	N = 6	N = 0
Amikacin	R	55	100	75	-	66.6	-
	I	25	0	25		16.6	
	S	20	0	0		16.6	
Ciprofloxacin	R	45	100	0	-	33.3	-
	I	35	0	0		-	
	S	20	0	100		66.6	
Imipenem	R	35	0	0	-	16.6	-
	I	30	0	25		16.6	
	S	35	100	75		66.6	
Gentamicin	R	80	100	75	-	83.3	-
	I	5	0	0		16.6	
	S	15	0	25		-	
Ceftazidime	R	55	100	50	-	50	-
	I	30	0	50		33.3	
	S	15	0	0		16.6	
Tobramycin	R	60	0	75	-	33.3	-
	I	30	100	0		16.6	
	S	10	0	25		50	
Piperacillin-Tazobactam	R	70	100	75	-	16.6	-
	I	30	0	25		66.6	
	S	0	0	0		16.6	
Cefepime	R	80	100	75	-	33.3	-
	I	10	0	25		16.6	
	S	10	0	0		50	
Collstln	R	60	0	50	-	33.3	-
	I	25	100	25		16.6	
	S	15	0	25		50	
Co-trimoxazole	R	85	100	75	-	33.3	-
	I	-	-	0		-	
	S	15	0	25		66.6	

R resistant, *I* intermediate, *S* sensitive

SHV and one strain had CTX). Coincidence of isolates that contained different types of ESBL genes and integron class 1 was 75–100%, which was statistically significant ($P > .05$).

Discussions

DA-NIs due to MDR bacteria are a serious threat to patient safety, being among of the most serious causes of morbidity, mortality and economic burden in developing countries such as Iran. Various studies have shown that the DA-NIs are a serious issue in Iran [13–16] But no studies had specifically addressed and evaluated the ESBL genes and mobile genetic elements such as integrons in *Enterobacteriaceae* as common agents of DA-NIs patients in Iran. It was found in this study that ESBL-producing *Enterobacteriaceae* were causative agents of 23% of DA-NIs in the region. Rosenthal et al. surveyed DA-NIs in 55 ICUs of eight developing countries and found that VAP posed the greatest risk (41%), followed by CVC-related bloodstream infections (30%) and CAUTI (29%). On the other hand, they reported *Enterobacteriaceae* were agents of about 27% of VAPs and 42% of CAUTIs [16]. In our study, overall 56% of *Enterobacteriaceae* were resistant to

Table 3 Coincidence of ESBL genes types and integron class 1 among *Enterobacteriaceae* isolated

ESBL types	Number	Coincidence with integron class 1	P value
GES, VEB, SHV	2 (5.71)	2 (100)	0.00
GES, CTX, SHV	3 (8.57)	3 (100)	0.00
VEB, CTX, SHV	4 (11.42)	3 (75)	0.00
CTX, SHV	10 (28.57)	8 (80)	0.01
GES, SHV	1 (2.85)	1 (100)	0.00
VEB, SHV	3 (8.57)	1 (100)	0.00
SHV	11 (31.42)	11 (100)	0.02
CTX	1 (2.85)	1 (100)	0.00

the 3rd generation of cephalosporin, and imipenem was the most effective antibiotic. Similar to the results of this study, Rosenthal et al. reported that 51% of *Enterobacteriaceae* isolates were resistant to ceftriaxone [16]. Salomao et al. reported that in five ICUs in three urban hospitals of Brazil during a three-year period, VAP rate was 20.9 per 1000 ventilator days, CAUTI rate was 9.6 per 1000 catheter days, and *Enterobacteriaceae* were agents of 22.8% of DA-NIs. *Enterobacteriaceae* in their study were resistant to ceftriaxone in 96.7% of the cases and resistance to ceftazidime was seen in 79.3% of the cases [17]. Guanche-Garcell in Cuba determined the incidence rate of DA-NIs to be 17.0% for VAP, 4.4% for CAUTI and 1% for CVC. They found that overall 51.7% of all DA-NIs were caused by *Enterobacteriaceae*. *Escherichia coli* was responsible for VAP and CAUTI for 15.4 and 53.8% of the cases respectively. VAP and CAUTI due to *Klebsiella* spp. were 23.1 and 15.4% respectively. The rate of VAP caused by *Enterobacteriaceae* in the mentioned studies was lower than the findings of this study.

ESBL *Enterobacteriaceae* pose unique challenges to infection control professionals and antibacterial-discovery scientists [18, 19]. In this study, prevalence of ESBL-related genes was; 94.3% for SHV, 48.6% for CTX, 22.9%for VEB and 17.14% for GES. β-Lactams not only are extensively used for treatment of common infections, but also frequently used as prophylaxis before surgery. *Enterobacteriaceae* are of clinical importance since they cause infections, especially in patients that use the devices in ICUs. ESBL-producing *Enterobacteriaceae* are often MDR, further limiting the therapeutic options. In the present study, Co-resistance with fluoroquinolones, aminoglycosides, trimethoprim, and cephalosporins were found in average in 33–80% of ESBL bacteria. Knowledge of the local epidemiology of ESBL DA-NIs in molecular level is very important. For an immunocompromised patient, such as patients admitted in ICUs with DA-NIs caused by ESBL-producing *Enterobacteriaceae*, administration of an ineffective antibiotic can be lethal. The rate of ESBL varies geographically but it is increasing

fast in the region; for example in our previous study on ESBL-Escherichia coli uropathogens of pediatrics in 2014, the rate of ESBL genes were SHV (44%), CTX (28%), VEB (8%), and GES (0%); but in this study, the rate of these genes were 16.6–100% among *E. coli* [20]. In addition, Khorshidi et al. in Kashan and Khosravi et al. in Ahvaz, reported the rates of bla-SHV to be about 50%, which is lower than the findings of this study [21, 22]. The prevalence of ESBL-producing *Enterobacteriaceae* in Iran has been reported in different rates by phenotypic confirmatory test.

For example Behroozi et al., reported that 21% of *E. coli* and 12% of *K. pneumonia* isolates were ESBL producers; on the other hand, Feizabadi et al. reported that 72% of *K. pneumonia* strains isolated from Tehran hospitals were ESBL producers. Also in our previous study on bacteria isolated from patients with chronic sinusitis, the rate of ESBL-producing bacteria was 28.75–37.03% among *Enterobacteriaceae* [12, 23, 24]. High prevalence of ESBL-producing *Enterobacteriaceae* that are agents of DA-NIS in ICUs, represent the rising problem of antibiotic resistance rate in the ICUs, which is caused by suboptimal infection control in hospitals and new mutations of resistant genes. Transmission of the genes of ESBL enzymes can occur by horizontal gene transfer. Integrons, as common genetic mobile elements, are associated with ESBL genes. In this study, the presence of class 1 integron varied from 80 to 100% among ESBL-producing species; also eight types of ESBL-producing *Enterobacteriaceae* were found. All these types significantly correlate with the incidence of integron class 1 ($p \geq 0.02$). Similar to these results, association of certain beta-lactamase genes with class 1 integrons by location of bla genes within integron platforms (blaVIM, blaIMP, blaGES, blaVEB, blaCTX-M-2/-9, and blaCMY) or by sharing the same plasmid context (blaTEM and blaSHV) among *Enterobacteriaceae*, has been previously reported in several studies [25–28].

Conclusions

The emergence of ESBL *Enterobacteriaceae* among DA-NIs is increasing in the Mazandaran province. The emergence of coincidence of different types of ESBL genes with integrons in 75–100% of strains is really dangerous and alarming for clinicians and healthcare safety managers. Due to the fact that prevalence of ESBL-producing strains can vary greatly from one ward to another, and even for a given ward in different points in time, therefore estimating regional and local ESBL agents of DA-NIs in molecular level in high-risk wards, at least once a year, could be useful in clinical decision-making of empiric therapy, especially for patients in ICUs.

Abbreviations

CAUTI: Catheter-associated urinary tract infections; CTX: Cefotaxime-beta lactamases; CVC: Central venous catheter; DA-NIs: Device associated nosocomial infections; ESBL: Extended-spectrum beta-lactamases; GES: Guyana Extended-Spectrum ß-lactamases; ICU: Intensive care unit; MIC: Minimum inhibitory concentration; NIs: Nosocomial infection; PCR: Polymerase chain reaction; SHV: Sulf-hydryl variable; VAP: Ventilator-associated pneumonia; VEB: Vietnam extended-spectrum β-lactamase

Acknowledgments

This article was a part of a specialty's thesis of Pediatric of Dr Azin Hajalibeig and was supported by the Vice-Chancellor for Research at Mazandaran University of Medical Sciences (Grant Number: 879).

Funding

Mohammad Sadegh Rezai received Research grants of Vice-Chancellor for Research at Mazandaran University of Medical Sciences with grant number 879.

Authors' contributions

Mohammad Sadegh Rezai and Masome Bagheri Nesami designed the project, collected data and wrote the manuscript. Gohar Eslami, Azin Hajalibeig, Fatemeh Ahangarkani and Attieh Nikkhah collected data. Alireza Rafiei carried out laboratory examinations. All authors read and approved the final manuscript.

Competing interests

The authors declare that they have no competing interests.

Author details

[1]Infection Diseases Research Center with Focus on Nosocomial Infection, Mazandaran University of Medical Sciences, Sari, Iran. [2]Molecular and Cell Biology Research Center, Department of Immunology, Faculty of Medicine, Mazandaran University of Medical Sciences, Sari, Iran. [3]Department of Clinical Pharmacy, Faculty of Pharmacy, Mazandaran University of Medical Sciences, Sari, Iran. [4]Student Research Committee, Antimicrobial Resistance Research Center, Mazandaran University of Medical Sciences, Sari, Iran. [5]Traditional and Complementary Medicine Research Center, Mazandaran University of Medical Sciences, Sari, Iran.

References

1. Blot S, et al. Influence of matching for exposure time on estimates of attributable mortality caused by nosocomial bacteremia in critically ill patients. Infect Control Hosp Epidemiol. 2005;26(4):352–6.
2. Maki DG, Tambyah PA. Engineering out the risk for infection with urinary catheters. Emerg Infect Dis. 2001;7(2):342.
3. Heyland DK, et al. The attributable morbidity and mortality of ventilator-associated pneumonia in the critically ill patient. Am J Respir Crit Care Med. 1999;159(4):1249–56.
4. Bradford PA. Extended-spectrum β-lactamases in the 21st century: characterization, epidemiology, and detection of this important resistance threat. Clin Microbiol Rev. 2001;14(4):933–51.
5. Pitout JD, Laupland KB. Extended-spectrum beta-lactamase-producing Enterobacteriaceae: an emerging public-health concern. Lancet Infect Dis. 2008;8(3):159–66.
6. White PA, McIver CJ, Rawlinson WD. Integrons and gene cassettes in the enterobacteriaceae. Antimicrob Agents Chemother. 2001;45(9):2658–61.
7. Ploy M-C, et al. Integrons: an antibiotic resistance gene capture and expression system. Clin Chem Lab Med. 2000;38(6):483–7.
8. Machado E, et al. Preservation of integron types among Enterobacteriaceae producing extended-spectrum β-lactamases in a Spanish hospital over a 15-year period (1988 to 2003). Antimicrob Agents Chemother. 2007;51(6):2201–4.
9. Collee J, Miles R, Watt B. Tests for identification of bacteria. In: Collee JG, Fraser AG, Marmion BP, editors. Practical medical microbiology. 14th ed. Edinburgh: Churchill Livingstone; 1996. p. 131–50.
10. Koneman E, Allen S, Janda W, Schreckenberger R, Winn W. Introduction to microbiology. In: Koneman EW, Alien SD, Janda WM, Schreckenberger RC, Winn W, editors. Part II; Guidelines for collection, transport, processing, analysis, and reporting of cultures from specific specimen sources, Color atlasand textbook of diagnostic microbiology. 5th ed. Philadelphia: Lippincott; 1997. p. 121–70.
11. Jarlier V, et al. Extended broad-spectrum β-lactamases conferring transferable resistance to newer β-lactam agents in Enterobacteriaceae: hospital prevalence and susceptibility patterns. Rev Infect Dis. 1988;10(4):867–78.
12. Rezai M-s, et al. Multidrug resistance pattern of bacterial agents isolated from patient with chronic sinusitis. Caspian J Intern Med. 2016;7(2):114–9.
13. Afhami S, et al. Ventilator-associated pneumonia in a teaching hospital in Tehran and use of the Iranian Nosocomial Infections Surveillance Software. East Mediterr Health J. 2013;19(10):883.
14. Askarian M, et al. Incidence of urinary tract and bloodstream infections in Ghotbeddin Burn Center, Shiraz 2000–2001. Burns. 2003;29(5):455–9.
15. Jahani-Sherafat S, et al. Device-associated infection rates and bacterial resistance in six academic teaching hospitals of Iran: findings from the International Nocosomial Infection Control Consortium (INICC). J Infect Public Health. 2015;8(6):553–61.
16. Rosenthal VD, et al. Device-associated nosocomial infections in 55 intensive care units of 8 developing countries. Ann Intern Med. 2006;145(8):582–91.
17. Salomao R, et al. Device-associated infection rates in intensive care units of Brazilian hospitals: findings of the International Nosocomial Infection Control Consortium. Rev Panam Salud Publica. 2008;24(3):195–202.
18. Behzadnia S, et al. Nosocomial infections in pediatric population and antibiotic resistance of the causative organisms in north of Iran. Iran Red Crescent Med J. 2014;16(2):e14562. doi:10.5812/ircmj.14562.
19. Saffar M, et al. Antibacterial susceptibility of uropathogens in 3 hospitals, Sari, Islamic Republic of Iran, 2002–2003. 2008.
20. Rezai MS et al. Characterization of Multidrug Resistant Extended-Spectrum Beta-Lactamase-Producing Escherichia coli among Uropathogens of Pediatrics in North of Iran. Biomed Res Int. 2015;2015. doi:10.1155/2015/309478.
21. Khorshidi A, et al. Prevalence of TEM1 & SHV1 genes in Kelebsiella pneumoniea with ESBL. J Mil Med. 2009;11(3):149–53.
22. Khosravi AD, Hoveizavi H, Mehdinejad M. Prevalence of Klebsiella pneumoniae Encoding Genes for Ctx-M-1, Tem-1 and Shv-1 Extended-Spectrum Beta Lactamases (ESBL) Enzymes in Clinical Specimens. Jundishapur J Microbiol. 2013;6(10):e8256. doi:10.5812/jjm.8256.
23. Behrooozi A, Rahbar M, Jalil V. Frequency of extended spectrum beta-lactamase (ESBLs) producing Escherichia coli and Klebseilla pneumonia isolated from urine in an Iranian 1000-bed tertiary care hospital. Afr J Microbiol Res. 2010;4(9):881–4.
24. Feizabadi MM, et al. Genetic characterization of ESBL producing strains of Klebsiella pneumoniae from Tehran hospitals. J Infect Dev Ctries. 2010;4(10):609–15.
25. Corkill JE, Anson JJ, Hart CA. High prevalence of the plasmid-mediated quinolone resistance determinant qnrA in multidrug-resistant Enterobacteriaceae from blood cultures in Liverpool, UK. J Antimicrob Chemother. 2005;56(6):1115–7.
26. Jones LA, et al. The aadB gene cassette is associated with blaSHV genes in Klebsiella species producing extended-spectrum β-lactamases. Antimicrob Agents Chemother. 2005;49(2):794–7.

6

Estimating the morbidity and mortality associated with infections due to multidrug-resistant bacteria (MDRB), France, 2012

M. Colomb-Cotinat[1]* , J. Lacoste[1], C. Brun-Buisson[2], V. Jarlier[3], B. Coignard[1] and S. Vaux[1]

Abstract

Background: A study based on 2007 data estimated that 386,000 infections due to multidrug-resistant bacteria (MDRB) occurred in Europe that year and 25,000 patients died from these infections. Our objective was to estimate the morbidity and mortality associated with these infections in France.

Methods: The MDRB considered were methicillin-resistant *Staphylococcus aureus* (MRSA), glycopeptide-resistant *enterococci*, third-generation cephalosporin-resistant (3GC-R) *Escherichia coli* and *Klebsiella pneumoniae*, carbapenem-resistant *Klebsiella pneumoniae*, *Acinetobacter* spp. and *Pseudomonas aeruginosa* (CR *P. aeruginosa*). The number of invasive infections (infections with bacteria isolated from blood or cerebrospinal fluid) due to MDRB, as reported by France to EARS-Net in 2012, was corrected for the coverage of our surveillance network and extrapolated to other body sites using ratios from the French healthcare-associated infections point prevalence survey and the literature. Mortality associated with MDRB infection was estimated using proportions from the literature. Methods and parameters were reviewed by a panel of experts.

Results: We estimate that 158,000 (127,000 to 245,000) infections due to MDRB occurred in 2012 in France (incidence: 1.48 to 2.85 per 1000 hospital days), including 16,000 invasive infections. MRSA, 3GC-R *E. coli* and *K. pneumoniae* were responsible for 120,000 (90,000 to 172,000) infections, i.e., 75% of the total. An estimated 12,500 (11,500 to 17,500) deaths were associated with these infections, including 2,700 associated with invasive infections. MRSA, 3GC-R *E. coli* and CR *P. aeruginosa* accounted for 88% of these deaths.

Conclusion: These first estimates confirm that MRSA, 3GC-R *Escherichia coli* and *Klebsiella pneumoniae* account for the largest portion of the morbidity and mortality of infections due to MDRB in France. These results are not directly comparable with the European study because the methodology used differs in many respects. The differences identified between our study and previous studies underline the need to define a standardised protocol for international assessments of the morbidity and mortality of antibiotic resistance. Estimating morbidity and mortality will facilitate communication and awareness in order to reinforce adherence and support of healthcare professionals and policy-makers to MDRB prevention programs.

Keywords: Antimicrobial resistance, Epidemiology, Morbidity, Mortality, Infection due to multidrug resistant bacteria, France

* Correspondence: Melanie.COLOMB-COTINAT@santepubliquefrance.fr
[1]Santé Publique France, The French Public Health Agency, F-94415 Saint-Maurice, France
Full list of author information is available at the end of the article

Background

Antibiotic resistance is a constantly evolving phenomenon and a threat to infection and disease control; it complicates patient management and treatment strategy and prolongs hospital stays. Nowadays, this international public health problem is recognised as one of the scourges of the 21st century [1].

Several studies have sought to estimate the morbidity and mortality of infections due to multidrug-resistant bacteria (MDRB). A joint report from the European Centre for Disease Prevention and Control (ECDC) and the European Medecines Agency (EMEA), published in 2009 and based on data from 2007 [2], estimated at approximately 386,000 the annual number of infections due to MDRB in Europe that year, including 42,500 cases (11%) of bloodstream infections. The number of deaths associated with these infections was estimated at more than 25,000. A report by the US Centers for Disease Control and Prevention (CDC) from 2013 [3] provided an overview of the annual morbidity and mortality of antibiotic-resistant infections in the United States, estimating their number at approximately 2 million and the number of deaths associated with these infections at 23,000. These two studies, although they used different methods and did not consider the same panel of microorganisms, both underlined the important morbidity and mortality of antibiotic resistance on public health.

No corresponding estimate has been so far available for France, despite its wealth of antibiotic-resistance surveillance networks. These networks focus on specific pathogens and sometimes on specific sources of samples [4, 5]. The data they provide are useful for assessing trends and detecting epidemics. Nonetheless, they do not provide an overall view of the MDRB morbidity and mortality nor do they permit simple communication on this topic.

The objective of this study conducted by Santé publique France (the French national public health agency) was to estimate for the first time the morbidity and mortality (number of cases and number of attributable deaths) of infections due to MDRB in France, in order to advocate for strategies to control and prevent them, to guide public health authorities in implementing these policies, and to support communication towards healthcare professionals and the general public.

Methods

Microorganisms selected

The MDRB considered in this study were defined using the following criteria:

- being associated with invasive infections, i.e., infections with a bacteria isolated from blood or cerebrospinal fluid [5];

- having a significant prevalence or having emerged recently;
- being included in a surveillance network in France;
- being multidrug-resistant (MDR) as defined in the European Antimicrobial Resistance Surveillance Network (EARS-Net) protocol [5].

We thus selected eight bacteria–antibiotic combinations:

- *Staphylococcus aureus* resistant to methicillin (MRSA);
- *Enterococcus faecium* and *E. faecalis* resistant to glycopeptides (GRE);
- *Escherichia coli* resistant to third-generation cephalosporins (3GC-R *E. Coli*);
- *Klebsiella pneumoniae* resistant to third-generation cephalosporins (3GC-R *K. pneumoniae*);
- *Pseudomonas aeruginosa* resistant to carbapenems (CR *P. aeruginosa*);
- *Klebsiella pneumoniae* resistant to carbapenems (CR *K. pneumoniae*);
- *Acinetobacter spp.* resistant to carbapenems (CR *Acinetobacter spp*).

According to the EARS-Net protocol, antibiotics considered for resistance were a) for MRSA: oxacillin, methicillin, flucloxacillin, cloxacillin, dicloxacillin and cefoxitin (and PCR mecA or PBP2a detection); b) for GRE: vancomycin; c) for 3GC-R *E.coli* and 3GC-R *K. pneumoniae*: cefotaxime, ceftriaxone, ceftazidime; d) for CR *P. aeruginosa*; imipenem, meropenem; e) for CR *K. pneumoniae*: imipenem, meropenem; f) for CR *Acinetobacter spp*: imipenem, meropenem, doripenem.

Streptococcus pneumoniae with reduced penicillin susceptibility was not considered as MDRB in accordance with generally accepted microbiological criteria [6].

Number of infections due to MDRB

To select the most frequently diagnosed infectious body sites for each of these MDRB, data from the 2012 point prevalence survey on healthcare-associated infections and antimicrobial use in French hospitals (2012 PPS) [7] were used. This survey, conducted every five years on a single day in nearly all French healthcare facilities collects standardised data about nosocomial infections. In 2012, data were collected for 91% of French hospital beds.

Based on this data, the following infectious body sites were selected, as there were the most frequent infections in the 2012 PPS:

- for all MDRB: invasive infections (bacteria isolated from blood or cerebrospinal fluid), urinary tract infections, skin and soft tissue infections, and surgical site infections;

- for all MDRB excluding GRE: respiratory tract infections;
- for MRSA only: bone and joint infections (does not include surgical site infections);
- for GRE only: gastrointestinal tract infections (gastro-intestinal and intra-abdominal infections).

The number of invasive infections for each MDRB was estimated from data transmitted by France to EARS-Net [5]. This European network collects resistance data of bacterial strains isolated from invasive infections (bacteria isolated from blood or cerebrospinal fluid). As duplicate isolates for the same patients had already been eliminated during data collection, the number of incident cases of invasive infections due to MDRB occurring each year in the network was directly estimated from the number of resistant strains isolated. For instance, there were 1005 strains of MRSA reported in EARS-Net for France in 2012, so the number of incident cases of invasive infections due to MRSA in 2012 in the French EARS network was estimated as 1005.

The number of incident cases of invasive infections was then corrected by taking into account the coverage of the EARS-Net network for France, estimated from the number of inpatient hospital days (HD) reported by hospitals whose laboratories had transmitted data to the network (secondary and tertiary care hospitals). The list of these hospitals was obtained from the Epibac network [8] and the total number of HD from the 2012 Health Facilities Annual Statistics (SAE) report [9]. The EARS-Net coverage was estimated by dividing the number of HD in the participating hospitals (N_1) by the total number of HD in all French secondary and tertiary care hospitals that same year provided by the same source (N_2). For instance, the number of cases of invasive infections due to MRSA in 2012 for France was estimated as 5574 (n_1). The incidence of patients with an invasive infection was also expressed as the number of cases per 1000 HD.

In order to estimate the number of cases with infections at other body sites, the ratio between the number of cases with infections at a given body site and the number of cases of invasive infections was calculated for each MDRB and each body site using data from the 2012 PPS. For instance, to evaluate the number of cases of urinary tract infections (UTI) due to MRSA in our study, we first calculated a specific ratio between the number of UTI due to MRSA reported in the 2012 PPS ($n = 103$) divided by the number of invasive infections due to MRSA reported in the 2012 PPS ($n = 105$). The specific ratio for UTI due to MRSA was $103/105 = 0.98$. We then multiplied the number of cases with invasive infections due to MRSA estimated in our study based on EARS-Net data ($n_1 = 5574$) by this ratio (0.98), to estimate the number of cases with urinary tract infections due to MRSA in France ($n_{11} = 5468$). The same approach was used for other body sites and MDRB.

In order to have intervals of plausibility around these estimates, we also estimated these ratios from a non-systematic review of the literature targeting French and European publications when available. Plausibility intervals were then calculated using high and low ratios estimated from the literature. Table 1 presents the ratios that were used, for each MDRB and body sites, to estimate the incidence of cases of non-invasive infections; ratios calculated from the French PPS 2012 were used as target values, and ratios excerpted from the literature as low and high values for intervals of plausibility.

The total number of infections due to MDRB was finally calculated by adding the number of infections obtained for each MDRB species and each body site considered.

Number of deaths associated with infections due to MDRB

For each infection due to MDRB and body site considered, the number of deaths was estimated by applying to the number of cases of infections estimated above the proportion of deaths associated with infection due to MDRB, based on a non-systematic review of the literature (Table 2) that focused on publications reporting proportions of deaths associated with infections due to MDRB considered. Results from French or European studies were used preferentially when available. The mortality indicator used in our study was therefore the number of deaths associated with MDRB infections as a whole, but not the number specifically associated with antibiotic resistance per se. Consequently, this study did not estimate the extra deaths relative to infections due to antibiotic-susceptible bacteria.

When a value for the associated mortality for a body site could not be found in the literature, it was estimated from the mortality associated with invasive infections (mainly bloodstream infections) for each of the MDRB studied, applying a correction factor from a US publication [10].

The total number of deaths associated with an infection due to MDRB was calculated by adding the number of associated deaths obtained for each MDRB and each body site studied.

We jointly validated the choices of the different parameters used in this study (ratios used to estimate the incidence of cases of non-invasive infections and associated mortality proportion) after a critical review with external experts, clinicians and microbiologists.

Figure 1 summarises the methodology used to estimate morbidity and mortality associated with infections due to MDRB in France.

Table 1 Ratios used to estimate the incidence of cases of non-invasive infections, France 2012

Body sites	PPS ratio	Ratios from the literature	
		Low value	High value
No. MRSA urinary tract infections/No. MRSA invasive infections	0.98 [7]	0.75 [11]	2.30 [12]
No. MRSA respiratory infections/No. MRSA invasive infections	2.37 [7]	1.25 [11]	2.50 [12]
No. MRSA skin and soft tissue infections and surgical site infections/No. MRSA invasive infections	4.17 [7]	4.90 [12]	5.25 [11]
No. MRSA bone and joint infections/No. MRSA invasive infections	0.79 [7]	b	1.38 [12]
No. GRE urinary tract infections/No. GRE invasive infections	4.33 [7]	2.33 [13]	3.44 [14]
No. GRE gastrointestinal tract infections /No. GRE invasive infections	2.65 [7]	1.89 [14]	b
No. GRE skin and soft tissue infections and surgical site infections/No. GRE invasive infections	1.46 [7]	4.67 [14]	5.00 [13]
No. 3GC-R *E. coli* urinary tract infections/No. 3GC-R *E. coli* invasive infections	5.50 [7]	2.30 [13]	b
No. 3GC-R *E. coli* respiratory tract infections/No. 3GC-R *E. coli* invasive infections	1.08 [7]	b	2.50 [13]
No. 3GC-R *E. coli* skin and soft tissue infections and surgical site infections/No. 3GC-R *E. coli* invasive infections	1.37 [7]	b	4.90 [13]
No. 3GC-R *K. pneumoniae* urinary tract infections/No. 3GC-R *K. pneumoniae* invasive infections	2.90 [7]	1.19 [15]	2.30 [13]
No. 3GC-R *K. pneumoniae* respiratory tract infections/No. 3GC-R *K. pneumoniae* invasive infections	2.55 [7]	1.19 [15]	2.50 [13]
No. 3GC-R *K. pneumoniae* skin and soft tissue infections and surgical site infections/No. 3GC-R *K. pneumoniae* invasive infections	0.82 [7]	0.33 [15]	4.90 [13]
No. CR *K. pneumoniae* urinary tract infections/No. CR *K. pneumoniae* invasive infections	2.71 [7]	3.00 [16]	3.10 [17]
No. CR *K. pneumoniae* respiratory tract infections/No. CR *K. pneumoniae* invasive infections	3.10 [7]	0.42 [17]	1.60 [16]
No. CR *K. pneumoniae* skin and soft tissue infections and surgical site infections/No. CR *K. pneumoniae* invasive infections	0.44[a]	0.28 [17]	0.60 [16]
No. CR *P. aeruginosa* urinary tract infections/No. CR *P. aeruginosa* invasive infections	2.11 [7]	b	11.30 [15]
No. CR *P. aeruginosa* respiratory tract infections/No. CR *P. aeruginosa* invasive infections	10.99 [7]	b	16.00 [15]
No. CR *P. aeruginosa* skin and soft tissue infections and surgical site infections/No. CR *P. aeruginosa* invasive infections	3.07 [7]	b	4.67 [15]
No. CR *Acinetobacter* urinary tract infections/No. CR *Acinetobacter* invasive infections	0.58[a]	0.32 [18]	0.83 [17]
No. CR *Acinetobacter* respiratory tract infections/No. CR *Acinetobacter* invasive infections	4.64 [7]	1.21 [18]	3.83 [17]
No. CR *Acinetobacter* skin and soft tissue infections and surgical site infections/No. CR *Acinetobacter* invasive infections	0.73[a]	0.29 [18]	1.17 [17]

[a]no 2012 PPS data for these infections because the prevalence of these MDRB is too low in France; the ratio value applied is the mean value of the 2 ratios from the literature

[b]no data in the literature for these infections; the value of the 2012 PPS ratio was applied

Results

Estimate of EARS-Net coverage, France

We estimate that in 2012 EARS-Net covered 18% of HD in secondary and tertiary care hospitals in France.

Number of infections due to MDRB

The number of infections due to MDRB was estimated at approximately 158,000 in France in 2012, for an incidence of 1.83 per 1,000 HD. Data from the literature enabled us to estimate a plausibility interval for the annual number of cases from 127,000 to 245,000 (incidence: 1.48 to 2.85 per 1,000 HD).

Most cases were infections caused by MRSA (33%; plausibility interval: 28 to 38%), 3GC-R *E. coli* (32%; 26 to 32%), CR *P. aeruginosa* (23%; 23 to 29%) or 3GC-R *K. pneumoniae* (10%; 6 to 10%). The other infections due

Table 2 Proportion of mortality associated with infections due to MDRB, France 2012

Body sites	Associated deaths (%)	Reference	Year of publication
MRSA invasive infections	9.8	[19]	2003
MRSA urinary tract infections	0.2	[10, 19]	1998
MRSA respiratory tract infections	7.0	[10, 19]	1998
MRSA skin and soft tissue infections and surgical site infections	1.4	[10, 19]	1998
MRSA bone and joint infections	9.8	d	
GRE invasive infections	25.0	[14]	2002
GRE urinary tract infections	9.0	[14]	2002
GRE gastrointestinal tract infections	3.0	[14]	2002
GRE skin and soft tissue infections and surgical site infections	6.0	[14]	2002
3GC-R *E. coli* invasive infections	18.0	[20]	2010
3GC-R *E. coli* urinary tract infections	0.0	[21]	2006
3GC-R *E. coli* respiratory tract infections	12.9	[10, 20]	1998
3GC-R *E. coli* skin and soft tissue infections and surgical site infections	2.6	[10, 20]	1998
3GC-R *K. pneumoniae* invasive infections	18.0	[20]	2010
3GC-R *K. pneumoniae* urinary tract infections	0.4	[10, 20]	1998
3GC-R *K. pneumoniae* respiratory tract infections	12.9	[10, 20]	1998
3GC-R *K. pneumoniae* skin and soft tissue infections and surgical site infections	2.6	[10, 20]	1998
CR *K. pneumoniae* invasive infections	37.0	[22]	2010
CR *K. pneumoniae* urinary tract infections	0.8	[10, 22]	1998
CR *K. pneumoniae* respiratory tract infections	26.4	[10, 22]	1998
3GC-R *K. pneumoniae* skin and soft tissue infections and surgical site infections	5.4	[10, 22]	1998
CR *P. aeruginosa* invasive infections	33.0	[23]	2010
CR *P. aeruginosa* urinary tract infections	0.8	[10, 23]	1998
CR *P. aeruginosa* respiratory infections	23.6	[10, 23]	1998
CR *P. aeruginosa* skin and soft tissue infections and surgical site infections	4.8	[10, 23]	1998
CR *Acinetobacter* invasive infections	36.5	[24]	2007
CR *Acinetobacter* urinary tract infections	0.8	[10, 24]	1998
CR *Acinetobacter* respiratory infections	26.1	[10, 24]	1998
CR *Acinetobacter* skin and soft tissue infections and surgical site infections	5.3	[10, 24]	1998

dno data could be found in literature, the fraction applied is therefore that estimated for invasive infections. Invasive infections: bacteria isolated from blood or cerebrospinal fluid

to MDRB considered accounted for less than 1% of all cases. Most infections were due to Gram-negative bacteria (67%; 62 to 71%).

Table 3 details the number and incidence rates of infections according to whether or not the infection was invasive. The total number of invasive infections due to MDRB was estimated at approximately 16,000 in 2012 (incidence: 0.185 per 1,000 HD), or 10% (6 to 13%) of all MDRB infections. Overall, 70% of the invasive infections were due to MRSA or 3GC-R *E. coli.*

Infections caused by MRSA were mostly skin and soft tissue and surgical site infections, which altogether accounted for 56% (42 to 45%) of MRSA infections, with an incidence of 0.318 (0.270 to 0.340) per 1,000 HD. Urinary tract infections accounted for most of the

3GC-R *E. coli* infections (40%; range 40 to 61%), with an incidence of 0.152 (0.364-0.364) per 1,000 HD, and respiratory tract infections for most of the CR *P. aeruginosa* infections (64%; range 48 to 64%), with an incidence of 0.274 (0.274 to 0.398) per 1,000 HD.

Number of deaths associated with infections due to MDRB

The number of deaths associated with infections due to MDRB in 2012 was estimated at 12,411 (11,422 to 17,470), of which approximately one fourth (2,800) were due to invasive infections. The corresponding incidence rate was estimated at 0.144 death per 1,000 HD (0.133 to 0.203).

More than half the deaths were associated with CR *P. aeruginosa* (53%; 54 to 58%) (Table 4). Infections caused

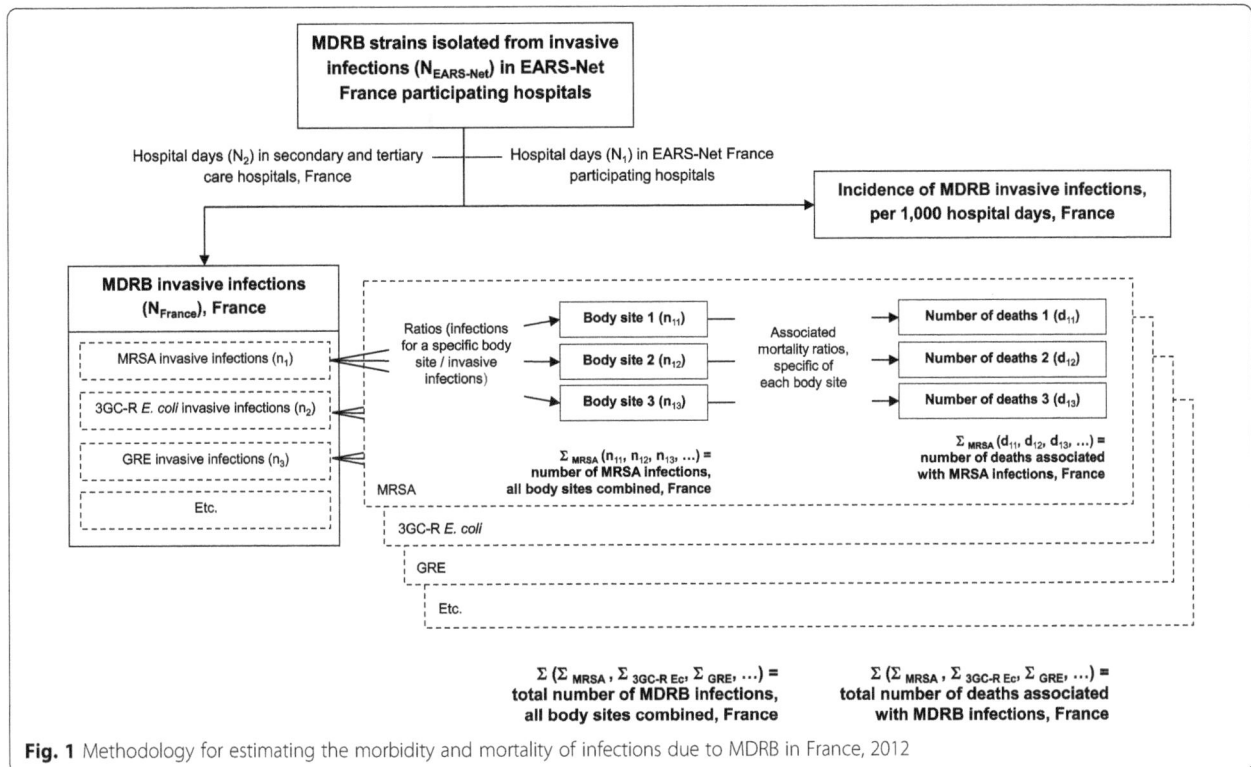

Fig. 1 Methodology for estimating the morbidity and mortality of infections due to MDRB in France, 2012

by MRSA and by 3GC-R *E.coli* were responsible for respectively 16% (15 to 18%) and 18% (16 to 20%) of deaths. Overall, Gram-negative bacteria infections accounted for 83% (82 to 84%) of the estimated total deaths.

Among the deaths associated with infections due to MDRB, 22% (16 to 24%) were due to invasive infections. This proportion was 11% (7 to 11%) for the CR *P. aeruginosa* infections, 24% (20 to 29%) for MRSA infections, and 51% (29 to 51%) for the 3GC-R *E. coli* infections.

Discussion

Our study quantifies for the first time the morbidity and mortality of infections due to MDRB in France. We thus estimate at approximately 158,000 (127,000 to 245,000) the number of infections due to MDRB occurring in 2012 in France, including nearly 16,000 (6 to 12%) invasive infections (bloodstream infections and meningitis), MRSA and the two major *enterobacteriaceae* species resistant to third-generation cephalosporins account for three quarters (70 to 75%) of the infections recorded. The annual number of deaths associated with these infections is estimated at 12,500 (11,500 to 17,500), including 2,800 (22%) due to invasive infections; MRSA, 3GC-R *E. coli* and CR *P. aeruginosa* account for 88% (90 to 92%) of these deaths. Most of the infections considered in this study are healthcare associated infections, and 20 to 30% of them can be considered avoidable [25].

These results underestimate the morbidity and mortality of infections due to antibiotic-resistant bacteria in France. Although our study covers a large panel of MDRB and the most frequent body sites, it does not include all bacteria resistant to antibiotics and all infection sites. For example, as only the most frequent infections in the 2012 PPS data were selected for each MDRB, gastro-intestinal tract infections due to *Enterobacteriacae* were not taken into account in our study.

We did not take into account patients with more than one MDRB. However, this bias in underestimating MDRB infections should be very limited. Indeed, according to data from the 2012 French PPS, only 39 patients among a total of 15,180 infected patients (0.2%) had two or more different MDRB (data not shown).

Furthermore, the extrapolation of EARS-Net data to France was calculated on the number of inpatient hospital days reported only by French secondary and tertiary care hospitals, as the laboratories participating in the EARS-Net network are located only in such institutions. This may have underestimated the incidence of MDRB infections, as cases occurring in other types of hospitals have being ignored. Conversely, taking into account all healthcare institutions in France would have greatly overestimated the incidence since it is based on the assumption that the burden of the antibiotic resistance is comparable in all institutions.

The estimates produced in this study are consistent with those from other French data sources, especially

Table 3 Annual number and incidence rate of infections due to MDRB, France 2012

| MDRB | Body site | Total number of cases (%) | | | Incidence per 1,000 HD | | |
| | | PPS ratio | Ratios from literature | | PPS ratio | Ratios from literature | |
			Low value	High value		Low value	High value
MRSA	Invasive inf.	5,574 (10.8%)	5,574 (11.5%)	5,574 (8.0%)	0.065	0.065	0.065
	Others	46,270 (89.2%)	42,852 (88.5%)	63,710 (92.0%)	0.538	0.498	0.741
	Total	51,844 (100%)	48,426 (100%)	69,284 (100%)	0.603	0.563	0.806
GRE	Invasive inf.	39 (10.6%)	39 (10.1%)	39 (8.3%)	<0.001	<0.001	<0.001
	Others	328 (89.4%)	345 (89.9%)	430 (91.7%)	0.004	0.004	0.005
	Total	367 (100%)	384 (100%)	469 (100%)	0.004	0.004	0.005
3GC-R *E. coli.*	Invasive inf.	5,690 (11.2%)	5,690 (17.4%)	5,690 (7.2%)	0.066	0.066	0.066
	Others	45,226 (88.8%)	27,028 (82.6%)	73,395 (92.8%)	0.526	0.314	0.854
	Total	50,916 (100%)	32,719 (100%)	79,085 (100%)	0.592	0.381	0.920
3GC-R *K. pneumoniae*	Invasive inf.	2,246 (13.8%)	2,246 (27.0%)	2,246 (9.3%)	0.026	0.026	0.026
	Others	14,068 (86.2%)	6,087 (73.0%)	21,789 (90.7%)	0.164	0.071	0.253
	Total	16,314 (100%)	8,333 (100%)	24,035 (100%)	0,190	0.097	0.280
CR *K. pneumoniae*	Invasive inf.	94 (13.8%)	94 (21.3%)	94 (15.9%)	0.001	0.001	0.001
	Others	589 (86.2%)	349 (78.7%)	500 (84.1%)	0.007	0.004	0.006
	Total	683 (100%)	443 (100%)	594 (100%)	0.008	0.005	0.007
CR *P. aeruginosa*	Invasive inf.	2,141 (5.8%)	2,141 (5.8%)	2,141 (3.0%)	0.025	0.025	0.025
	Others	34,616 (94.2%)	34,616 (94.2%)	68,442 (97.0%)	0.403	0.403	0.796
	Total	36,757 (100%)	36,757 (100%)	70,583 (100%)	0.428	0.428	0.821
CR *Acinetobacter spp*	Invasive inf.	111 (14.4%)	111 (35.5%)	111 (14.6%)	0.001	0.001	0.001
	Others	660 (85.6%)	202 (64.5%)	647 (85.4%)	0.008	0.003	0.008
	Total	771 (100%)	313 (100%)	758 (100%)	0.009	0.004	0.009
Total invasive inf.		15,895 (10.1%)	15,895 (12.5%)	15,895 (6.5%)	0.185	0.185	0.185
TOTAL		157,652 (100%)	127,375 (100%)	244,808 (100%)	1.834	1.481	2.847

Invasive infections: bacteria isolated from blood or cerebrospinal fluid

Table 4 Number of deaths associated with infections due to MDRB, France 2012

MDRB	Number of deaths associated with MDRB						Incidence per 1,000 HD			
	PPS ratios		Ratios from literature				PPS ratios	Ratios from literature		
			Low value		High value			Low value	High value	
Gram +										
MRSA	2,236	(18.0%)	1,855	(16.2%)	2,711	(15.5%)	0.026	0.022	0.032	
GRE	31	(0.3%)	31	(0.3%)	36	(0.2%)	<0.001	<0.001	<0.001	
Subtotal Gram +	2,268	(18.3%)	1,886	(16.5%)	2,747	(15.7%)	0.026	0.022	0.032	
Gram -										
3GC-R *E. coli.*	2,020	(16.3%)	2,020	(17.7%)	3,584	(20.5%)	0.023	0.023	0.042	
3GC-R *K. pneumoniae*	1,217	(9.8%)	779	(6.8%)	1,436	(8.2%)	0.014	0.009	0.017	
CR *K. pneumoniae*	116	(0.9%)	49	(0.4%)	80	(0.5%)	0.001	0.001	0.001	
CR *P. aeruginosa*	6,610	(53.3%)	6,610	(57.9%)	9,464	(54.2%)	0.077	0.077	0.110	
CR *Acinetobacter spp*	180	(1.4%)	78	(0.7%)	159	(0.9%)	0.002	0.001	0.002	
Subtotal Gram -	10,143	(81.7%)	9,536	(83.5%)	14,723	(84.3%)	0.118	0.111	0.171	
TOTAL	12,411	(100%)	11,422	(100%)	17,470	(100%)	0.144	0.133	0.203	

from the BMR-RAISIN network [4], where between 4,000 and 5,000 cases of MRSA bloodstream infections and 4,000 to 9,000 cases of bloodstream infections due to extended-spectrum beta-lactamase (ESBL)-producing *enterobacteriaceae* — mostly with *E. coli* and *K. pneumoniae* — were estimated to occur in France in 2013.

The results of our study should also be examined in light of previous studies published in other countries. Nonetheless they are not directly comparable because the methodology used differs in many respects.

The European study [2] estimated there were more than 386,000 annual infections due to MDRB in Europe, and attributed 25,000 extra deaths to them. The EARS-Net data used for that European estimate date back to 2007, while the French study used more recent data (2012). Trends in the epidemiology of MDRB between 2007 and 2012, especially major changes for MRSA and 3GC-R enterobacteriaceae [5], may thus explain some of these differences. Indeed, Ears-Net data show the spread of 3GC-R resistance in *E. coli*, with a four-fold increase from 2.5% in 2007 to 10% in 2012.

In addition, the European study sought to examine the morbidity and mortality of MDRB associated with hospital-acquired infections only. This study considered only a fraction of all bloodstream infections, by correcting their incidence reported by EARS-Net by a factor derived from national prevalence studies to take into account only those of nosocomial origin, e.g., only 65.6% of MRSA bloodstream infections and 58.9% of 3GC-R *E. coli* bloodstream infections (ECDC, unpublished data). Moreover, the panels of infections and MDRB species considered in the present study were more complete than those of the European study, which did not include three MDRB from our panel (CR *K. pneumoniae*,

Acinetobacter spp. and GR *Enterococcus faecalis*) and one infection site (bone and joint infections for MRSA).

Another major difference between the two studies is related to the correction of the EARS-Net data to estimate the number of cases for the entire country. The European study estimated the incidence of invasive infections due to resistant bacteria in France from the median incidence of invasive infections observed in all EU/EEA countries. The percentage of resistance in species from the EARS-Net data was then applied (ECDC, unpublished data). Our estimates are therefore more precise because they are based on actual national surveillance and hospital data.

Finally, the estimates of the number of deaths from the European study cannot be compared to our results because the associated mortality proportion used in our study differs for some MDRB.

The 2013 CDC report [3] used surveillance data collected between 2009 and 2011 to estimate that there were more than 2 million infections due to antibiotic-resistant microorganisms that year in the United States. The same limitations raised for the European study apply when comparing the CDC results with ours, because the US considered more bacteria-antibiotic combinations than our study did, e.g. infections with *Salmonella*, *Shigella*, tuberculosis, and even *Candida*. The CDC also used a different methodology to calculate the number of deaths, which limits the comparisons still further. It applied the same proportion of deaths — 6.5% — to infections with carbapenemase-producing *enterobacteriaceae*, MDR *Acinetobacter*, ESBL-producing *enterobacteriaceae*, GRE, and MDR *P. aeruginosa*. This figure, derived from a study published in 2009 [26], is an estimate of the overall mortality associated with nosocomial infections due to MDRB. Instead, we used MDR-specific and site-specific mortality ratios for each type of infection, which appears more appropriate, in view of the great variability of associated mortality rates between different infections due to MDRB and body sites.

The specifications of the European study, the CDC American study and our Santé publique France study have been summarised in three additional tables (Additional file 1: Tables a, b, c). The differences in these studies underline the need to define a standardised protocol for international assessments of the morbidity and mortality of antibiotic resistance. Only results from studies based on such a protocol, which could be promoted for example by the ECDC or WHO as part of the global action plan on antimicrobial resistance recently adopted by the World Health Assembly [1], will allow valid comparisons between countries.

We decided here to assess the overall mortality associated with infections due to MDRB and not specifically that associated with antibiotic resistance. Several publications have already reported the excess mortality associated with resistance alone. A study of two matched cohorts of patients [27] showed that the 30-day mortality associated with 3GC-R E. coli bloodstream infections was 2.5 times greater (confidence interval: 0.9-6.8) than that associated with susceptible strains. A meta-analysis of 16 studies [28] also showed a significant increased risk in the mortality associated with bloodstream infections due to ESBL-producing Enterobacteriaceae, almost twice as high as that observed for susceptible Enterobacteriaceae (pooled RR: 1.85; confidence interval: 1.39-2.47).

Several studies suggest that infections due to MDRB do not replace those with susceptible bacteria, but add to them (the so-called "Boyce effect"), thus increasing the total morbidity and mortality of infection from a given bacterium. This characteristic was initially described for MRSA [29], and more recently for 3GC-R E. coli [30], two bacteria that account for two thirds of the cases of infections due to MDRB and more than one third of the deaths estimated in our study. A substantial fraction — and if the Boyce effect also applies to other MDRB, the majority — of the deaths we estimate should therefore be considered as excess mortality compared with those associated with infections by susceptible bacteria.

Our estimates are accompanied by uncertainty. To overcome this limit, for morbidity estimates, each PPS-based ratio was assigned a lower and an upper plausibility value, provided by the literature. The number of deaths was calculated by multiplying this ratio with the value of the morbidity estimates and their plausibility intervals, allowing presenting a plausibility interval for mortality estimates too. The numbers of deaths and plausibility intervals for deaths were estimated with these morbidity estimates and their plausibility intervals multiplied with mortality ratio provided by the literature. Part of uncertainty on the mortality estimates is taken into account through these plausibility intervals. However, uncertainty around proportions of deaths remain because of lack of sufficient-sized studies leaded in Europe on MDRB infections mortality.

Conclusions

The results of our study confirm that multidrug-resistance to antibiotics is a major public health problem in France. The morbidity and mortality associated with infections due to MDRB is particularly important for MRSA and 3GC-R Enterobacteriaceae. Surveillance of resistance to these bacteria therefore remains an important priority. The number of infections due to emerging highly resistant bacteria is still limited in France, probably due to the measures implemented to prevent cross-transmission.

The number of cases of infections and the number of deaths associated with infections due to MDRB calculated in this study are indicators that should facilitate communication and awareness of both healthcare professionals and the general public. Repeat this study in a few years with data from the next French PPS study, which will occur in 2017, and EARS-Net data, would provide trends estimations.

Additional studies remain to be conducted, for example to assess the projected morbidity and mortality of antibiotic resistance in France according to several scenarios based on incidence rates and efficacy of control programmes. It is equally important to assess the economic costs (of medical care, of measures to control dissemination in hospitals, and to the community) of infections due to MDRB in order to reinforce the adherence of healthcare professionals and policy-makers to prevention programmes.

Additional file

Additional file 1: Tables a, b, c. Table a, table b, table c have been added as supplementary material. **Table a** presents the methodology, parameters and main results of 3 studies estimating the morbidity and mortality of multidrug-resistant bacteria infections : the European study, the US study and our French study. **Table b** compares the ratios used for estimating the incidence of non-invasive infections in the European study and Santé publique France study. **Table c** compares the ratios used for estimating mortality associated with infections due to MDRB in the European study and Santé publique France study [31–34]. (PDF 285 kb)

Abbreviations

3GC-R E. coli: Escherichia coli resistant to third-generation cephalosporins; 3GC-R K. pneumoniae: Klebsiella pneumoniae resistant to third-generation cephalosporins; 3GC-R: Third-generation cephalosporin-resistant; CDC: US Centers for disease control and prevention; CR Acinetobacter spp: Acinetobacter spp. resistant to carbapenems; CR K. pneumoniae: K. pneumoniae resistant to carbapenems; CR P. aeruginosa: Pseudomonas aeruginosa resistant to carbapenems; EARS-Net: European antimicrobial resistance surveillance network; ECDC: European centre for disease prevention and control; ESBL: Extended-spectrum beta-lactamase producing enterobacteriaceae; EU/EEA countries: European union and European economic area countries; GRE: *Enterococcus faecium* and *E. faecalis* resistant to glycopeptides; HD: Inpatient hospital days; MDR: Multidrug resistant; MDRB: Multidrug resistant bacteria; MRSA: Methicillin-resistant *Staphylococcus aureus*; PPS 2012: Point prevalence survey of healthcare-associated infections and antimicrobial use in French hospitals in 2012

Acknowledgments
We thanks Jean Carlet, Lidia Kardas, Lucie Léon, Jean-Christophe Lucet, Camille Pelat, Cécile Sommen, Dieter Van Cauteren, Yazdan Yazdanpanah for validation of methodology and parameters used for morbidity and mortality estimations.

Funding
No external funding was received for this study.

Authors' contributions
All authors contributed to the interpretation of the results, the revision of the draft manuscript and approved the final version. MCC conducted the data analysis and wrote the manuscript; JL was involved in the data analysis; CBB and VJ were involved in the validation of parameters used for morbidity and mortality estimations; SV and BC conceived and designed the study and were involved in the validation of parameters used for morbidity and mortality estimations.

Competing interests
The authors declare that they have no competing interests.

Author details
[1]Santé Publique France, The French Public Health Agency, F-94415 Saint-Maurice, France. [2]Assistance publique-hôpitaux de Paris, CHU Henri Mondor, F-94000 Créteil, France. [3]Sorbonne Universités, UPMC Univ Paris 06, Inserm, Centre d'Immunologie et des Maladies Infectieuses, UMR 1135 & APHP, CHU Pitié-Salpêtrière, Laboratoire de Bactériologie-Hygiène, F-75013 Paris, France.

References
1. World Health Organization (WHO). Global action plan on antimicrobial resistance. WHO. 2015. http://apps.who.int/gb/ebwha/pdf_files/WHA68/A68_ACONF1Rev1-en.pdf. Accessed 27 May 2016.
2. European Centre for Disease prevention and Control (ECDC), European Medicine Agency (EMEA). The bacterial challenge: time to react. ECDC. 2009. http://www.ecdc.europa.eu/en/publications/Publications/0909_TER_The_Bacterial_Challenge_Time_to_React.pdf. Accessed 27 May 2016.
3. Centers for disease control and prevention (CDC). Antibiotic resistance threats in the United State. 2013. http://www.cdc.gov/drugresistance/threat-report-2013/. Accessed 27 May 2016.
4. Arnaud I, Jarlier V. The BMR-Raisin working group. Surveillance des bactéries multirésistantes dans les établissements de santé en France, Réseau BMR-Raisin, résultats 2013. Institut de veille sanitaire. 2015. http://www.invs.sante.fr/Publications-et-outils/Rapports-et-syntheses/Maladies-infectieuses/2015/Surveillance-des-bacteries-multiresistantes-dans-les-etablissements-de-sante-en-France. Accessed 27 May 2016.
5. European Centre for Disease prevention and Control (ECDC). Antimicrobial resistance surveillance in Europe, annual report of the European Antimicrobial Resistance Surveillance Network (Ears-Net). ECDC. 2014. http://ecdc.europa.eu/en/publications/_layouts/forms/

6. Magiorakos AP, Srinivasan A, Carey RB, Carmeli Y, Falagas ME, Giske CG, et al. Multidrug-resistant, extensively drug-resistant and pandrug-resistant bacteria: an international expert proposal for interim standard definitions for acquired resistance. Clin Infect Dis. 2012; doi: 10.1111/j.1469-0691.2011.03570.x
7. Thiolet JM, Vaux S, Lamy M, Gauthier A, Barret AS, Leon L, et al. Enquête nationale de prévalence des infections nososcomiales et des traitements anti-infectieux en établissements de santé, France, mai-juin 2012. Institut de veille sanitaire. 2013. http://www.invs.sante.fr/Publications-et-outils/Rapports-et-syntheses/Maladies-infectieuses/2013/Enquete-nationale-de-prevalence-des-infections-nosocomiales-et-des-traitements-anti-infectieux-en-etablissements-de-sante-France-mai-juin-2012. Accessed 13 June 2016.
8. Institut de Veille Sanitaire (InVS). Infections invasives d'origine bactérienne, Réseau EPIBAC. Institut de veille sanitaire. 2015. http://www.invs.sante.fr/Dossiers-thematiques/Maladies-infectieuses/Maladies-a-prevention-vaccinale/Infections-invasives-d-origine-bacterienne-Reseau-EPIBAC/Methodes-de-la-surveillance. Accessed 27 May 2016.
9. Données administratives et statistiques sur les établissements de santé. Ministère des Affaires sociales et de la santé, Direction de la recherche, des études, de l'évaluation et des statistiques, Paris. 2015. http://drees.social-sante.gouv.fr/etudes-et-statistiques/opendata/etablissements-de-sante-sociaux-et-medico-sociaux/article/la-statistique-annuelle-des-etablissements-sae.
10. Martone WJ, Jarvis WR, Edwards JR, Culver DH, Haley RW. Incidence and nature of endemic and epidemic nosocomial infections. In: Benett J, Brachman P, editors. Hospitals infections. Philadelphia: Lippincott-Raven; 1998. p. 461–76.
11. Gavalda L, Masuet C, Beltran J, Garcia M, Garcia D, Sirvent JM, et al. Comparative cost of selective screening to prevent transmission of methicillin-resistant Staphylococcus aureus (MRSA), compared with the attributable costs of MRSA infection. Infect Control Hosp Epidemiol. 2006; doi: 10.1086/507968.
12. Kallen AJ, Mu Y, Bulens S, Reingold A, Petit S, Gershman K, et al. Health care-associated invasive MRSA infections, 2005–2008. JAMA. 2010; doi: 10.1001/jama.2010.1115.
13. Kanerva M, Ollgren J, Hakanen AJ, Lyytikainen O. Estimating the burden of healthcare-associated infections caused by selected multidrug-resistant bacteria Finland, 2010. Antimicrob Resist Infect Control. 2012; doi: 10.1186/2047-2994-1-33.
14. Carmeli Y, Eliopoulos G, Mozaffari E, Samore M. Health and economic outcomes of vancomycin-resistant enterococci. Arch Intern Med. 2002;162:2223–8.
15. The Brooklyn Antibiotic Resistance Task Force. The cost of antibiotic resistance: effect of resistance among Staphylococcus aureus, Klebsiella pneumoniae, Acinetobacter baumannii, and Pseudmonas aeruginosa on length of hospital stay. Infect Control Hosp Epidemiol. 2002; doi: 10.1086/502018.
16. Jain R, Walk ST, Aronoff DM, Young VB, Newton DW, Chenoweth CE, et al. Emergence of Carbapenemase producing Klebsiella Pneumoniae of Sequence type 258 in Michigan, USA. Infect Dis Rep. 2013; doi: 10.4081/idr.2013.e5.
17. Perez F, Endimiani A, Ray AJ, Decker BK, Wallace CJ, Hujer KM, et al. Carbapenem-resistant Acinetobacter baumannii and Klebsiella pneumoniae across a hospital system: impact of post-acute care facilities on dissemination. J Antimicrob Chemother. 2010; doi: 10.1093/jac/dkq191.
18. Livermore DM, Hill RL, Thomson H, Charlett A, Turton JF, Pike R, et al. Antimicrobial treatment and clinical outcome for infections with carbapenem- and multiply-resistant Acinetobacter baumannii around London. Int J Antimicrob Agents. 2010; doi: 10.1016/j.ijantimicag.2009.09.014.
19. Cosgrove SE, Sakoulas G, Perencevich EN, Schwaber MJ, Karchmer AW, Carmeli Y. Comparison of mortality associated with methicillin-resistant and methicillin-susceptible Staphylococcus aureus bacteremia: a meta-analysis. Clin Infect Dis. 2003; doi: 10.1086/345476.
20. Marchaim D, Gottesman T, Schwartz O, Korem M, Maor Y, Rahav G, et al. National multicenter study of predictors and outcomes of bacteremia upon hospital admission caused by Enterobacteriaceae producing extended-spectrum beta-lactamases. Antimicrob Agents Chemother. 2010; doi: 10.1128/AAC.00565-10.
21. Ena J, Arjona F, Martinez-Peinado C, Lopez-Perezagua MM, Amador C. Epidemiology of urinary tract infections caused by extended-spectrum beta-

Publication_DispForm.aspx?List=4f55ad51-4aed-4d32-b960-af70113dbb90&ID=1205. Accessed 27 May 2016.

lactamase-producing Escherichia coli. Urology. 2006; doi: 10.1016/j.urology.
2006.08.1075.

22. Mouloudi E, Protonotariou E, Zagorianou A, Iosifidis E, Karapanagiotou A,
Giasnetsova T, et al. Bloodstream infections caused by metallo-beta-
lactamase/Klebsiella pneumoniae carbapenemase-producing K. pneumoniae
among intensive care unit patients in Greece: risk factors for infection and
impact of type of resistance on outcomes. Infect Control Hosp Epidemiol.
2010; doi: 10.1086/657135.

23. Suarez C, Pena C, Gavalda L, Tubau F, Manzur A, Dominguez MA, et al.
Influence of carbapenem resistance on mortality and the dynamics of
mortality in Pseudomonas aeruginosa bloodstream infection. Int J Infect Dis.
2010; doi: 10.1038/srep11715.

24. Grupper M, Sprecher H, Mashiach T, Finkelstein R. Attributable mortality of
nosocomial Acinetobacter bacteremia. Infect Control Hosp Epidemiol.
2007; doi: 10.1086/512629.

25. Bonnal C, Mourvillier B, Bronchard R, de Paula D, Armand-Lefevre L,
L'heriteau F, et al. Prospective assessment of hospital-acquired bloosdstream
infections: how many may be preventable? Qual Saf Health Care. 2010;
doi: 10.1136/qshc.2008.030296.

26. Roberts RR, Hota B, Ahmad I, Scott RD, Foster SD, Abbasi F, et al. Hospital
and societal costs of antimicrobial-resistant infections in a Chicago teaching
hospital: implications for antibiotic stewardship. Clin Infect Dis. 2009; doi: 10.
1086/605630.

27. de Kraker ME, Wolkewitz M, Davey PG, Koller W, Berger J, Nagler J, et al.
Burden of antimicrobial resistance in European hospitals: excess mortality
and length of hospital stay associated with bloodstream infections due to
Escherichia coli resistant to third-generation cephalosporins. J Antimicrob
Chemother. 2011; doi: 10.1093/jac/dkq412.

28. Schwaber MJ, Carmeli Y. Mortality and delay in effective therapy associated
with extended-spectrum beta-lactamase production in Enterobacteriaceae
bacteraemia: a systematic review and meta-analysis. J Antimicrob
Chemother. 2007; doi: 10.1093/jac/dkm318.

29. Boyce JM, White RL, Spruill EY. Impact of methicillin-resistant
Staphylococcus aureus on the incidence of nosocomial staphylococcal
infections. J Infect Dis. 1983;148:763.

30. de Kraker ME, Jarlier V, Monen JC, Heuer OE, van de Sande N, Grundmann
H. The changing epidemiology of bacteraemias in Europe: trends from the
European Antimicrobial Resistance Surveillance System. Clin Microbiol Infect.
2013; doi: 10.1111/1469-0691.12028.

31. Huang SS, Johnson KM, Ray GT, Wroe P, Lieu TA, Moore MR, et al.
Healthcare utilization and cost of pneumococcal disease in the United
States. Vaccine. 2011;29(18):3398–412. doi:10.1016/j.vaccine.2011.02.088.

32. Hoban DJ, Doern GV, Fluit AC, Roussel-Delvallez M, Jones RN. Worldwide
prevalence of antimicrobial resistance in Streptococcus pneumoniae,
Haemophilus influenzae, and Moraxella catarrhalis in the SENTRY
antimicrobial surveillance program, 1997–1999. Clin Infect Dis. 2001;32
Suppl 2:S81–93. doi:10.1086/320181.

33. Schwaber MJ, Navon-Venezia S, Kaye KS, Ben-Ami R, Schwartz D, Carmeli Y.
Clinical and economic impact of bacteremia with extended- spectrum-beta-
lactamase-producing Enterobacteriaceae. Antimicrob Agents Chemother.
2006;50(4):1257–62. doi:10.1128/AAC.50.4.1257-1262.2006.

34. Carmeli Y, Troillet N, Karchmer AW, Samore MH. Health and economic
outcomes of antibiotic resistance in Pseudomonas aeruginosa. Arch Intern
Med. 1999;159(10):1127–32. doi:10.1001/archinte.159.10.1127.

7

High rates of multidrug resistance among uropathogenic *Escherichia coli* in children and analyses of ESBL producers from Nepal

Narayan Prasad Parajuli[1,3*], Pooja Maharjan[1], Hridaya Parajuli[1], Govardhan Joshi[1], Deliya Paudel[1], Sujan Sayami[2] and Puspa Raj Khanal[3]

Abstract

Background: Emergence of Extended-spectrum beta-lactamase producing *Escherichia coli* causing urinary tract infections (UTI) among pediatric patients is an increasing problem worldwide. However, very little is known about pediatric urinary tract infections and antimicrobial resistance trend from Nepal. This study was conducted to assess the current antibiotic resistance rate and ESBL production among uropathogenic *Escherichia coli* in pediatric patients of a tertiary care teaching hospital of Nepal.

Methods: A total of 5,484 urinary tract specimens from children suspected with UTI attending a teaching hospital of Nepal over a period of one year were processed for the isolation of bacterial pathogens and their antimicrobial susceptibility testing. *Escherichia coli* ($n = 739$), the predominant isolate in pediatric UTI, was further selected for the detection of ESBL-production by phenotypic combination disk diffusion test.

Results: Incidence of urinary tract infection among pediatric patients was found to be 19.68% and *E coli* (68.4%) was leading pathogen involved. Out of 739 *E coli* isolates, 64.9% were multidrug resistant (MDR) and 5% were extensively drug resistant (XDR). Extended spectrum beta lactamase (ESBL) was detected in 288 (38.9%) of the *E coli* isolates.

Conclusion: Alarming rate of drug resistance among pediatric uropathogens and high rate of ESBL-producing *E. coli* was observed. It is extremely necessary to routinely investigate the drug resistance among all isolates and formulate strict antibiotics prescription policy in our country.

Keywords: Urinary tract infection, Children, *E coli*, ESBL, Nepal

Background

Urinary tract infection (UTI) is among the most common causes of febrile illness in children requiring antimicrobial treatment [1]. Worldwide, an estimated 8% of girls and 2% of boys experience at least one episode of UTI by the age of seven years and recurrence occurs in 12-30% of them within a year [2]. Pediatric UTI in many instances, remain under-diagnosed because of the absence of specific symptoms and signs, particularly in infants and young children [2, 3]. Therefore, accurate diagnosis and appropriate use of antimicrobials for treatment and prevention of urinary tract infections (UTIs) is vital to reduce the burden and also to prevent the possible long-term consequences [4].

Escherichia coli have been recognised as the most common pathogen accounting for majority of urinary tract infections in children [5]. Antimicrobial therapy, usually of traditional antibiotics, is commonly prescribed to treat urinary tract infections in pediatric patients. However, increased rates acquired resistance in *E. coli* has made usual antibiotics less acceptable choice for empirical therapy in recent years [1]. The most common mechanism associated with acquired resistance in *E. coli* and other *Enterobacteriaceae* is the production of hydrolytic enzymes called β-lactamases [6, 7]. Extended-spectrum β-lactamase (ESBL), a major beta lactamase enzyme,

* Correspondence: narayan.parajuli@iom.edu.np
[1]Department of Clinical Laboratory Services, Manmohan Memorial Medical College and Teaching Hospital, P.O.B.: 15201Swayambhu, Kathmandu, Nepal
[3]Department of Laboratory Medicine, Manmohan Memorial Institute of Health Sciences, Kathmandu, Nepal
Full list of author information is available at the end of the article

has the ability to hydrolyze oxyimino-cephalosporins, and monobactams but not cephamycins or carbapenems and inhibited in-vitro by inhibitors such as clavulanic acid, sulbactam and tazobactam [8]. Since their evolution in 1983, more than 300 types of ESBLs have been identified in various members of the family *Enterobacteriaceae* and other non-enteric organisms [3, 6]. The infections associated with these ESBL producing isolates are difficult to treat because of their resistance towards beta lactam agents and also due to the emergence of co-existing resistance determinants such as aminoglycosides and fluoroquinolones [7]. Moreover, emergence of ESBL producing bacteria, particularly *E. coli* and *K. pneumoniae* causing pediatric urinary tract infections is a worldwide concern [9]. Options for the treatment of such multidrug resistant (MDR) gram negative bacterial infections are generally limited, and very few antibiotics are approved for use in children [10].

In Nepal, pediatric UTIs are usually treated empirically because of the unavailability of standard therapeutic guidelines and local susceptibility data [11, 12]. Knowledge of the etiological agent of UTIs and their antimicrobial resistance patterns in our setting may help clinicians in choosing the appropriate antimicrobial treatment. Moreover, most of the studies on pediatric urinary tract infections caused by multidrug resistant and ESBL producing bacteria have been reported from western world [10, 13], but the same from South Asian region including Nepal are scarce on the published literature [14]. In this perspective, the present study was designed to investigate the clinical isolates of multi-drug resistant and ESBL producing *Escherichia coli* causing urinary tract infections in children visiting a tertiary care teaching hospital in Nepal.

Methods
Study design and setup
A cross-sectional study was carried out for 1 year (June 2015 - May 2016) in the department of Microbiology and Pediatric Medicine, Manmohan Memorial Medical College and Teaching Hospital (MMCTH), a tertiary care hospital with 500 patient beds in Kathmandu, the capital city of Nepal. Study hospital is a referral center with medical, surgical, gynecological, pediatric, geriatric and other specialties.

Inclusion and exclusion criteria
During the study period, children up to 14 years of age presented to the pediatric outpatient department or admitted to pediatric inpatient ward with a clinical diagnosis of UTI were included. The clinical diagnosis of UTI was made by respective unit pediatrician in the presence of fever and/or any of the symptoms such painful micturition, increased frequency, burning micturition, or suprapubic pain/flank pain. Those children who had previous known history of antimicrobial therapy within 48 h prior to attending the

hospital and samples which grew more than one type of organism was considered as contaminated and hence, excluded from the study.

Laboratory methods
A total of 5,484 non-repetitive urine specimens (Midstream, Suprapubic, Catheter aspirated and Clean catch) representing urinary tract infections in pediatric patients (0-14 years) were processed semi-quantitatively by inoculating 0.001 ml of the specimen (by using a calibrated wire loop) onto the cystine lactose electrolyte deficient (CLED) agar for the isolation and identification of significant uropathogens [15]. The inoculated plates were incubated for 24 h at 37 °C in aerobic atmosphere. Growth of a single organism with a count of $\geq 10^5$ colony-forming units (CFU)/ml were considered to represent the infection and were identified using appropriate routine identification methods including colony morphology, Gram-stain, and an in-house set of biochemical tests [15]. *Escherichia coli*, the predominant uropathogen, was selected for the determination of antimicrobial susceptibility as well as identification of the multidrug resistant (MDR), extensively drug resistant (XDR) and extended spectrum beta lactamase (ESBL) producing isolates.

Antimicrobial susceptibility testing
The susceptibility of bacterial isolates against different antibiotics was tested by the disk diffusion method [modified Kirby-Bauer method] on Mueller Hinton agar (Hi-Media, India) following standard procedures recommended by the Clinical and Laboratory Standards Institute (CLSI), Wayne, USA [16]. Antibiotics that were tested in our study include Ampicillin (AMP 25 µg), Amoxycillin clavulanate (AMC20/10 µg), Aztreonam (30 µg) Gentamycin (GEN10µg), Ciprofloxacin (CIP5µg), Levofloxacin (LEV5µg) trimethoprim sulfamethoxazole/cotrimoxazole (COT30µg), Cephalexin (CN30 µg), Cefixime (CFM5µg), Ceftriaxone (CTR30µg), Ceftazidime (CAZ30µg), Piperacillin tazobactam (PIT 100/10 µg), Imipenem (IMP 10 µg), Meropenem (MRP 10 µg) Tigecycline (TGC30µg), and Colistin sulphate (CT10µg) (HiMedia Laboratories, India). Interpretations of antibiotic susceptibility results were made according to the zone size interpretative standards of CLSI [16]. *Escherichia coli* ATCC 25922 was used as a control organism for antibiotic susceptibility testing.

Identification of Multidrug Resistant (MDR), Extensive Drug Resistant (XDR) and potential ESBL *Escherichia coli*
MDR and XDR isolates were identified according to the combined guidelines of the European Centre for Disease Prevention and Control (ECDC) and the Centers for Disease Control and Prevention (CDC) [17]. In this study, the isolate resistant to at least one antimicrobial from three different group of first line drugs tested was

regarded as multidrug resistant (MDR). Extensively drug resistant (XDR) isolates were identified when the isolates are resistant to at least one agent in all but two or fewer antimicrobial categories (i.e., bacterial isolates remain susceptible to only one or two categories).

Isolates of *E. coli* were examined for their susceptibility to third generation cephalosporins by using Ceftazidime (30 µg) and Cefotaxime (30 µg) disks. If the zone of inhibition (ZOI) was ≤25 mm for Ceftriaxone, ≤22 mm for Ceftazidime and/or ≤27 mm for Cefotaxime, the isolate was considered a potential ESBL producer as recommended by CLSI and further tested by confirmatory methods [16].

Confirmatory test of ESBL
Isolates considered potential ESBL producers by initial screening were emulsified with nutrient broth to adjust the inoculum density equal to that of 0.5 Mac Farland turbidity standards. Combination Disk test (CDT), as recommended by the CLSI, was performed in all isolates presumed to be ESBL producers. In this test, Ceftazidime (30 µg) disks alone and in combination with clavulanic acid (Ceftazidime + clavulanic Acid, 30/10 µg) disks, were applied onto a plate of Mueller Hinton Agar (MHA) which was inoculated with the test strain and then incubated in ambient air for 16-18 h of incubation at 35 ± 2 °C. Isolate that showed increase of ≥ 5 mm in the zone of inhibition of the combination discs in comparison to that of the Ceftazidime disk alone was considered an ESBL producer [16].

Data analysis
The information regarding patient's profile and the results were entered into a computer program. Data analysis was carried out using the Statistical Package for Social Sciences [SPSS^{TM}] version 20.0 [IBM, Armonk, NY, USA] and presented in percentage base distribution. Data with p value of less than 0.05 (CI-95%) was regarded as significant.

Ethical consideration
Written approval was taken from Institutional Review Committee of Manmohan Memorial Institute of Health Sciences (MMIHS) after submitting and presenting research proposal. Written informed consent was taken

from every patient or their guardians before enrollment into the study.

Results
Patient demographics
During the study period, a total of 5,484 representative specimens of urinary tract from pediatric patients suspected with urinary tract infections were processed. Among total clinical specimens, 1079 (19.68%) were found with growth of at least one significant pathogen confirming urinary tract infection (UTI). Female (659, 61.0%) were most affected group of patients in both inpatient and outpatient department ($p < 0.005$). Maximum number of cases was found in the children of age group 1 to 4 years (Table 1). *Escherichia coli* (n =739, 68.5%) was the most common organism isolated from urinary tract infections in pediatric group in this study.

Antimicrobial resistance pattern of *E. coli*
High level of drug resistance was noted in *E. coli* isolates. Among 739 *E. coli* isolated, highest resistance (87% each) were to ampicillin and cephalexin, followed by ciprofloxacin (78%), cefixime (71%) and levofloxacin (67%) respectively. Very few isolates (5%) were resistant to imipenem whereas entire strains revealed high susceptibility (100% each) towards colistin and tigecycline (Table 2).

Multidrug resistant (MDR) and Extensive drug resistant (XDR) isolates
Among total 739 *E. coli* isolates subjected for antimicrobial susceptibility testing, 480 (64.9%) isolates were found multidrug resistant (MDR) and 37 (5.0%) isolates were extensive drug resistant (XDR). MDR isolates were resistant to ampicillin (100%), amoxicillin clavulanate (84.7%), cephalexin (81.6%) and ciprofloxacin (80.6%) respectively. However, MDR isolates were susceptible towards amikacin (87%), imipenem (92%) and piperacillin tazobactam (81%). Although the number of XDR isolates was low, they were completely resistant to all antibiotics except colistin and tigecycline (Table 2).

Table 1 Pediatric patients with Urinary tract infections ($N = 1079$)

Patients with Urinary tract infections							
Age Group	Male (%)	Female (%)	p	Outpatient (%)	Inpatient (%)	p	Cc
<1	87	129	0.352	54	162	0.001	0.014
1 to 4	129	141	0.001	119	151	0.004	0.104
5 to 9	118	238	0.004	248	108	0.007	0.083
10 to 14	86	151	0.193	151	86	0.001	0.029
Total	420	659		572	507		

Cc Contingency coefficient

Table 2 Antibiotic susceptibility of MDR, XDR and ESBL *E coli* isolates

Antibiotics	No. of resistant isolates (%)			
	Total isolates (%)	MDR ($n = 480$)%	XDR ($n = 37$)%	ESBL ($n = 288$)%
Ampicillin	645(87)	480(100)	37(100)	288(100)
Amoxicillin-clavulanate	355(48)	407(84.7)	37(100)	288(100)
Piperacillin-tazobactam	244(33)	91(19)	37(100)	78(27)
Cephalexin	645(87)	392(81.6)	37(100)	265(92)
Cefixime	525(71)	312(65)	37(100)	288(100)
Ceftazidime	333(45)	306(64)	37(100)	288(100)
Ceftriaxone	333(45)	306(64)	37(100)	288(100)
Aztreonam	318(43)	294(61)	37(100)	288(100)
Imipenem	37(5)	37(8)	37(100)	28(10)
Gentamycin	244(33)	130(27)	37(100)	118(41)
Amikacin	103(14)	64(13)	37(100)	52(18)
Ciprofloxacin	576(78)	387(80.6)	37(100)	225(78)
Levofloxacin	495(67)	245(51)	37(100)	155(54)
Cotrimoxazole	310(42)	158(33)	37(100)	141(49)
Tigecycline	0(0)	0(0)	0(0)	0(0)
Colistin	0(0)	0(0)	0(0)	0(0)

ESBL *E coli* and their susceptibility pattern

Extended spectrum beta lactamase (ESBL) enzyme was detected in 288(38.9%) *E. coli* isolates. Penicillins, cephalosporins and monobactam group of antibiotics were appeared completely ineffective (100% resistance) against ESBL producers. However, ESBL producing *E coli* strains were susceptible to reserve class of antibiotics including imipenem (90%), colistin (100%) and tigecycline (100%) (Table 2).

Discussion

To the best of our knowledge, this report represents the first description of ESBL producing uropathogenic *E. coli* involved in pediatric cases of urinary tract infections from our country, Nepal. Urinary tract infections are the most common infections in children and *E. coli* being leading pathogenic agent in these infections; it was our matter of interest. There was no previous report before this study to estimate the most common pathogen and its resistant pattern in pediatrics patients with urinary tract infection in our hospital.

The incidence of urinary tract infection based on significant bacterial growth among pediatric patients in this study was 19.6% and *E. coli* (68.5%) was the predominant pathogen. Similar rates have been previously reported from nearby hospitals [11, 12] and from studies of other countries [18–22]. Concurrently, significantly more females (61.0%) were found with UTI corroborating with other similar studies [12, 19, 20]. In our study, children of age group 1-4 years were found with highest number of UTI cases (contingency coefficient 0.104). Similar study

from nearby hospital also reported that children less than six years of age were found UTI prone [11]. Urinary tract infection was significantly more prevalent in the female children of age group 1-4 and 5-9 years and also, more inpatients were found with UTI ($p < 0.05$). The higher rates of UTI in this age group might be due to immune status, sanitation, and ascending infection with fecal flora.

The high prevalence of ESBL-producing uropathogenic *E. coli* (38.9%) among children is reported in this study. In addition, this study also documents the enhanced resistance of ESBL producing *E. coli* to other antimicrobial groups like aminoglycosides and fluoroquinolones. Indeed, variations in the prevalence rates of ESBL-producing *E. coli* isolates in children around the globe and even among different hospitals within a country have been reported. Our prevalence rate of ESBL producing *E coli* (38.9%) is close to the findings reported by other studies in different parts of Asian region including Shettigar et al. (37.7%) from India [22], Pourakbari et al. (37%) and Rezai et al. (30.5%) from Iran [21, 23], Moore et al. (44%) from Cambodia [19] and Kizilca et al. (41.4%) from Turkey [24]. Extremely higher rates of ESBL *E coli* have also been reported, notably by Chinnasami et al. (83%) from India [25], Masud et al. (53.8%) from Bangladesh [20] and Shah et al. (50.9%) from Pakistan [18]. The increased rate of ESBL-producing bacteria causing infection in community as well as hospital settings constitutes an undeniable trend. Worldwide, pediatric UTIs due to ESBL-producing bacteria are an important part of this problem because they limit therapeutic choices and increases morbidity of infection [26]. However, lower rates of ESBL-producing *E.*

coli were also reported, particularly from developed countries including 9.3% from USA [27], 10.2% from Korea [28], 14% from Taiwan [26], 14.1% from Lebanon [5] and 20.2% from Turkey [29]. These variations in the rate of ESBL producing strains of E coli among UTI cases might be attributable to the geographical difference, local antibiotic prescribing policy, the extensive use of broad spectrum antibiotics especially third generation cephalosporins and endemicity of drug resistance pathogens in the locality.

ESBL producing bacteria causing infections in children may have various complications and adverse outcomes [30]. ESBL producers are non susceptible to aminopenicillins and ureidopenicillins as well as extended-spectrum β-lactam agents like second- and third-generation cephalosporins. Use of these agents as the first choice for the treatment of urinary tract infections may lead to the inappropriate treatment and predispose to long term renal complications [24]. Therefore, antimicrobial therapy in infections with ESBL producing organism is really challenging. Published reports showed that ESBL- producing strains causing UTI in children associated with prior hospitalization, beta-lactam therapy, catheterization, underlying co-morbidity and infancy [24].

In this study, multidrug resistant (MDR) and extensively drug resistant E coli were found 64.9% and 5.0% respectively. Increasing pattern of resistance of urinary tract pathogens against common antibiotics in Nepal have also been reported by other researchers [12, 31] but MDR rates and drug resistance pattern among pediatric isolates from Nepal was not available. It is observed that ampicillin, cephalexin, ciprofloxacin and cefixime were poorly effective against uropathogenic E coli. Only 13% of the isolates were found susceptible to all the antibiotics tested. Cephalosporin, the commonly prescribed antibiotic as empirical therapy in pediatric and adults, resistance to this group of antibiotics was found high. Almost 45% of E coli isolates were resistant to at least one cephalosporin and monobactam. Similar rates of antimicrobial resistance was documented in the study from Bangladesh [20], Iran [32] and India [14]. However, compared to previous reports from Nepal, we observed a considerable increase in resistance against penicillins, aminoglycosides, quinolones and ceftriaxone [12, 31]. Lower rates of resistance among the pediatric isolates causing UTI have been documented in western countries [33].

Higher resistance to penicillins third generation cephalosporins in this study has been attributable to ESBL production among gram negative isolates. In ESBL producing isolates, augumentins (combined with beta lactamase inhibitor) such as amoxicillin clavulanate or piperacillin tazobactam can be used as alternative antimicrobials [34]. However, in this study, alarming state of resistance was observed among ESBL producers towards amoxicillin clavulanate (100%) and piperacillin tazobactam (27%). In

the case when UTI is caused by an ESBL producing bacteria in children, the broadest-spectrum antibiotic agents such as carbapenems are recommended [35] but they are only useful in hospitalized patients. In this study, too, carbapenems were found effective to the ESBL isolates. Nevertheless, for pediatric UTIs in our setting, cotrimoxazole, amoxicillin clavulanate, ciprofloxacin and amikacin can still be used as first line therapy. Furthermore, other non carbapenem groups of antibiotics in UTIs due to ESBL-producing strains have also been described [36, 37]. ESBL stable cephamycins, fosfomycin and nitrofurantoin were shown effective for UTIs caused by ESBL-producing strains but their clinical utility as monotherapy is controversial [38–40]. In addition, ESBLs usually confer resistance to other classes of antibiotics, such as quinolones and trimethoprim/sulfamethoxazole, therefore susceptibility testing of these agents is important [23]. In this study, entire MDR isolates were resistant to ampicillin and 33% isolates were resistant to cotrimoxazole, 19% to piperacillin tazobactam and 8% to imipenem whereas no isolates were found to be resistant to colistin and tigecycline. Similarly, all XDR isolates were resistant to most of the antimicrobials tested whereas colistin and tigecycline were the most effective regimens against XDR isolates. Similar rate of resistance has been documented by Ansari et al. [41] but their study included E coli isolates from all age groups.

The level of drug resistance in uropathogenic E coli among pediatric patient in this study is a serious issue. Previous reports have suggested that higher resistance is likely to be occurring in the communities with higher proportion of young children and high antibiotic consumption [42]. In Nepal, higher antimicrobial pressure for community infections and inappropriate therapeutic guidelines for pediatric patients might be attributable to this menacing scenario [12, 31]. Resistance to the broad spectrum cephalosporins, fluoroquinolones and aminoglycosides among the ESBL producing E.coli isolates in this study necessitates the use of carbapenem as alternative choice for pediatric UTIs. Although we found carbapenems as the most effective agent against the ESBL but the high rate of resistance from similar studies is of special concern [41]. Furthermore, the genes associated with antibiotic resistance usually reside in plasmid and may transfer antibiotic resistance to other wild strains of bacteria [20]. Therefore, evidence based therapy with broad spectrum antibiotics for serious or critical cases to prevent bacterial resistance is extremely needful. Aminoglycosides, amoxicillin clavulanate and trimethoprim sulfamethoxazole/cotrimoxazole would be useful alternatives as empirical antibiotics for children suspected with UTIs in our scenario.

Limitations of the study

This study has a number of limitations. We could not evaluate the risk factors and outcome of pediatric UTI cases in our setting. Further cohort studies with antimicrobial therapy and outcome would generate more significant results. Antimicrobial susceptibility testing by dilution methods and determination of minimum inhibitory concentration (MIC) of therapeutic antibiotics would be helpful for treatment and monitoring of the drug resistant infections. Due to unavailability of resources, we could not detect the genotype of ESBLs among *E coli* isolates. Further investigations with larger patient population and multiple centers would generate more significant ideas.

Conclusion

We found the menacing state of drug resistance in almost all of the *E coli* isolates included in this study. Childhood UTIs caused by ESBL-producing *E. coli* has been emerged as a serious problem in our setting. Aminoglycosides and carbapenems can be used as alternative regimens for serious infections caused by MDR *E coli*. Furthermore, it is extremely necessary to formulate a strict antibiotics prescription policy and prudent use antibiotics in our country.

Abbreviation

ASM: American Society for Microbiology; ATCC: American Type Culture Collection; CDT: Combined Disk Test; CLSI: Clinical and Laboratory Standard Institute; *E coli: Escherichia coli;* ESBL: Extended spectrum beta-lactamases; MDR: Multidrug resistant; MHA: Mueller Hinton Agar; MIC: Minimum inhibitory concentration; UTI: Urinary tract infection; XDR: Extensive drug resistant

Acknowledgements

We are deeply thankful to all the patients participating in this study. Our special thanks go to all the laboratory staffs, management and officials of Manmohan Memorial Teaching Hospital Kathmandu for providing the opportunity to carry out this research work.

Funding

No monetary funding support has been received for this study.

Authors' contributions

NPP conceived the design of the study, reviewed the literature and performed the laboratory investigations. PM, HP and GJ performed the laboratory tests and helped in manuscript preparation. SS identified the clinical cases, DP and PRK guided the necessary laboratory tests. NPP prepared the manuscript with the guidance of PRK. All authors read the manuscript and approved.

Competing interests

The authors declare that they have no competing interests.

Author details

[1]Department of Clinical Laboratory Services, Manmohan Memorial Medical College and Teaching Hospital, P.O.B.: 15201Swayambhu, Kathmandu, Nepal. [2]Department of Pediatrics, Manmohan Memorial Medical College and Teaching Hospital, Kathmandu, Nepal. [3]Department of Laboratory Medicine, Manmohan Memorial Institute of Health Sciences, Kathmandu, Nepal.

References

1. Zorc JJ, Kiddoo DA, Shaw KN. Diagnosis and management of pediatric urinary tract infections. Clin Microbiol Rev. 2005;18(2):417–22.
2. Desai DJ, Gilbert B, McBride CA. Paediatric urinary tract infections: Diagnosis and treatment. Aust Fam Physician. 2016;45(8):558–63.
3. Robinson JL, Le Saux N. Management of urinary tract infections in children in an era of increasing antimicrobial resistance. Expert Rev Anti Infect Ther. 2016;14(9):809–16.
4. Hay AD, Sterne JA, Hood K, Little P, Delaney B, Hollingworth W, Wootton M, Howe R, MacGowan A, Lawton M, et al. Improving the Diagnosis and Treatment of Urinary Tract Infection in Young Children in Primary Care: Results from the DUTY Prospective Diagnostic Cohort Study. Ann Fam Med. 2016;14(4):325–36.
5. Hanna-Wakim RH, Ghanem ST, El Helou MW, Khafaja SA, Shaker RA, Hassan SA, Saad RK, Hedari CP, Khinkarly RW, Hajar FM, et al. Epidemiology and characteristics of urinary tract infections in children and adolescents. Front Cell Infect Microbiol. 2015;5:45.
6. Paterson DL, Bonomo RA. Extended-spectrum beta-lactamases: a clinical update. Clin Microbiol Rev. 2005;18(4):657–86.
7. Livermore DM. Current epidemiology and growing resistance of gram-negative pathogens. Korean J Intern Med. 2012;27(2):128–42.
8. Bradford PA. Extended-spectrum beta-lactamases in the 21st century: characterization, epidemiology, and detection of this important resistance threat. Clin Microbiol Rev. 2001;14(4):933–51. table of contents.
9. Sedighi I, Arabestani MR, Rahimbakhsh A, Karimitabar Z, Alikhani MY. Dissemination of extended-spectrum beta-lactamases and quinolone resistance genes among clinical isolates of uropathogenic escherichia coli in children. Jundishapur J Microbiol. 2015;8(7):e19184.
10. Uyar Aksu N, Ekinci Z, Dundar D, Baydemir C. Childhood urinary tract infections caused by ESBL-producing bacteria: Risk factors and empiric therapy. Pediatr Int. 2016. 0.1111/ped.13112. (Epub ahead of print).
11. Rai GK, Upreti HC, Rai SK, Shah KP, Shrestha RM. Causative agents of urinary tract infections in children and their antibiotic sensitivity pattern: a hospital based study. Nepal Med Coll J. 2008;10(2):86–90.
12. Singh SD, Madhup SK. Clinical profile and antibiotics sensitivity in childhood urinary tract infection at Dhulikhel Hospital. KUMJ. 2013;11(44):319–24.
13. Flokas ME, Detsis M, Alevizakos M, Mylonakis E. Prevalence of ESBL-producing Enterobacteriaceae in paediatric urinary tract infections: A systematic review and meta-analysis. J Infect. 2016;73(6):547–57.
14. Sharma S, Kaur N, Malhotra S, Madan P, Ahmad W, Hans C. Serotyping and antimicrobial susceptibility pattern of escherichia coli isolates from urinary tract infections in pediatric population in a tertiary care hospital. J Pathog. 2016;2016:2548517.
15. Isenberg HD. Clinical Microbiology Procedures Handbook. 2nd edition. Washington DC: ASM press; 2004.
16. Performance Standards for Antimicrobial Disk Susceptibility Tests.2012. Clinical and Laboratory Standards Institute. 2012, M02-A11 (Approved Standard—Eleventh Edition).
17. Magiorakos AP, Srinivasan A, Carey RB, Carmeli Y, Falagas ME, Giske CG, Harbarth S, Hindler JF, Kahlmeter G, Olsson-Liljequist B, et al. Multidrug-resistant, extensively drug-resistant and pandrug-resistant bacteria: an international expert proposal for interim standard definitions for acquired resistance. Clin Microbiol Infect. 2012;18(3):268–81.
18. Shah Samin Ullah AAG. Islam Rehman Gohar: etiology and antibiotic resistance pattern of community-acquired urinary tract infections in children. KJMS. 2015;8(3):428.
19. Moore CE, Sona S, Poda S, Putchhat H, Kumar V, Sopheary S, Stoesser N, Bousfield R, Day N, Parry CM. Antimicrobial susceptibility of uropathogens isolated from Cambodian children. Paediatr Int Child Health. 2016:1–5. [Epub ahead of print].

20. Masud MR, Afroz H, Fakruddin M. Prevalence of extended-spectrum beta-lactamase positive bacteria in radiologically positive urinary tract infection. Springer Plus. 2014;3:216.

21. Pourakbari B, Ferdosian F, Mahmoudi S, Teymuri M, Sabouni F, Heydari H, Ashtiani MT, Mamishi S. Increase resistant rates and ESBL production between E. coli isolates causing urinary tract infection in young patients from Iran. Braz J Microbiol. 2012;43(2):766–9.

22. Shettigar SCG, Roche R, Nayak N, Anitha KB, Soans S. Bacteriological profile, antibiotic sensitivity pattern, and detection of extended-spectrum β-lactamase in the isolates of urinary tract infection from children. J Child Health. 2016;3(1):5.

23. Rezai MS, Salehifar E, Rafiei A, Langaee T: Characterization of Multidrug Resistant Extended-Spectrum Beta-Lactamase-Producing Escherichia coli among Uropathogens of Pediatrics in North of Iran. 2015, 2015:309478

24. Kizilca O, Siraneci R, Yilmaz A, Hatipoglu N, Ozturk E, Kiyak A, Ozkok D. Risk factors for community-acquired urinary tract infection caused by ESBL-producing bacteria in children. Pediatr Int. 2012;54(6):858–62.

25. Balaji Chinnasami SS. Kanimozhi Sadasivam, Sekar Pasupathy Pathogens Causing Urinary Tract Infection in Children and their in vitro Susceptibility to Antimicrobial Agents- A Hospital Based Study. Biomed Pharmacol J. 2016;9(1):7.

26. Wu CT, Lee HY, Chen CL, Tuan PL, Chiu CH. High prevalence and antimicrobial resistance of urinary tract infection isolates in febrile young children without localizing signs in Taiwan. J Microbiol Immunol Infect=Wei mian yu gan ran za zhi. 2016;49(2):243–8.

27. Degnan LA, Milstone AM, Diener-West M, Lee CK. Extended-spectrum beta-lactamase bacteria from urine isolates in children. J Pediatr Pharmacol Ther. 2015;20(5):373–7.

28. Han SB, Lee SC, Lee SY, Jeong DC, Kang JH. Aminoglycoside therapy for childhood urinary tract infection due to extended-spectrum beta-lactamase-producing Escherichia coli or Klebsiella pneumoniae. BMC Infect Dis. 2015;15:414.

29. Dotis J, Printza N, Marneri A, Gidaris D, Papachristou F. Urinary tract infections caused by extended-spectrum betalactamase-producing bacteria in children: a matched casecontrol study. Turk J Pediatr. 2013;55(6):571–4.

30. Lee B, Kang SY, Kang HM, Yang NR, Kang HG, Ha IS, Cheong HI, Lee HJ, Choi EH. Outcome of antimicrobial therapy of pediatric urinary tract infections caused by extended-spectrum beta-lactamase-producing enterobacteriaceae. Infect Chemother. 2013;45(4):415–21.

31. Sharma A, Shrestha S, Upadhyay S, Rijal P. Clinical and bacteriological profile of urinary tract infection in children at Nepal Medical College Teaching Hospital. Nepal Med Coll J. 2011;13(1):24–6.

32. Mirsoleymani SR, Salimi M, Shareghi Brojeni M, Ranjbar M, Mehtarpoor M. Bacterial pathogens and antimicrobial resistance patterns in pediatric urinary tract infections: a four-year surveillance study (2009-2012). Int J Pediatr. 2014;2014:126142.

33. Stultz JS, Doern CD, Godbout E. Antibiotic resistance in pediatric urinary tract infections. Curr Infect Dis Rep. 2016,18(12):40.

34. Ramphal R, Ambrose PG. Extended-spectrum beta-lactamases and clinical outcomes: current data. Clin Infect Dis. 2006;42 Suppl 4:S164–172.

35. Dalgic N, Sancar M, Bayraktar B, Dincer E, Pelit S. Ertapenem for the treatment of urinary tract infections caused by extended-spectrum beta-lactamase-producing bacteria in children. Scand J Infect Dis. 2011;43(5):339–43.

36. Park SH, Choi SM, Chang YK, Lee DG, Cho SY, Lee HJ, Choi JH, Yoo JH. The efficacy of non-carbapenem antibiotics for the treatment of community-onset acute pyelonephritis due to extended-spectrum beta-lactamase-producing Escherichia coli. J Antimicrob Chemother. 2014;69(10):2848–56.

37. Asakura T, Ikeda M, Nakamura A, Kodera S. Efficacy of empirical therapy with non-carbapenems for urinary tract infections with extended-spectrum beta-lactamase-producing Enterobacteriaceae. Int J Infect Dis. 2014;29:91–5.

38. Tasbakan MI, Pullukcu H, Sipahi OR, Yamazhan T, Ulusoy S. Nitrofurantoin in the treatment of extended-spectrum beta-lactamase-producing Escherichia coli-related lower urinary tract infection. Int J Antimicrob Agents. 2012;40(6):554–6.

39. Veve MP, Wagner JL, Kenney RM, Grunwald JL, Davis SL. Comparison of fosfomycin to ertapenem for outpatient or step-down therapy of extended-spectrum beta-lactamase urinary tract infections. Int J Antimicrob Agents. 2016;48(1):56–60.

40. Lepeule R, Ruppe E, Le P, Massias L, Chau F, Nucci A, Lefort A, Fantin B. Cefoxitin as an alternative to carbapenems in a murine model of urinary tract infection due to Escherichia coli harboring CTX-M-15-type extended-spectrum beta-lactamase. Antimicrob Agents Chemother. 2012;56(3):1376–81.

41. Ansari S, Nepal HP, Gautam R, Shrestha S, Neopane P, Gurung G, Chapagain ML. Community acquired multi-drug resistant clinical isolates of Escherichia coli in a tertiary care center of Nepal. Antimicrob Resist Infect Control. 2015;4:15.

42. Bryce A, Hay AD, Lane IF, Thornton HV, Wootton M, Costelloe C. Global prevalence of antibiotic resistance in paediatric urinary tract infections caused by Escherichia coli and association with routine use of antibiotics in primary care: systematic review and meta-analysis. BMJ. 2016;352:i939.

8

30-day readmission, antibiotics costs and costs of delay to adequate treatment of Enterobacteriaceae UTI, pneumonia, and sepsis

Marya D. Zilberberg[1]*, Brian H. Nathanson[2], Kate Sulham[3], Weihong Fan[3] and Andrew F. Shorr[4]

Abstract

Background: Enterobacteriaceae are common pathogens in pneumonia, sepsis and urinary tract infection (UTI). Though rare, carbapenem resistance (CRE) among these organisms complicates efforts to ensure adequate empiric antimicrobial therapy. In turn this negatively impacts such outcomes as mortality and hospital costs. We explored proportion of total costs represented by antibiotics, 30-day readmission rates, and per-day costs of inadequate antimicrobial coverage among patients with Enterobacteriaceae pneumonia, sepsis and/or UTI in the context of inappropriate (IET) vs. appropriate empiric (non-IET) therapy and carbapenem resistance (CRE) vs. susceptibility (CSE).

Methods: We conducted a retrospective cohort study in the Premier Research database (2009–2013) of 175 US hospitals. We included all adult patients admitted with a culture-confirmed UTI, pneumonia, or sepsis as principal diagnosis, or as a secondary diagnosis in the setting of respiratory failure. Patients with hospital acquired infections or transfers from other acute facilities were excluded. IET was defined as failure to administer an antibiotic therapy in vitro active against the culture-confirmed pathogen within 2 days of admission.

Results: Among 40,137 patients with Enterobacteriaceae infections (54.2% UTI), 4984 (13.2%) received IET. CRE (3.1%) was more frequent in patients given IET (13.0%) than non-IET (1.6%, $p < 0.001$). The proportions of total costs represented by antibiotics were similar in IET and non-IET (3.3% vs. 3.4%, $p = 0.01$), and higher among the group with CRE than CSE (4.2% vs. 3.4%, $p < 0.001$). The 30-day readmission rates were higher in both IET than non-IET (25.6% vs. 21.1%, $p < 0.001$) and CRE than CSE (29.7% vs. 21.5%, p < 0.001) groups. Each additional day of inadequate therapy cost an additional $766 (95% CI $661, $870, $p < 0.001$) relative to adequate treatment.

Conclusions: In this large US cohort of Enterobacteriaceae infections, the cost of antibiotics was a small component of total costs, irrespective of whether empiric treatment was appropriate or whether a CRE was isolated. In contrast, each extra day of inadequate treatment added >$750 to hospital costs. Both CRE and IET were associated with an increased risk of readmission within 30 days.

Keywords: Enterobacteriaceae, Costs, Readmission, Sepsis, Pneumonia, UTI

* Correspondence: evimedgroup@gmail.com
[1]EviMed Research Group, LLC, PO Box 303, Goshen, MA 01032, USA
Full list of author information is available at the end of the article

Background

Antimicrobial resistance remains a growing threat to public health and a vexing challenge to clinicians. Rates of in vitro susceptibility for most commonly utilized antibiotics continue to decline for both gram-positive and gram-negative organisms [1]. This is particularly problematic among such gram-negative pathogens as *Pseudomonas aeruginosa*, *Acinetobacter baumannii* and various Enterobacteriaceae [1–7]. Since prompt appropriate treatment is critical for treatment success, this rise in the risk of inappropriate empiric therapy (IET) associated with resistant organisms is a harbinger of potentially worse outcomes [8–17]. Exposure to IET is associated with longer durations of hospitalizations and greater healthcare costs, independent of its impact on mortality [18, 19]. Despite the link between inappropriate therapy and worsened outcomes, multiple obstacles preclude clinicians from effectively targeting these resistant organisms. These challenges include difficulty with risk stratification, concern about promoting further resistance through prescribing unnecessarily broad empiric coverage, and the acquisition costs of potentially active, newer antimicrobials. However, the trade-offs between these pathways have not been fully explored. For example, in a representative cohort of patients, on balance, does each day of exposure to inadequate antimicrobial treatment cost more than the potential savings from using less active but cheaper medications, which are more likely to be inadequate? Or what proportion of the overall hospital bill is attributable to antimicrobials and how, if at all, does it differ between patients given appropriate and inappropriate empiric treatment? Answering these questions may lend a broader perspective to the debate of risks and benefits of broad-spectrum treatment when warranted than simply focusing on acquisition costs.

Enterobacteriaceae represent frequent pathogens in multiple common infections such as urinary tract infection (UTI), sepsis and pneumonia. Not surprisingly, the rising prevalence of carbapenem resistant Enterobacteriaceae (CRE) heightens the risk for the clinician to prescribe IET, which, in turn, increases mortality [20]. The full economic impact of IET in this setting, however, is less well understood. Although in a prior study IET was associated with an approximately 5-day increase in length of stay (LOS) and a $10,000 increase in costs, other important economic outcomes have not been examined in this population [20]. Hence, we sought to explore the direct costs associated with antibiotics prescribed and also those attributable to delaying adequate treatment. We further examined rates of hospital readmission at 30-days in the setting of an index hospitalization with Enterobacteriaceae (both carbapenem susceptible [CSE] and CRE) in UTI, sepsis and/or pneumonia.

Methods

We conducted a multi-center retrospective cohort study of patients admitted to the hospital with a UTI + sepsis (referred to throughout the paper as "UTI"), pneumonia and/or sepsis in the Premier Research database for the years 2009–2013. The aim of the current analysis was to quantify 30-day readmission rates, antibiotics cost as an absolute value and as a proportion of the total hospital costs, as well as the incremental daily contribution of delays in adequate antimicrobial treatment to increasing total hospital costs.

Because this study utilized an already existing HIPAA-compliant fully de-identified data, it was exempt from IRB review.

Patient population

The current analysis was performed on a cohort previously described [20]. Briefly, patients were included if they were adults (age ≥ 18 years) hospitalized with Enterobacteriaceae UTI, pneumonia, and/or sepsis (cultured from a urinary, respiratory or blood source). UTI, pneumonia, and sepsis were identified via combinations of previously published ICD-9-CM codes [20–25]. In order to eliminate confounding cost calculations and isolate infection-related costs, only patients with community-onset (present on admission) infection were included. To differentiate infection from colonization, we further required subjects to be treated with an antibiotic beginning within the first two hospital days and continued for ≥3 consecutive days, or until discharge [22–24]. Patients were followed until death in or, if discharged alive from the hospital, for an additional 30 days for evidence of hospital readmission.

To establish the attributable per-day costs of inadequate antimicrobial coverage (defined as each day of not receiving an antimicrobial the pathogen is susceptible to), we analyzed a subgroup of the cohort who had the following characteristics: 1) They survived the hospitalization; 2) They, at some point during the hospitalization, received adequate coverage for their infection. Since our "appropriate/inappropriate" definition applies only to the empiric treatment period, we refer to "adequate/inadequate" treatment as a period that encompasses both, empiric and definitive time frames.

Data source

Premier Research database, an electronic laboratory, pharmacy and billing data repository for years 2009 through 2013, contains ~15% of all hospitalizations nationwide. In addition to patient age, gender, race/ethnicity, principal and secondary diagnoses and procedures, the database contains a date-stamped log of all medications, laboratory tests, and diagnostic and therapeutic services charged to the patient or their insurer. We used data from 176 US institutions who submit microbiology data into the database. Eligible time began only following the commencement of microbiology data submission by each institution.

Baseline variables

For a full description of baseline variable, please, refer to the previously published study [20]. Briefly, patient factors included demographic variables and comorbid conditions. The Charlson comorbidity index (CCI) score was computed as a measure of the burden of chronic illness, while ICU admission, mechanical ventilation and vasopressor use served as markers for disease severity. Hospital-level characteristics examined included geographic region, size, teaching status, and urbanicity.

Microbiology and treatment variables and definitions

Urinary, blood and/or respiratory cultures had to be obtained within the first 2 days of hospitalization.

The following organisms were defined as Enterobacteriaceae of interest:

1. *Escherichia coli*
2. *Klebsiella pneumoniae*
3. Klebsiella oxytoca
4. *Enterobacter cloacae*
5. *Enterobacter aerogenes*
6. *Proteus mirabilis*
7. *Proteus spp.*
8. *Serratia marcescens*
9. *Citrobacter freundii*
10. *Morganella morganii*
11. *Providencia spp.*

CRE were defined as one of the above organisms where susceptibility testing yielded an "intermediate" or "resistant" result to at least one of the four carbapenems: imipenem, meropenem, ertapenem or doripenem.

IET was present if the antibiotic administered for the infection did not cover the organism based on reported in vitro information, or if appropriate coverage did not begin within 2 days of the positive culture being obtained.

The costs of antibiotics examined pertained to any antibiotics administered during the given hospitalization, regardless of whether they were used to treat the index infection or other infections.

Statistical analyses

The complete details of statistical analyses of the cohort have been described previously [20]. For the current analyses, the following was also done.

To assign costs to the delay in appropriate empiric treatment, we categorized LOS into 3 groups: 1). number of days until the first index culture (the "pre" time), 2). number of days after the index culture until the first

appropriate antibiotic (the period of interest), and 3). number of days after the first appropriate antibiotic until hospital discharge (the "post" time). It was important to adjust for the "pre" and "post" times so that the costs associated with these time periods were not attributed to the wrong period. The model structure was a generalized linear model with a logarithmic link to account for the skew in total costs (the outcome variable). In addition to the 3 time variables, other variables included all the other predictors known by hospital day 2 (i.e., all demographics, comorbidities, healthcare-associated (HCA) status, and a large number of treatments such as mechanical ventilation, vasopressor use, dialysis, inotropes, opioids, etc. as done in prior modeling [20]).

All inference tests were two-tailed, and a p value <0.05 was deemed a priori to represent statistical significance. All analyses were performed in Stata/MP 13.1 for Windows (StataCorp LP, College Station, TX).

Results

Among 37,694 patients presenting to the hospital with a UTI, pneumonia or sepsis, who met the inclusion criteria and had treatment data, 4984 (13.2%) received IET. The prevalence of CRE was low. Specifically CRE accounted for 13.0% of cases within the IET cohort and 1.6% in non-IET groups ($p < 0.001$). Complete baseline, infection, treatment and hospital characteristics and outcomes of the entire population are available in an earlier publication and are reproduced in the Additional file 1: Table S1 (20). Briefly, with the exception of race (more likely black in the IET group than non-IET), and comorbidity burden (greater in IET than non-IET), other demographic variables were largely similar between the groups. Sepsis and UTI among those receiving IET were slightly less and pneumonia slightly more frequent upon admission. Except for the greater prevalence of mechanical ventilation among IET than the non-IET group (21.3% vs. 15.5%, $p < 0.001$), acute illness severity did not differ based on ICU admission or administration of vasopressors as a function of initial therapy appropriateness. Unadjusted hospital mortality was higher in patients receiving IET than non-IET (10.6% vs. 8.6%, $p < 0.001$) in both infection types. Both unadjusted LOS and costs were significantly higher in the IET group than in the group receiving non-IET. These relationships generally held irrespective of the infection type (Additional file 1: Table S1) (20).

The total median unadjusted antibiotics costs did not exceed $750 in any of the infection types, with the aggregated median antibiotic cost in the IET group higher than in the non-IET ($602, IQR [$230, $1422] vs. $441, IQR [$206, $919], $p < 0.001$) (Table 1). The highest proportion of the median total costs of hospitalization due to antibiotic costs reached 4.1% in the setting of appropriate treatment in pneumonia (Table 1). Across all

Table 1 Unadjusted hospital resource utilization outcomes

| | Non-IET | | IET | | |
	N = 32,710		N = 4984		
Antibiotics costs, $	Mean/Median	SD/IQR	Mean/Median	SD/IQR	P-value
UTI					
Mean	779	1486	1333	2655	<0.001
Median	405	190, 844	586	226, 1332	<0.001
Sepsis					
Mean	958	2496	1736	3840	<0.001
Median	478	226, 1007	731	310, 1782	<0.001
Pneumonia					
Mean	887	1106	918	1202	<0.001
Median	552	269, 1067	459	183, 1148	0.098
Any					
Mean	845	1844	1381	2909	<0.001
Median	441	206, 919	602	230, 1422	<0.001
Antibiotics costs as a fraction of total hospital costs	Mean/Median	SD/IQR	Mean/Median	SD/IQR	P-value
UTI					
Mean	4.5%	4.4%	5.0%	5.2%	<0.001
Median	3.4%	1.9%, 5.8%	3.5%	1.8%, 6.4%	0.066
Sepsis					
Mean	4.3%	4.2%	4.3%	5.1%	0.923
Median	3.2%	1.8%, 5.5%	3.0%	1.4%, 5.3%	<0.001
Pneumonia					
Mean	5.3%	4.4%	4.6%	4.3%	<0.001
Median	4.1%	2.3%, 7.0%	3.2%	1.7%, 6.0%	<0.001
Any					
Mean	4.5%	4.4%	4.7%	5.0%	0.028
Median	3.4%	1.9%, 5.8%	3.3%	1.6%, 6.0%	0.012
30-day readmission	Rate	N at risk	Rate	N at risk	P-value
UTI	20.8%	16,028	24.8%	2194	<0.001
Sepsis	20.6%	9097	26.7%	1191	<0.001
Pneumonia	23.8%	3521	25.8%	294	0.204
Any	21.1%	28,646	25.6%	4279	<0.001

IET inappropriate empiric therapy, SD standard deviation, UTI urinary tract infection, IQR interquartile range

infection types, though, the fraction of median hospital costs represented by antibiotic acquisition varied significantly between the IET and non-IET populations. Despite this statistical difference, the absolute difference in costs was trivial from a financial perspective. Specifically, for IET and non-IET patients, this proportion was 3.3% and 3.4%, respectively (Table 1).

30-day readmission rates were high for all infection types (> 20%). More importantly, rates of readmission were significantly higher in those given IET compared to non-IET (25.6% vs. 21.1%, p < 0.001) (Table 1).

The sub-cohort of patients analyzed to assess the daily attributable cost of receiving inadequate antimicrobial coverage consisted of 27,953 patients who survived their index hospitalizations and at some point during their hospital stay received adequate treatment. The vast majority of them (78.5%) received such treatment as soon as infection was suspected and the culture obtained. In the remaining 21.5%, the mean (SD) duration of delay to appropriate therapy was 1.8 (1.1) days. In an adjusted analysis, each day's delay in instituting adequate therapy added $766 (95% confidence interval $661, $870, p < 0.001) to the total cost of hospitalization. This represents 3.5% of the total mean daily hospital cost and is similar in magnitude to the actual direct costs for antibiotic acquisition.

Discussion

In this study, we show that regardless of the appropriateness of initial antibiotic treatment, antibiotic costs represented less than 3.5% of the total hospital costs. We also demonstrate that the prevalence of 30-day readmission among the survivors of a hospitalization with an Enterobaceriaceae UTI, pneumonia and/or sepsis was over 20%, with those given initially inappropriate therapy facing a significantly higher risk for readmission.

Importantly, each additional day of inadequate therapy (among survivors) was associated with an appreciable cost of $766/day, and this cost became evident as soon as infection was suspected and culture obtained. Taken together, these results suggest that the additive costs of IET are high and independent of many confounders. Furthermore, there are hidden costs related to IET. Specifically, the attributable costs related to the delay in adequate therapy are similar in size to the costs for a day on a general medical floor in the US, while the increased rate of readmissions represents a potential for lost revenue to medical institutions, as the federal agencies may not reimburse for such readmissions. In other words, the total true costs of inappropriate therapy extend beyond the impact on the index event. In this sense our findings are novel in that they reveal that initial antibiotic treatment decisions have substantial downstream consequences that are important both for the patient and the healthcare institution.

To the best of our knowledge, this is the first study to address concerns around the costs of antibiotic therapy, including broad-spectrum agents available during the study timeframe, as empirical coverage for serious infections. The considerable expense associated with delay to adequate therapy may act to countervail fiscal concerns regarding the expenses associated with some of the newer therapies in appropriately targeted patients, particularly given that the median expenditures on antibiotics comprise less than 4% of the overall hospital costs. Put another way, acquisition costs must be viewed in the totality of the cost for hospitalization and potential readmission. The most expensive antibiotic may not be the one with the highest price but the one that is used as inappropriate initial therapy.

Under the best of all possible circumstances, a clinician would be able to order a bedside test to establish with a high degree of certainty, both the pathogen and its antimicrobial susceptibility profile before administering treatment. Unfortunately, such technologies remain only on the horizon, and even when available will raise concerns of overtreatment [26]. Many clinicians currently advocate for a probabilistic approach to risk stratification to guide the use of broad-spectrum antibiotic therapy [27]. The usefulness of such Bayesian approaches is limited in clinical practice for a pathogen like CRE, which, although rare (under 1.3% of all Enterobacteriaceae infections in the current study), raises the risk of IET significantly. In other words, a low pre-test probability (as displayed by the low prevalence of CRE) limits the conclusions that can be definitively drawn from such mathematical approaches. However, if a predictive test could identify with a high degree of confidence patients who do not require broad-spectrum coverage, its combination with molecular diagnostics could identify more precisely a more limited population that would require safeguarding with broader antimicrobials. Such bracketing of eligibility for newer agents along with the high cost of treating inadequately may both offset the concerns for draining the pharmacy budgets and improve patient outcomes. This hypothesis, however, requires exploration in future research.

Our novel result of the cost associated with each day's delay to adequate coverage complements prior work. Zhang and coworkers in patients with sepsis recently reported that each hour's delay in appropriate antimicrobial treatment is associated with a 0.1-day's add-on to the post-infection onset hospital LOS [19]. While such an increment does not seem substantial, over days of delay this LOS increases dramatically. Our data build on this finding by calculating the actual costs associated with such delays and therefore serve to reinforce the point that the most expensive antibiotic is the one used inappropriately or for rescue therapy, irrespective of its acquisition cost.

Our cost calculation brings out the following important point: each additional day of inadequate therapy for an Enterobaceriaceae UTI, pneumonia or sepsis contributes as much to the total cost of the hospitalization as the total price of all antibiotics administered during the given hospitalization. Given the known improvement in the chances of survival with immediate appropriate treatment, this serves as further compelling evidence to start broadly and de-escalate as necessary [12, 14, 16].

Our study has a number of strengths and limitations. As a large multicenter cohort it is representative of US institutions, and thus has broad generalizability. Although susceptible to bias, particularly selection bias, we dealt with it by setting a priori enrollment criteria and definitions for the main exposures and outcomes. Though some misclassification is possible, particularly in the face of relying on administrative coding for case definition, the main exposure (IET) and outcomes (30-day readmission, antibiotics costs) are minimally susceptible to misclassification. At the same time, in at least some of the identified cases Enterobacteriaceae might have represented colonization, rather than a true infection. Finally, we did not examine how specific antibiotic regimens contribute to the costs of the hospitalization, so it remains unknown how much of those costs can be attributed to the newer more expensive agents. However, it may be assumed that those patients who received appropriate empiric treatment were more likely than those treated inappropriately to get the newer agents, particularly in the setting of CRE. At the same time, the time frame of the study predates coming to market of any of the newer broad-spectrum anti-gram-negative agents, and our analysis may need to be repeated when those data become available.

Conclusions

Hospitalizations with Enterobacteriaceae are costly, and specific antibiotic agent choice exerts less impact on overall costs than antibiotic appropriateness. Given many lines of evidence that document that IET is detrimental to survival, it becomes a clinical imperative to adopt strategies and protocols that maximize rates of appropriate therapy. We demonstrate that concerns about the costs of broader-spectrum antibiotics, at least those available at the time of the analysis, appear unwarranted, since the total antimicrobial costs comprise only a modest proportion of total costs of hospitalization and must also be weighed against the potential for a no-pay event, such as a hospital readmission. Finally, the fact that each additional day of inadequate treatment is roughly equivalent in cost to the total per-patient cost of all antimicrobials administered is a reason to pause to reconsider these now clearer trade-offs in clinical decision-making. If other investigations confirm our findings, there may be a need for a paradigm shift to account for failure to cover serious infections appropriately.

Abbreviations

CCI: Charlson comorbidity index; CRE: Carbapenem resistant enterobacteriaceae; CSE: Carbapenem susceptible enterobacteriaceae; HCA: Healthcare-associated; HIPAA: Healthcare insurance portability and accountability act; ICD-9-CM: International classification of diseases, version 9, clinical modification; ICU: Intensive care unit; IET: Inappropriate empiric therapy; IQR: Interquartile range; IRB: Institutional review board; LOS: Length of stay; UTI: Urinary tract infection

Acknowledgements
Not applicable.

Funding
This study was funded by a grant from The Medicines Company.

Sponsor role
Although Ms. Sulham and Ms. Fan are employees of the sponsor and participated in the study as co-investigators, the larger sponsor had no role in study design, data analysis or interpretation or publication decisions.

Guarantor
Dr. Zilberberg takes responsibility for the content of the manuscript, including the data and analysis.

Disclosure
This study was funded by The Medicines Company, Parsippany, NJ, USA. The data from this study will in part be presented at the ECCMID 2017 meeting. I certify that all coauthors have seen and agree with the contents of the manuscript. I certify that the submission is not under review by any other publication.

Authors' contributions
MDZ, KS, WF and AFS contributed substantially to the study design, data interpretation, and the writing of the manuscript. BHN had full access to all of the data in the study and takes responsibility for the integrity of the data and the accuracy of the data analysis. He contributed substantially to the study design, data analysis, and the writing of the manuscript. No one other than the listed authors participated in the study design, analysis, interpretation or manuscript drafting or revision. All authors read and approved the final manuscript.

Competing interests
Dr. Zilberberg is a consultant to The Medicines Company. Her employer, EviMed Research Group, LLC, has received research grant support from The Medicines Company.
Dr. Nathanson is an employee of OptiStatim, LLC, who received grant support from EviMed Research Group, LLC, for conducting the analyses.
Ms. Fan and Ms. Sulham are employees of and stockholders in The Medicines Company.
Dr. Shorr is a consultant to and has received research grant support from The Medicines Company.
Drs. Zilberberg and Shorr have received grant support and/or have served as consultants to Merck, Tetraphase, Pfizer, Astellas, Shionogi and Theravance.

Author details
[1]EviMed Research Group, LLC, PO Box 303, Goshen, MA 01032, USA. [2]OptiStatim, LLC, Longmeadow, MA, USA. [3]The Medicines Company, Parsippany, NJ, USA. [4]Washington Hospital Center, Washington, DC, USA.

References
1. Centers for Disease Control and Prevention. Antibiotic resistance threats in the United States, 2013. Available at http://www.cdc.gov/drugresistance/threat-report-2013/pdf/ar-threats-2013-508.pdf#page=59 Accessed January 8, 2016.
2. National Nosocomial Infections Surveillance. (NNIS) system report. Am J Infect Control. 2004;32:470.
3. Obritsch MD, Fish DN, MacLaren R, Jung R. National surveillance of antimicrobial resistance in *Pseudomonas aeruginosa* isolates obtained from intensive care unit patients from 1993 to 2002. Antimicrob Agents Chemother. 2004;48:4606–10.
4. Zilberberg MD, Shorr AF. Secular trends in gram-negative resistance among urinary tract infection hospitalizations in the United States, 2000-2009. Infect Control Hosp Epidemiol. 2013;34:940–6.

5.   Zilberberg MD, Shorr AF. Prevalence of multidrug-resistant *Pseudomonas aeruginosa* and carbapenem-resistant Enterobacteriaceae among specimens from hospitalized patients with pneumonia and bloodstream infections in the United States from 2000 to 2009. J Hosp Med. 2013;8:559–63.

6.   CDDEP: The Center for Disease Dynamics, Economics and Policy. Resistance Map: *Acinetobacter baumannii* Overview. Available at https://www.cddep.org/research-area/gram-negative/. Accessed 8 Jan 2016.

7.   Zilberberg MD, Kollef MH, Shorr AF. Secular trends in *Acinetobacter baumannii* resistance in respiratory and blood stream specimens in the United States, 2003 to 2012: a survey study. J Hosp Med. 2016;11:21–6.

8.   Micek ST, Kollef KE, Reichley RM, et al. Health care-associated pneumonia and community-acquired pneumonia: a single-center experience. Antimicrob Agents Chemother. 2007;51:3568–73.

9.   Iregui M, Ward S, Sherman G, et al. Clinical importance of delays in the initiation of appropriate antibiotic treatment for ventilator-associated pneumonia. Chest. 2002;122:262–8.

10. Alvarez-Lerma F. ICU-acquired pneumonia study group. Modification of empiric antibiotic treatment in patients with pneumonia acquired in the intensive care unit. Intensive Care Med. 1996;22:387–94.

11. Zilberberg MD, Shorr AF, Micek MT, Mody SH, Kollef MH. Antimicrobial therapy escalation and hospital mortality among patients with HCAP: a single center experience. Chest. 2008;134:963–8.

12. Dellinger RP, Levy MM, Carlet JM, Bion J, Parker MM, Jaeschke R, Reinhart K, Angus DC, Brun-Buisson C, Beale R, Calandra T, Dhainaut JF, Gerlach H, Harvey M, Marini JJ, Marshall J, Ranieri M, Ramsay G, Sevransky J, Thompson BT, Townsend S, Vender JS, Zimmerman JL, Vincent JL. Surviving sepsis campaign: international guidelines for management of severe sepsis and septic shock: 2008. Crit Care Med. 2008;36:296–327.

13. Kollef MH, Sherman G, Ward S, Fraser VJ. Inadequate antimicrobial treatment of infections: a risk factor for hospital mortality among critically ill patients. Chest. 1999;115:462–74.

14. Garnacho-Montero J, Garcia-Garmendia JL, Barrero-Almodovar A, Jimenez-Jimenez FJ, Perez-Paredes C, Ortiz-Leyba C. Impact of adequate empirical antibiotic therapy on the outcome of patients admitted to the intensive care unit with sepsis. Crit Care Med. 2003;31:2742–51.

15. Harbarth S, Garbino J, Pugin J, Romand JA, Lew D, Pittet D. Inappropriate initial antimicrobial therapy and its effect on survival in a clinical trial of immunomodulating therapy for severe sepsis. Am J Med. 2003;115:529–35.

16. Ferrer R, Artigas A, Suarez D, Palencia E, Levy MM, Arenzana A, Pérez XL, Sirvent JM. Effectiveness of treatments for severe sepsis: a prospective, multicenter, observational study. Am J Respir Crit Care Med. 2009;180:861–6.

17. Zilberberg MD, Shorr AF, Micek ST, Vazquez-Guillamet C, Kollef MH. Multi-drug resistance, inappropriate initial antibiotic therapy and mortality in gram-negative severe sepsis and septic shock: a retrospective cohort study. Crit Care. 2014;18(6):596.

18. Shorr AF, Micek ST, Welch EC, Doherty JA, Reichley RM, Kollef MH. Inappropriate antibiotic therapy in gram-negative sepsis increases hospital length of stay. Crit Care Med. 2011;39:46–51.

19. Zhang D, Micek ST, Kollef MH. Time to appropriate antibiotic therapy is an independent determinant of postinfection ICU and hospital lengths of stay in patients with sepsis. Crit Care Med. 2015;43:2133–40.

20. Zilberberg MD, Nathanson BH, Sulham K, Fan W, Shorr AF. Carbapenem resistance, inappropriate empiric treatment and outcomes among patients hospitalized with Enterobacteriaceae urinary tract infection, pneumonia and sepsis. BMC Infect Dis. in press

21. Meddings J, Saint S, McMahon LF. Hospital-acquired catheter-associated urinary tract infection: documentation and coding issues may reduce financial impact of Medicare's new payment policy. Infect Control Hosp Epidemiol. 2010;31:627–33.

22. Rothberg MB, Pekow PS, Priya A, et al. Using highly detailed administrative data to predict pneumonia mortality. PLoS One. 2014;9(1):e87382.

23. Rothberg MB, Haessler S, Lagu T, et al. Outcomes of patients with healthcare-associated pneumonia: worse disease or sicker patients? Infect Control Hosp Epidemiol. 2014;35(Suppl 3):S107–15.

24. Rothberg MB, Zilberberg MD, Pekow PS, et al. Association of guideline-based antimicrobial therapy and outcomes in healthcare-associated pneumonia. J Antimicrob Chemother. 2015;70:1573–9.

25. Martin GS, Mannino DM, Eaton S, Moss M. The epidemiology of sepsis in the United States from 1979 through 2000. N Engl J Med. 2003;348:1546–54.

26. Zilberberg MD, Shorr AF. Impact of prior probabilities of MRSA as an infectious agent on the accuracy of the emerging molecular diagnostic tests: a model simulation. BMJ Open. 2012;2(6)

27. Shorr AF, Zilberberg MD. Role for risk-scoring tools in identifying resistant pathogens in pneumonia: reassessing the value of healthcare-associated pneumonia as a concept. Curr Opin Pulm Med. 2015;21:232–8.

9

Urinary pathogenic bacterial profile, antibiogram of isolates and associated risk factors among pregnant women in Ambo town, Central Ethiopia: a cross-sectional study

Yonas Alem Gessese[1*†], Dereje Leta Damessa[2†], Mebratenesh Mengistu Amare[1], Yonas Hailesilassie Bahta[1], Assalif Demisew Shifera[1], Fikreslasie Samuel Tasew[3] and Endrias Zewdu Gebremedhin[4]

Abstract

Background: Urinary tract infection (UTI) is a well-known bacterial infection posing serious health problem in pregnant women. A study was conducted in pregnant women with the objectives of estimating prevalence of UTI, determining antibiogram of the bacterial isolates and assessment of the potential risk factors associated with UTI.

Methods: A cross-sectional study design was used to collect 300 mid-stream urine samples from pregnant women from March 2016 to December, 2016. Samples were inoculated into Cysteine Lactose Electrolyte Deficient medium (CLED). Colonies from CLED were subcultured onto MacConkey and Blood agar plates. A standard agar disc diffusion method was used to determine antimicrobial susceptibility. Chi-square (X^2) test & logistic regression were used to show associations between UTI and explanatory variables & identify the predictors of UTI, respectively.

Results: The age of pregnant women enrolled in this study ranges from 16 to 46 years (mean ± standard deviation = 25 ± 4.7 years).The overall prevalence of UTI in pregnant women was 18.7% (95% confidence interval [CI]: 14.4–23.54%).The prevalence of symptomatic and asymptomatic UTI was 20.4% (95% CI: 13.09–29.46%) and 17.8% (95% CI: 12.70–23.83%) respectively. The predominant bacteria identified were E. coli (46.4%), S. aureus (14.3%), coagulase negative Staphylococci [CoNS] (14.3%) and Proteus species (10.6%). Majority of Gram-negative bacteria isolates were resistant to ampicillin (70%), ceftriaxon (66%), gentamicin (68%) and nitrofurantoin (64%) while 75–100% of the Gram positive isolates were resistance to ampicillin. Multiple drug resistance was observed in all of the isolates. Multivariable logistic regression revealed that the odds of acquiring UTI was 4.78 times higher in pregnant women earning monthly income of ≤500 Ethiopian Birr (21.18 USD) as compared to those earning monthly income >2001 Ethiopian Birr [84.79 USD] (P = 0.046). Similarly, the risk of UTI was higher in those who eat raw meat (OR = 2.04, 95% CI: 1.09, 3.83, P = 0.026) and had previous UTI history (OR = 2.29, 95% CI = 1.15–4.56, P = 0.019) as compared to those who eat cooked meat and had no previous history of UTI.

(Continued on next page)

* Correspondence: alemg577@gmail.com
†Equal contributors
[1]Department of Medical Laboratory Sciences, Ambo University, College of Medicine and Health Sciences, Ambo, Ethiopia
Full list of author information is available at the end of the article

(Continued from previous page)

Conclusions: The prevalence & antimicrobial resistance of uropathogens was high. Health education, continuous surveillance of UTI and their antimicrobial resistance pattern are essential to reduce the consequence of symptomatic and asymptomatic bacteriuria and multi-drug resistant bacteria in pregnant women.

Keywords: Uropathogens, Pregnant women, Prevalence, Antibiogram, Multidrug resistance, Risk factors, Central Ethiopia

Background

Urinary tract infection (UTI) is an infection caused by the presence and growth of microorganisms anywhere in the urinary tract. It is usually due to bacteria from the digestive tract which climb the opening of the urethra and begin to multiply to cause infection. In contrast to men, women are more susceptible to UTI [1, 2], and this is mainly due to short urethra, absence of prostatic secretion, pregnancy and ease of contamination of the urinary tract with fecal flora [3].

Urinary tract infection is a common health problem among pregnant women [4]. Asymptomatic bacteriuria (ASB) is a common bacterial infection of the urinary tract requiring medical treatment in pregnancy. Diagnosis and treatment of ASB is important as approximately 20–40% of pregnant women [5, 6], if untreated during pregnancy, symptomatic UTI will develop. Treatment of UTI is important in keeping with the goal of safe motherhood initiative; that women safely go through pregnancy and childbirth and produce healthy babies. Untreated ASB is a risk factor for acute cystitis (40%) and pyelonephritis (25–30%) in pregnancy and could lead to adverse obstetric outcomes such as prematurity, low-birth weight, and higher fetal mortality rates [5, 7, 8].

Urinary tract infection is mostly caused by Gram-negative aerobic bacilli found in gastrointestinal tract. The most common are: *E. coli, Klebsilla pneumoniae, Enterobacter, Citrobacter, Proteus mirabilis,* and *P. aeruginosa*. Other common pathogens include: *Staphylococcus epidermidis, Staphylococcus saprophyticus, Enterococcus* species and *Serratia* species which presumably result in UTI following colonization of the genito-urinary tract [9]. *E.coli* (60–70%), *Klebsiella* species (10%), *Proteus* species(5–10%) and *Pseudomonas* species (2–5%) are the dominant Gram-negative bacteria causing UTI. Among Gram-positive bacteria pathogens *Streptococcus* species and *Staphylococcus* species are frequently isolated from cases of UTIs [10, 11].

Microbial drug resistance is a major problem in treating infectious diseases worldwide. It is aggravated by the increased use of muddled empirical treatments, mainly in economically developing countries like Ethiopia [12]. Recently, UTI has become more complicated and difficult to treat because of appearance of uropathogens resistant to the commonly used antimicrobial agents [13]. In Ethiopia, there are indications on the misuse of

antimicrobial drugs by health care providers, unskilled practitioners, and drug consumers. Studies in Ethiopia show that antimicrobial drug resistance seriously affects the management of bacterial infections leading to increased mortality, morbidity and cost of treatment [14].

The prevalence of UTI is increased by several factors. Poor socioeconomic status is reported to be a major risk factor with indigent patients having a five-fold increased risk [15]. Other risk factors include increased age, high parity, poor perineal hygiene, history of recurrent UTI, diabetes mellitus, anatomic or functional urinary tract abnormality, and increased frequency of sexual activity [16].

The aims of the present study were to isolate and identify the predominant pathogenic bacteria causing UTI, evaluation of the antimicrobial susceptibility pattern of the isolates and identification of potential risk factors of UTI.

Methods
Study area

The study was conducted at Ambo town public health facilities from March 2016 to December 2016. Ambo, the capital city of West Shoa Zone, is located 112 Km to the West of Addis Ababa. The health facilities or institutions are one of the biggest health care hospital and health centers in the Zone and provide services to about 61,900 (31,655 males and females 30,245) inhabitants in and around the town.

Study population

The study population was those pregnant women attending antenatal clinic (ANC) at Ambo hospital, Ambo Health Center and Awaro Health Center during the study period and who did not initiate antimicrobial drug therapy for at least in the preceding 2 weeks prior to sample collection.

Study design

A cross-sectional study was conducted on urine samples collected from pregnant women (both outpatients and inpatients) attending antenatal clinic (ANC) at Ambo hospital, Ambo Health Center and Awaro Health Center from March, 2016 to December, 2016. A detail history and complete clinical examination was carried out for each sampled pregnant women. For each selected pregnant women, information on socio-demographic factors (age, religion, pregnancy category, gestational stage, level of income, level of education, habit of raw meat eating, water source, previous UTI history) and clinical data were obtained by using structured questionnaires.

Sample size determination

The required sample size was determined using single population formula $N = Z^2 (P \times q)/d^2$ [17]. Considering: prevalence (P) of 18.8% (prevalence of culture proven pregnant women with UTI previously reported from Hawasa, Ethiopia [7] where: N = the required sample size, Z = Z score for 95% confidence interval (1.96), d = tolerable error (5%), $q = 1-P = 1-0.188 = 0.812$. The calculated sample size ($n = 234$) was raised to 300 to consider for non-responses.

Sampling methods

The list of pregnant women (sampling frame) was obtained from ANC health institutions. Study participants were selected using simple random sampling technique. The calculated sample size was proportionally distributed to Ambo hospital ($n = 220$), Ambo ($n = 50$) and Awaro ($n = 30$) Health Centers.

Operational definitions
Asymptomatic UTI
It is the presence of significant bacteria ($\geq 10^5$ cfu/ml) in two consecutive clean-voided mid-stream urine specimen in a patient without signs or symptoms.

Symptomatic UTI
It is defined as a condition whereby a patient has one or more of the following signs or symptoms with other recognized cause: fever (temperature, > 38 °C), urgency, frequency, dysuria, suprapubic pain or flank pain and a urine culture positive for 10^5 or more microorganisms per milliliter.

Midstream urine
A specimen obtained from the middle part of urine flow.

Sample collection, uropathogen isolation & identification
A total of 300 mid-stream urine (MSU) samples were collected from pregnant women attending antenatal clinic in the study period. Ten to fifteen milliliter of freshly void midstream urine samples were used for microscopic investigation & culture media inoculation. Urine samples were stored in a cool ice box at 2–8 °C within 4 h of collection [1]. In the laboratory, urine samples were centrifuged at 1500 RPM for 5 min. After centrifugation a drop of the sediment was placed on the grease free slide, covered with cover slip and examined under the microscope using the high power objective lens (40X). Reporting system for microscopic identification was at high magnification using power field for pus cells, red blood cells (RBCs), epithelial cells, casts, crystals, yeast cells [18].

Standard loop technique was used to place 0.001 ml of urine for inoculation on Cysteine lactose electrolyte deficient medium, Blood agar, MacConkey agar and incubated at 37 °C for 24 h [1, 7]. The numbers of colonies were counted to quantify organisms. Diagnosis of UTI is defined on the basis of significant colony count of $\geq 10^5$ cfu/ml for Gram-negative and Gram-positive bacteria [7]. Growths on the culture media were identified by using bacterial growth characteristics (morphology), Gram staining [19, 20] and general biochemical tests [21, 22].

Antimicrobial susceptibility testing (AST) of uropathogens
The antimicrobial susceptibility testing of all isolates was done using commercial disks following the standard disk diffusion method recommended by the National Committee for Clinical Laboratory Standards [23].The drugs that were tested include, Amoxicillin-Clavulinic acid (AMC, 30 μg), Ampicillin (AMP, 30 μg), Ciprofloxacin (CPR, 5 μg), Norfloxacin (NOR, 10 μg), Gentamicin (GM, 10 μg), Erythromycin (E, 15 μg), Ceftriaxon (CRO, 10 μg), Nitrofurantoin (NIT, 300 μg) and Sulfamethoxazole-trimethoprim (SXT, 1.25 μg). All the antimicrobials used for the study were purchased from Oxoid Ltd. Bashing store, USA.

Statistical analysis
Data from laboratory investigation and questionnaire survey was entered into Microsoft Excel Spreadsheet. The coded data was processed and analyzed using STATA version 11.0 for Windows (Stata Corp., USA). Descriptive statistics was used to summarize the data.. Chi-square test was used to assess differences in the proportions of culture positive and negative participants. The prevalence of UTI was calculated. To determine predictors of bacteriuria, odds ratios were calculated using likelihood estimation technique. Independent variables (age, level of education, monthly income, parity, residence, raw meat consumption habit, raw milk consumption habit, washing habit and previous history of UTI) which are non-collinear and with P-values ≤ 0.25 in univariable logistic regression analysis were further tested via multivariable logistic regression in order to get adjusted odds ratios and significant predictors of UTI in pregnant women. P-value of <0.05 was considered statistically significant.

Results
The age of pregnant women enrolled in this study ranges from 16 to 46 years with a mean age of 25 years (Standard Deviation [SD] = 4.7).

Overall prevalence

From 300 urine samples, 56 (18.7%) (95% CI: 14.4–23.54%) were culture positive with colony count of more than 10^5 cfu/ml. Of the culture positive urine samples, 39 (69.6%) and 17 (30.4%), were Gram-negative and Gram-positive bacteria, respectively. The most predominant isolate was *E. coli* 26 (66.7% of the Gram-negatives, 46.4% of all isolate). Microscopic examination of urine samples indicated the presence of pus cells in 56 (18.7%), leukocyturia in 87 (29%) and nitrite positive cases in 8 (2%) of samples examined.

From 300 pregnant women seven bacterial species of UTI were isolated in which *E. coli* ($n = 26$) was the predominant bacteria followed by *S. aureus* and coagulase negative *Staphylococci* [CoNS] ($n = 8$).

The prevalence of symptomatic and asymptomatic UTI was 20.4% (95% CI: 13.09–29.46%) and 17.8% (95% CI: 12.70–23.83%) respectively (Table 1).

Of the 56 bacterial isolates, 37 (66.1%) were from urban dwellers and the remaining 19 (33.9%) were from periurban and rural areas. Monthly income, raw meat consumption habit and previous history of UTI are significantly associated with prevalence of UTI ($P < 0.05$). Two hundred twelve (71%) of study participants had income level of 501–1000 Ethiopian birr (21.23–42.37 USD) and below. On the basis of their lifestyle about 115, 38.3%, had a habit of eating raw meat. About 18 (32.1%) of positive pregnant women had previous history of UTI (Table 2).

Antimicrobial susceptibility pattern of bacterial uropathogens

Bacterial uropathogen isolates from patients with UTIs revealed the presence of high levels of single and multiple

antimicrobial resistances against commonly prescribed drugs. Gram-negative isolates showed higher resistance pattern in comparison to Gram-positive for most of commonly prescribed antibiotics. *E. coli*, which is the predominant cause of UTI, showed high percentage of resistance to ampicillin and gentamycin, and low resistance to ciprofloxacin and amoxicillin-clavulinic acid (Table 3).

Multiple drug resistance patterns of the isolates

Multiple drug resistances (MDR) i.e., resistance to two or more antimicrobial drugs, was found in all uropathogens isolated (100%). All isolates of Gram-negative and Gram-positive bacteria were resistant to at least two antimicrobials. There were no isolates sensitive to all antibiotics tested.

Associated risk factors

Univariable logistic regression analysis showed significant association between prevalence of UTI and income level ($P = 0.046$), residential place ($P = 0.029$), raw meat consumption ($P = 0.04$) and previous history of UTI ($P = 0.028$) (Table 4).

Multivariable logistic regression revealed that the odds of acquiring UTI in pregnant women with monthly income of ≤500 Ethiopian Birr (≤21.18 USD) is 4.78 times higher than those pregnant women earning greater than 2001 Ethiopian Birr (>84.79 USD) (95% CI of OR = 1.03–22.21, $P = 0.046$). Similarly, the risk of UTI infection is twice and 2.04 times higher in those who eat raw meat (95% CI of OR = 1.09–3.83, $P = 0.026$) and had previous history UTI infection (OR = 2.29, 95% CI of OR = 1.15–4.56, $P = 0.019$), respectively, as compared to those who eat cooked meat and had no previous history of UTI (Table 4).

Discussion

The present study revealed that 18.7% of the pregnant women had UTIs during their pregnancy. *E. coli* was the most commonly isolated uropathogen. The overall prevalence of UTI in pregnant women in this study is comparable to the prevalence of UTI reported in Hawasa, Southern Ethiopia (18.8%) [7], but higher than the reports from Tikur Anbessa Specialized Hospital, Addis Ababa, Ethiopia (11.6%) [18]. The present prevalence of UTI in pregnant women was lower than the prevalence figure reported from Ghana (29.9%) [24]. This variation may be explained by the differences in the environmental conditions, methodology adopted & characteristics of study populations such as social and food habits and the standard of personal hygiene [25]. The prevalence of bacteriuria among symptomatic and asymptomatic pregnant women was 20.4% and 17.8% respectively. This finding is higher than the studies done in Sudan and Tanzania [26, 27].

Table 1 Overall and bacterial level of prevalence of UTI in symptomatic and asymptomatic pregnant women in Ambo Hospital, Ambo and Awaro Health Centers from March 2016 to December 2016 ($n = 300$)

Isolated Bacteria	Prevalence		Total positive N (%)
	Symptomatic (103) Number positive (%)	Asymptomatic (197) Number positive (%)	
E. coli	9 (8.7)	17 (8.6)	26 (8.7)
S. aureus	1(1.0)	7 (3.6)	8 (2.7)
CoNS	4 (3.9)	4 (2.0)	8 (2.7)
Proteus mirabilis	2 (1.9)	1(0.5)	3 (1.0)
Proteus Spp	1(1.0)	2 (1.0)	3 (1.0)
Klebsiella pneumoniae	0(0.0)	2 (1.0)	2 (0.7)
Klebsiella Spp	0 (0)	2 (1.0)	2 (0.7)
Citrobacter Spp	3 (2.9)	0 (0.0)	3 (1.0)
Streptococcus Spp	1 (1.0)	0(0.0)	1(0.3)
Total	21 (20.4)	35 (17.8)	56 (18.7)

Table 2 Socio-demographic characteristics of study participants in Ambo Hospital, Ambo and Awaro health centers ($n = 300$)

Socio-demographic variables	Bacterial Culture (%)		Total	X^2	p-value
	Positive = 56 (18.7)	Negative = 244 (81.3)			
Age in years					
15–24	27 (18)	126 (82)	153	1.359	0.51
25–34	25 (19)	109 (81)	134		
35–44	4 (31)	9 (69)	13		
Gestation stage					
Second trimester	23 (16)	120 (84)	143	1.201	0.27
Third trimester	33 (21)	124 (79)	157		
Pregnancy Category					
Primiparous	25 (18)	113 (82)	138	0.051	0.82
Multiparous	31 (19)	131 (81)	162		
Employment					
Employed	17 (17)	86 (83)	103	0.483	0.49
Unemployed	39 (20)	158 (80)	197		
Residency					
Urban	37 (17)	187 (83)	224	5.096	0.08
Rural	10 (20)	40 (80)	50		
Periurban	9 (35)	17 (65)	26		
Education					
Illiterate	10 (20)	41 (80)	51	0.170	0.98
Primary school	20 (19)	85 (81)	105		
Secondary school	13 (19)	55 (81)	68		
University	13 (17)	63 (83)	76		
Income/month					
<500	32 (19)	85 (81)	117	14.079	0.007
501–1000	18 (25)	77 (75)	95		
1001–1500	3 (8)	36 (92)	39		
1501–2000	1 (9)	22 (91)	23		
>2001	2 (15)	24 (85)	26		
Eat raw meat					
Yes	28 (24)	87 (76)	115	3.965	0.046
No	28 (15)	157 (85)	185		
Drink raw milk					
Yes	14 (18)	63 (82)	77	0.016	0.90
No	42 (19)	181 (81)	223		
Eat raw vegetable					
Yes	19 (24)	61 (76)	80	1.857	0.17
No	37 (17)	183 (83)	220		
Water source					
Others	2 (9)	20 (91)	22	3.418	0.18
Spring water	6 (32)	13 (68)	19		
Tap water	48 (19)	211 (81)	259		

Table 2 Socio-demographic characteristics of study participants in Ambo Hospital, Ambo and Awaro health centers (*n* = 300) (*Continued*)

Socio-demographic variables	Bacterial Culture (%)		Total	X^2	*p*-value
	Positive = 56 (18.7)	Negative = 244 (81.3)			
UTI history					
Yes	18 (27)	48 (73)	66	4.128	0.04
No	38 (16)	196 (84)	234		

In this study, Gram-negative bacteria isolates were more prevalent (69.6%) than Gram-positive bacteria isolates (30.4%). This finding is in line with studies done in Dire Dawa where 73.1% of the isolates were Gram-negative [28]. The present finding was lower than the report from India [29, 30]. The high rate of isolation of Gram-negative uropathogens could be due to the presence of unique structure in Gram-negative bacteria which help for attachment to the uro-epithelial cells and prevent bacteria from urinary lavage, allowing for multiplication and tissue invasion [31].

E. coli was the most frequent etiological agent of UTI, which accounts for up to 46.4% of isolated cases. The present finding is in agreement with the finding from Gondar [1]. It is also consistent with findings from India & Tanzania [27, 32]. It is higher than the finding in Dire Dawa [28]. *E. coli* was considered as the most prominent uro-pathogenic bacteria due to a number of virulence factors specific for colonization and invasion of the urinary epithelium, [31]. It is also associated with microorganisms ascending from the peri-urethral areas contaminated by fecal flora due to the close proximity to the anus and warm, moist environment [3, 33].

In this study, *S. aureus* and CoNS were the second predominant spps of UTI bacteria which accounts each for up to 14.3% of isolated cases. The present finding of isolation of *S. aureus* as a uropathogen, was in line with the studies done in Gondar university teaching hospital

and Tikur Anbesa specialized teaching hospital [1, 18].It is curious that *S aureus* is a common cause of ASB in regions that practice female genital mutilation [34]. Ethiopia, like other Sub-Saharan African countries, practices female genital mutilation. Coagulase Negative Staphylococci, *S. saprophyticus*, isolated in our study is lower than the study done in Gondar university teaching hospital and Dire Dawa, Ethiopia [1, 28].

Proteus spp. was also etiological agent for UTI which accounts for about 10.7% of isolated cases. This finding is in line with the study done in Kenya [10]. The high prevalence of *Proteus* spp. in the study area might be due to the high prevalence of *S. mansoni*. Bacteriuria with a prevalence of 10% was reported in Tanzania [35] among persons infected with *Schistosoma*.

This study revealed a higher percentage of resistance to commonly prescribed antimicrobial drugs. In this study, most isolates of Gram-negative bacteria showed resistance to ampicillin (70%), ceftriaxon (66%), gentamicin (68%) and nitrofurantoin (64%). This study is in line with the finding from Dire Dawa [28]. However, this finding disagrees from the study done in Addis Ababa in which most Gram negative isolates showed high susceptibility to gentamicin and nitrofurantoin [18]. In this study, *E. coli* isolates showed high resistance to ampicillin (62%) and gentamicin (62%). The present finding is slightly similar with the finding from Dire Dawa in which *E.coli*

Table 3 Antimicrobial resistance pattern of Gram-negative and Gram-positive bacteria isolated from asymptomatic and symptomatic pregnant women in Ambo Hospital, Ambo and Awaro Health Centers from March 2016 to December 2016

Antimicrobial Agents	Number of Resistant Urinary isolates (%)						
	Gram-Negative Isolates				Gram-Positive Isolates		
	E.coli (*n* = 26)	*Proteus* Spp (*n* = 6)	*Klebsiella*Spp (*n* = 4)	*Citobacter*Spp (*n* = 3)	*S.aureus* (*n* = 8)	CoNS (*n* = 8)	*Streptococcus*Spp (*n* = 1)
Ampicillin	16(62)	6(–)	4(–)	2(–)	6(–)	6(–)	1(–)
Ciprofloxacin	1(–)	0(–)	1(–)	0(–)	0((–)	4(–)	0(–)
Norfloxacin	1(–)	0(–)	1(–)	0(–)	2(–)	1(–)	0(–)
Gentamicin	16(62)	4(–)	3(–)	2(–)	2(–)	1(–)	1(–)
Ceftriaxone	10(–)	5(–)	3(–)	2(–)	5(–)	2(–)	0(–)
Amoxicillin-Clavulanic acid	1(–)	1(–)	1(–)	1(–)	2(–)	0(–)	0(–)
Nitrofurantion	6(–)	–	–	1(–)	2(–)	0(–)	1(–)
Sulfamethoxazole -trimethoprim	4(–)	2(–)	0(–)	1(–)	1(–)	1(–)	1(–)

Table 4 Results of logistic regression analysis of potential risk factors associated with prevalence of UTI in pregnant women in Ambo Hospital, Ambo and Awaro Health Centers

Variables	Category	Univariable		Multivariable	
		OR (95% CI)	p-value	OR (95% CI)	p-value
Age in years	15–24	2.07(0.14, 1.68)	0.25	1.86 (0.12, 2.44)	0.42
	25–34	1.94(0.15, 1.81)	0.30	1.51 (0.15, 2.96)	0.59
	35–44	1.00		1.00	
Level education	Illiterate	1.00			
	Primary	1.04 (0.41, 2.25)	0.93		
	Secondary	1.03 (0.39, 2.43)	0.95		
	Tertiary	1.18 (0.34, 2.11)	0.72		
Income level	<500	4.52 (1.01, 20.22)	0.049	4.78 (1.03, 22.21)	0.046
	501–1000	2.81 (0.61, 12.97)	0.19	2.72 (0.56, 13.27)	0.22
	1001–1500	1.00 (0.12, 6.44)	1.00	1.06 (0.16, 7.00)	0.96
	1501–2000	1.83 (0.05, 6.44)	0.63	0.67 (0.06, 8.27)	0.76
	>2001	1.00		1.00	
Residency	Periurban	1.00		1.00	
	Rural	2.68 (0.15, 0.90)	0.029	2.18 (0.18, 1.20)	0.11
Religion	Orthodox	1.00		1.79 (0.16, 2.03)	0.38
Pregnancy category	Primiparous	1.00	–		
	Multiparous	1.07 (0.60, 1.92)	0.82		
Employment	Employed	1.00			
	Unemployed	1.25 (0.67, 2.34)	0.49		
Eat Raw Meat	Yes	1.84 (1.02, 3.30)	0.042	2.04 (1.09, 3.83)	0.026
	No	1.00		1.00	
Vegetable Eat	Yes	0.65 (0.35, 1.21)	0.18	1.38 (0.37, 1.43)	0.35
	No	1.00		1.00	
Drink Raw Milk	Yes	1.04 (0.54, 2.04)	0.90		
	No	1.00			
Drink Raw Milk	Yes	1.04 (0.54, 2.04)	0.90		
	No	1.00			
Water Source	Others	1.00		1.00	
	Spring water	4.62 (0.81, 26.45)	0.09	3.85 (0.61, 24.38)	0.15
	Tap water	2.28 (0.51, 10.06)	0.28	2.49 (0.47, 13.31)	0.29
Washing Habit	Yes	1.29 (0.43, 3.90)	0.65		
	No	1.00			
UTI History	Yes	2.04 (1.08, 3.86)	0.028	2.29 (1.15, 4.56)	0.019
	No	1.00		1.00	
UTI symptom	Yes	1.02 (0.53, 1.81)	0.94		
	No	1.00			

OR odd ratio, CI confidence interval, Others River water, Wells water

showed high resistance to ampicillin [28]. The high resistance rate of *E.coli* to gentamicin contradicts with the finding from Gondar [1].*E.coli* exhibited unusual high rate of resistance to nitrofurantoin. This finding is higher than the finding from Dessie area, northeast Ethiopia. But, the finding from Dire dawa is higher than the present finding [20, 28]. High level of resistance of *Proteus* species to ampicillin (100%), gentamicin (67%) and ceftriaxone (83%) were exhibited in the study area. In this study, resistance of *Proteus* species to ampicillin is in line with the finding from Dire Dawa. However, the present finding disagrees with the finding from Dire Dawa in which all *Proteus* species were susceptible to ceftriaxon and gentamicin [28].

Among Gram-positive bacteria evaluated for antimicrobial drug resistance, *S. aureus* showed resistance to ampicillin (75%) and ceftriaxon (63%), while CoNS *(S. saprophyticus)* showed resistance to ampicillin (75%).

On the other hand, low levels of resistances were detected to ciprofloxacin, norfloxacin and amoxicillin-clavulanic acid as compared with the previous reports from Ethiopia [1, 7, 18, 28], Nigeria [36], Ghana [24] and Tanzania [27, 37]. The low level of resistance observed for these drugs might be related to the relative inaccessibility and the high prices compared to other antimicrobial drugs. Thus, these drugs could be considered as alternative options in the empirical treatment of UTIs.

All bacterial isolates of the current study showed resistance to at least two antimicrobials (MDR) and no isolate was susceptible to all antimicrobials tested. This correlates with the study conducted in Gondar university teaching hospital, Niger Delta University and Yanagoa, Nigeria [1, 36, 38]. However, this finding is higher than the report from Tikur Anbesa specialized hospital [18].The high prevalence of MDR reported in this study might be due to the unrestricted availability and high rate of use of non-prescribed drugs. It could also be related to the rapid spread of resistant bacteria and high prevalence of misuse of antimicrobial drugs such as self-medication, unnecessary use, failure to adhere to standard treatment guideline and inadequate or absence of antimicrobial drug resistance surveillance program [14, 39].

In the present study, although higher prevalence of UTI was found in pregnant women of 15–24 years old (9.3%) as compared to 25–34 years (8%) and 35–44 years (1.3%) the difference was not statistically significant. This suggests that UTI is distributed in pregnant women of all age groups. This finding disagrees with the study done in Addis Ababa [40] and Jimma [13].

Univariable logistic regression analysis showed significant difference in the prevalence of UTI with respect to residential place, in that pregnant women living in peri-urban and rural areas are at higher risk of UTI as compared to pregnant women living in urban areas. This might be due to the relatively poor hygienic practices in periurban and rural areas [41, 42] and geographical difference [25].

The frequency of UTI was higher among pregnant women who had family monthly income of less than 500 (<21.19 USD) and 501–1000 Ethiopian Birr (21.22–42.37 USD). In accordance with the current finding, a study from Bahir Dar [2] also showed that pregnant women who had low income level were more likely to have bacteriuria. The significant association between low level of income and high frequency of UTI in pregnant women could be due to the negative influence of low income on the nutrition and immune status of pregnant women.

Pregnant women who eat raw meat are twice more likely to be infected by urinary tract bacteria as compared to those pregnant women who don't consume raw meat (Adjusted OR = 2.04, 95% CI: 1.09, 3.83, $P = 0.026$). This indicates that raw animal meat might be the source of these urinary tract bacterial infections. Handling or ingestion of meat was the primary source of resistant *E. coli* among the human subjects. Potential origins of *E. coli* contamination could include human or food animal sources. Transfer of *E. coli* results from contamination during food processing or preparation and reflects human-to-human transmission by food [43]. Raw meat sold in supermarkets, restaurants and other outlets may place pregnant women at risk of UTIs. When animals are slaughtered and their meat is processed for sale, the meat can be contaminated with these bacteria [44].

The prevalence of UTI among the study participants with previous history of UTI was significantly higher than those without previous history of UTI. This result agrees with report from Bahir Dar [2] and Gonder [45], but disagrees with the report from Hawassa [46] and Sudan [26]. The reasons for the high prevalence among pregnant women with previous history of UTI might be due to the presence of antimicrobial resistant strains contributing for recurrent (relapsing) infections and failures of drugs in destroying the bacteria [46].

The main limitations of this cross sectional health institution based study is that equal number of study participants from urban, periurban and rural areas were not included and hence this might limit inference of the results to the general population of the area.

Conclusions

The study revealed an overall high prevalence of UTI in pregnant women. *E. coli* were the most predominant bacterial isolates followed by *S. aureus* and CoNS. A large number of the isolates were resistant to the commonly used antimicrobial drugs. Low level of resistances were detected against ciprofloxacin, norfloxacin and amoxicillin-clavulanic acid and hence could be used as empirical therapy for UTI in the study area. Multi-drug resistant urinary tract bacteria are widespread in pregnant women of the study area. Low level of income, raw meat consumption and previous history of urinary tract infection are significant predictors of UTI in pregnant women. Health education, continuous and collaborative surveillance of UTI and antimicrobial resistance pattern are essential to reduce the consequence of symptomatic and asymptomatic bacteriuria and multi-drug resistant bacteria in pregnant women.

Abbreviations

ANC: Antenatal care; ASB: Asymptomatic bacteriuria; AST: Antimicrobial susceptibility test; CFU: Colony forming unit; CI: Confidence interval; CLED: Cysteine lactose electrolyte deficient; CLSI: Clinical Laboratory Standard Institute; CoNS: Coagulase negative *staphylococcus*; *E. coli*: *Escherichia coli*; MDR: Multiple Drug Resistance; MHA: Muller hinton agar; NCCLS: National Committee for Clinical Laboratory Standard; OR: Odds ratio; RPM: Revolutions per minute; STATA: South Texas Art Therapy Association; UTI: Urinary tract infection

Acknowledgements

We thank health workers of Ambo Hospital, Ambo and Awaro Health Centers for their active cooperation during sample collection. We would like to extend our heartfelt thanks and appreciation to the study participants.

Funding

This study was fully supported by Ambo University, Ambo, Ethiopia. The sponsor of the study had no role in the study design, data collection, data analysis or interpretation, but did review this report prior to submission for publication. The corresponding author had full access to all data in the study and had final responsibility for the decision to submit for publication.

Authors' contributions

YAG design & co-directed the project, supervised bacteria isolation & prepared the manuscript. DLD co-directed the project, supervised bacteria isolation & antimicrobial susceptibility. MMA performed antimicrobial susceptibility & supervised urine sample collection. YHB assisted with bacterial isolation. ADS involved in bacteria isolation. FST involved in assisting antimicrobial susceptibility testing. EZG involved in the design, data analysis & manuscript preparation. All authors read and approved the final version of the manuscript.

Competing interests

The authors declare that they have no competing interests.

Author details

[1]Department of Medical Laboratory Sciences, Ambo University, College of Medicine and Health Sciences, Ambo, Ethiopia. [2]West Shewa Health Bureau, Ambo District Health Office, Awaro Health Center, Ambo, Ethiopia. [3]Ethiopian Public Health Institute, Addis Ababa, Ethiopia. [4]Department of Veterinary Laboratory Technology, Ambo University, College of Agriculture and Veterinary Sciences, Ambo, Ethiopia.

References

1. Alemu A, Moges F, Shiferaw Y, Tafesse K, Kassu A, Anagaw B, Agegn A. Bacterial profile and drug susceptibility pattern of UTI in pregnant women at University of Gondar teaching hospital. Ethiop J Health Sci. 2012;25(5): 197. doi: 10.1186/1756-0500-5-197.

2. Emiru T, Beyene G, Tsegaye W, Melaku S. Associated risk factors of UTI among pregnant women at Felege Hiwot referral hospital, Bahir Dar. BMC Res Notes. 2013;6(2):292. doi: 10.1186/1756-0500-6-292.

3. Tazebew D, Getenet B, Selabat M, Wondewosen T. Urinary bacterial profile and antibiotic susceptibility pattern among pregnant women in north West Ethiopia. Ethiop J of Health Sci. 2012;22(2):121–8.

4. Mittal P, Wing DA: Urinary tract infections in pregnancy. Clin Perinatol 2005, 32:749-7641. PubMed Abstract | Publisher Full Text.

5. Alfred AO, Chiedozie I, Martin DU. Pattern of asymptomatic bacteriuria among pregnant women attending an antenatal clinic at a private health facility in Benin, South Nigeria. Ann Afr Med. 2013;12(3):160–4.

6. Dash M, Sahu S, Mohanty I, Narasimham MV, Turuk J, Sahu R. Prevalence, risk factors and antimicrobial resistance of asymptomatic bacteriuria among antenatal women. Basic ClinReprodSci. 2013;2(2):92–6.

7. Tadesse E, Teshome M, Merid Y, Kibret B, Shimelis T. Asymptomatic urinary tract infection among pregnant women attending the antenatal clinic of Hawassa referral hospital, southern Ethiopia. BMC Res Notes. 2014;7:155. doi: 10.1186/1756-0500-7-155.

8. Connolly A, Thorp J. Urologic clinic of North America. 1999;26:776–87.

9. Ade-Ojo IP, Oluyege AO, Adegun PT, Akintayo AA, Aduloju OP, Olofinbiyi BA. Prevalence and antimicrobial susceptibility of asymptomatic significant bacteriuria among new antenatal enrollees in Southwest Nigeria. Intl Res J Microbiol. 2013;4(8):197–203.

10. Fred NW, Gichuhi JW, Mugo NW. Prevalence of UTI, microbial etiology, and antibiotic sensitivity pattern among antenatal women presenting with lower abdominal pains at Kenyatta National Hospital, Nairobi, Kenya. J Sci and Tech. 2015;3(6) doi: 10.11131/2015/101115.

11. Matuszkiewicz-Rowinska J, Małyszko J, Wieliczko M. Urinary tract infections in pregnancy: old and new unresolved diagnostic and therapeutic problems. Archives of Med Sci. 2015;11(1):67–77.

12. Kabew G, Abebe T, Miheret A. A retrospective study on prevalence and antimicrobial susceptibility patterns of bacterial isolates from urinary tract infections in Tikur Anbessa specialize teaching hospital, Addis Ababa, Ethiopia. Ethiop J Health Devel. 2011;27(2):112–7.

13. Beyene G, Tsegaye W. Bacterial Uropathogens in UTI and antibiotic susceptibility pattern in Jimma University specialized hospital. Ethiop J Health Sci. 2011;21(2):141–6.

14. DACA (2009). Antimicrobials use, resistance and containment baseline survey syntheses of findings, august 2009, Addis Ababa, Ethiopia.

15. Haider G, Zehra N, Munir A, Haider A. Risk factors of UTI in pregnancy. J Pak Med Assoc. 2010;60(3):213–6.

16. Ezechi OC, Gab-Okafor CV, Oladele DA, Kalejaiye OO, Oke BO, Ekama SO, Audu RA, Okoye RN, Ujah IA. Prevalence and risk factors of asymptomatic bacteriuria among pregnant Nigerians infected with HIV. J Matern Fetal Neonatal Med. 2013;26(4):402–6.

17. Israel GD. Sampling the evidence of extension program impact. Program evaluation and organizational development, IFAS. University of Florida: PEOD-5; 1992.

18. Assefa A., Asrat D., Woldeamanuel Y., G/Hiwot Y., Abdella A., and Melesse T. (2008). Bacterial profile and drug susceptibility pattern of UTI in pregnant women at Tikur Anbessa specialized hospital. Ethiop Med J, 46 (3), 227-235.

19. Maji SK, Maity C, Halder SK, Paul T, Kundu PK, Mondal KC. Studies on drug sensitivity and bacterial prevalence of UTI in tribal population of PaschimMedinipur, West Bengal, India. Jundishapur J Microbiol. 2012; 6(1):42–6.

20. Abejew AA, Denboba AA, Mekonnen AG. Prevalence and antibiotic resistance pattern of urinary tract bacterial infections in Dessie area. BMC Res Notes. 2014;7:687. doi: 10.1186/1756-0500-7-687.

21. Rizvi M., Khan F., Shukla I., Malik A. and Shaheen (2011). Rising prevalence of antimicrobial resistance in urinary tract infections during pregnancy: necessity for exploring newer treatment options. J Lab Physicians, 3 (2), 98-103.

22. Mgbakogu RA, Eledo BO. Polymicrobial agents and antibiotic profile of urinary tract infections among pregnant women in Anambra state, Nigeria. Advances in Life Sci and Tech. 2015;35(38):224–36.

23. National Committee for Clinical Laboratory Standards (Clinical Laboratory Standard Instituetes). (2012). Performance of standard for antimicrobial disk susceptibility tests: approved standards. M2-A7. PA, USA: NCCL, 32 (1), Villanova.

24. Afriyie DK, Gyansa-Lutterodt M, Amponsah SK, Asare G, Wiredu V, Wormenor E, Bugyei KA. Susceptibility pattern of uropathogens to

ciprofloxacin at the Ghana police hospital. Pan Afr Med. 2015;22(87) https://doi.org/10.11604/pamj.2015.22.87.6037.

25. Shaifali I, Gupta U, Mahmood SE, Ahmed J. Antibiotic susceptibility patterns of urinary pathogens in female outpatients. North Am J Med Sci. 2012;4(4): 163–9.

26. Hamdan ZH, Ziad AM, Ali SK, Adam I. Investigating epidemiology of UTI and antibiotics sensitivity among pregnant women Khartoum hospital. Ann ClinMicrobiol and Antimicrobials. 2011;10(2) doi: 10.1186/1476-0711-10-2.

27. Masinde A, Gumodoka B, Kilonzo A, Mshana SE. Prevalence of urinary tract infection among pregnant women at Bugando medical Centre, Mwanza, Tanzania. Tanzan J Health Res. 2009;11(3):154–9.

28. Derese B, Kedir H, Teklemariam Z, Weldegebreal F, Balakrishnan S. Bacterial profile of UTI and antimicrobial susceptibility pattern among pregnant women attending at antenatal Clinic in Dil Chora Referral Hospital, Dire Dawa, eastern Ethiopia. TherClin Risk Manag. 2016;12(1): 251–60.

29. Sibi G, Kumari P, Kabungulundabungi N. Antibiotic sensitivity pattern from pregnant women with urinary tract infection in Bangalore, India. Asian Pac J Trop Med. 2014;S1:S116–20. doi: 10.1016/S1995-7645(14)60216-9.

30. Hisano M, Bruschini H, Nicodemo AC, Gomes CM, Lucon M, Srougi M. The bacterial spectrum and antimicrobial susceptibility in female recurrent UTI. Urology. 2015;86(3):492–7.

31. Lavigne JP, Boutet-Dubois A, Laouini D, Combescure C, Bouziges N, Mares P, andSotto A. Virulence potential of E. coli strains causing asymptomatic bacteriuria during pregnancy. J ClinMicrobiol, 2011. 2011;49(11):3950–3.

32. Mandira M, Snehashis K, SandipKumar M, Shreya B, Biplab G, Somajita C. Phylogenetic background of E. coli isolated from asymptomatic pregnant women from Kolkata, India. J Infect Devel Countries. 2015;9(7):720–4.

33. Ramos NL, Sekikubo M, Dzung DT, Kosnopfel C, Kironde F, Mirembe F, Brauner A. Uropathogenic E. coli isolates from pregnant women in different countries. J ClinMicrobiol. 2012;50(11):3569–74.

34. NM Gilbert, VP O'Brien, S Hultgren, G Macones, WG Lewis, AL Lewis (2013). Urinary tract infection as a preventable cause of pregnancy complications: opportunities, challenges, and a global call to action. Global Adv Health Med. 2013;2(5):59-69. DOI: 10.7453/gahmj.2013.061.

35. Forsyth DM, Bradley DJ. The consequences of bilharziasis; medical and public health importance in north-west Tanzania. Bull WHO. 1966;34:715–35.

36. Onanuga A, Selekere TL. Virulence and antimicrobial resistance of common urinary bacteria from asymptomatic students of Niger Delta University, Amassoma, Bayelsa state, Nigeria. J Pharm and Bioallsci. 2016;8(1):29–33.

37. Rasamiravaka T, Shaistasheila HS, Rakotomavojaona T, Rakoto-Alson AO, andRasamindrakotroka A. Changing profile & increasing antimicrobial resistance of uropathogenic bacteria in Madagascar. Med Mal Infect. 2015; 45(5):173–6.

38. Onanuga A, Awhowho GO. Antimicrobial resistance of Staphylococcus aureus strains from patients with urinary tract infections in Yenagoa, Nigeria. J Pharm and Bioallsci. 2012;4(3):226–30.

39. Gebrekirstos NH, Workneh BD, Gebregiorgis YS, Misgina KH, Weldehaweria NB, Weldu MG, Belay HS. Non-prescribed antimicrobial use and associated factors among customers in drug retail outlet in central zone of Tigray, northern Ethiopia: a cross-sectional study. 2017;6: 70. doi: 10.1186/s13756-017-0227-7.

40. Getachew K, Tamirat A, Adane M. A retrospective study on prevalence and antimicrobial susceptibility patterns of bacterial isolates from UTIs in Tikur Anbessa specialize teaching hospital, Addis Ababa, Ethiopia. Ethiop J of Health Devel. 2013;27(2):111–7.

41. Demilie T, Beyene G, Melaku S, Tsegaye W. Diagnostic accuracy of rapid urine dipstick test to predict UTI among pregnant women in Felege Hiwot referral hospital, Bahir Dar, Ethiopia. BMC Res Notes. 2014;29(7): 481. doi: 10.1186/1756-0500-7-481.

42. Al-Badr A, Al-Shaikh G. Recurrent UTIs Management in Women. Sultan Qaboos Universal Med J. 2013;13(3):359–67.

43. Vincent C, Boerlin P, Daignault D, Dozois CM, Dutil L, Galanakis C, Reid-Smith RJ, Tellier P, Tellis PA, Ziebell K, Manges AR. Food reservoir for E. coli causing UTIs. Emerg Infect Dis. 2010;16(1):88–95.

44. Nordstrom L, Liu Cindy M, Lance B, Price LB. Foodborne urinary tract infections: a new paradigm for antimicrobial-resistant foodborne illness. J. Front Microbiol. 2013;4(29) doi: 10.3389/fmicb.2013.00029.

45. Gizachew Y, Daniel A, Yimtubezinash W, Chandrashekhar GU. Urinary tract infection, bacterial etiologies, drug resistance profile and associated risk factors in diabetic patients attending Gondar University hospital, Gondar, Ethiopia. Europ J ExperBiol. 2012;2(4):889–98.

46. Mucheye G, Mulugeta K, Yared M, Yenework S, Moges T, Martha A. E. coli isolated from patients suspected for urinary tract infections in Hawassa referral hospital, southern Ethiopia, an institution based cross sectional study. J. Microbiol Res. 2013;1(1):009–15.

10

An observational case study of hospital associated infections in a critical care unit in Astana, Kazakhstan

Dmitriy Viderman[1,3], Yekaterina Khamzina[1], Zhannur Kaligozhin[2], Makhira Khudaibergenova[2], Agzam Zhumadilov[2], Byron Crape[1] and Azliyati Azizan[1*] (ORCID)

Abstract

Background: Hospital Associated infections (HAI) are very common in Intensive Care Units (ICU) and are usually associated with use of invasive devices in the patients. This study was conducted to determine the prevalence and etiological agents of HAI in a Surgical ICU in Kazakhstan, and to assess the impact of these infections on ICU stay and mortality.

Objective: To assess the rate of device-associated infections and causative HAI etiological agents in an ICU at the National Research Center for Oncology and Transplantation (NRCOT) in Astana, Kazakhstan.

Methods: This retrospective, observational study was conducted in a 12-bed ICU at the NRCOT, Astana, Kazakhstan. We enrolled all patients who were admitted to the ICU from January, 2014 through November 2015, aged 18 to 90 years of age who developed an HAI.

Results: The most common type of HAI was surgical site infection (SSI), followed by ventilator-associated pneumonia (VAP), catheter-related blood stream infection (BSI) and catheter-associated urinary tract infection (UTI). The most common HAI was SSI with *Pseudomonas aeruginosa* as the most common etiological agent. The second most common HAI was VAP also with *P. aeruginosa* followed by BSI which was also associated with *P. aeruginosa* (in 2014) and *Enterococcus faecalis*, and *Klebsiella pneumoniae* (in 2015) as the most common etiological agents causing these infections.

Conclusion: We found that HAI among our study population were predominantly caused by gram-negative pathogens, including *P. aeruginosa*, *K. pneumoniae*, and *E. coli*. To our knowledge, this is the only study that describes ICU-related HAI situation from a country within the Central Asian region. Many developing countries such as Kazakhstan lack surveillance systems which could effectively decrease incidence of HAIs and healthcare costs for their treatment. The epidemiological data on HAI in Kazakhstan currently is underrepresented and poorly reported in the literature. Based on this and previous studies, we propose that the most important interventions to prevent HAI at the NRCOT and similar Healthcare Institutions in Kazakhstan are active surveillance, regular infection control audits, rational and effective antibacterial therapy, and general hygiene measures.

Keywords: Intensive care unit (ICU), Hospital associated infections (HAI), Surgical site infections (SSI), Ventilator associated pneumonia (VAP), Blood stream infections (BSI), Urinary tract infections (UTI)

* Correspondence: azliyati.azizan@nu.edu.kz
[1]Nazarbayev University School of Medicine (NUSOM), 5/1 Kerey and Zhanibek Khans Street, Astana, Kazakhstan010000
Full list of author information is available at the end of the article

Background

HAI influence the quality of health care and are a major source of adverse outcomes during health care delivery [1, 2]. HAI greatly increase morbidity and mortality of patients and healthcare costs [3]. The burden of HAI in developing countries is significant, whereby the incidence can be up to 15% of total hospitalized patients, and up to 50% among ICU patients [4]. HAI are challenging to treat because the etiological agents frequently develop multidrug, extensively drug and pandrug-resistance [5]. HAI have a big economic impact on healthcare by extending ICU stay, hospital stay, and increasing the need for invasive procedures. The most common HAI are primary bloodstream infections (BSI), ventilator-associated pneumonia (VAP), urinary tract infections (UTI) and surgical site infections (SSI), with SSI being the most prevalent in some studies [2, 6]. Prevention programs for HAI which could result in positive cost-benefit ratios typically originate with laboratory data from the clinical microbiology laboratory; this provides information regarding the causative pathogenic organisms causing the HAI [6].

The incidence of HAI in ICUs is about 2 to 5 times higher than those in general inpatient departments due to many associated risk factors [1, 7]. Furthermore, antimicrobial resistance rates in ICU are much greater than in general departments [7]. In order to reduce incidence of HAI, surveillance analysis is an essential step to identify problems and implement interventions [8]. National surveillance data form the basis for prevention and control of HAI in developed countries such as the USA and Australia, but this is rarely available in many developing countries, including Kazakhstan [9]. A recent systematic meta-analysis of the burden of HAI in Southeast Asia found that the most common HAI pathogens were mostly gram-negative bacilli, and were predominantly *Pseudomonas aeruginosa*, *Klebsiella* species and *Acinetobacter baumannii*; these findings are similar to those reported for many other developing countries [9]. According to the National Healthcare Safety Network (NHSN) report in 2013, ICU-related central-line associated BSI continued to decrease, whereas urinary catheter-associated tract infection rates increased in the majority of ICU types [10]. Several studies conducted in developing countries similar to ours, reported their findings in the literature; one study from Kuwait reported that their VAP rate was 4.0 per 1000 mechanical ventilator days, the central line–associated BSI rate was 3.5 per 1000 central line days, and the catheter-associated urinary tract infection (CAUTI) rate was 3.3 per 1000 urinary catheter days [11]. Another study from Ecuador showed that device associated HAIs rates in their ICUs were higher than the United States CDC/NSHN rates and similar to International Nosocomial

Infection Control Consortium (INICC) international rates [12].

In an effort to evaluate the local HAI situation in Kazakhstan, we conducted an observational case study to assess incidence of the different types of HAI over a period of two years in 2014 and 2015. Our goal was to investigate if the patterns regarding type of HAI cases and the etiological agents were consistent from year to year, therefore we performed an analysis and comparison of data from at least two years. The data from the study was retrospectively analyzed in our effort to identify the causative HAI bacterial pathogens. We aimed to assemble and analyze epidemiological data associated with four different types of device associated HAI in an ICU at the National Research Center for Oncology and Transplantation (NRCOT) in Astana, Kazakhstan. The information summarized here will form the basis for a much larger surveillance study that could guide decisions regarding appropriate and potentially more efficacious use of prophylactic control within the ICU. This study could also guide the establishment of a national surveillance program to control and prevent HAI in hospitals in Kazakhstan and worldwide.

Methods

This retrospective, observational study was conducted from January 2014 through January 2016 in a 12 bed ICU at the National Research Center for Oncology and Transplantation (NRCOT), which is a 280-bed hospital in Astana, Kazakhstan. We undertook this pilot study comparing HAI cases and causative agents over a two year period to assess the current local infection control practices. We hope to understand from this study if intervention in the future would be appropriate to improve upon the current HAI scenario. The main change between 2014 and 2015 was access to better diagnostic capabilities within the hospital laboratory, though there are future plans to implement an improved HAI prevention program. This was considered by us to be a "retrospective" study because data analysis on the most part was done after these were collected (even though the staff collected the data during the patients' ICU visit). A standard screening protocol for HAI was used [13]. We tested all patients who spent more than 48 h in the ICU (whereby, all patients with less than 48 h stay in the ICU were excluded from this study). Samples for microbiological culture and analysis were obtained from patients who presented with HAI symptoms. Blood count, blood biochemistry, and blood coagulation tests were performed on all suspected patients who were at high risk of developing HAI following guidelines provided by the Healthcare Infection Control Practices Advisory Committee [14]. Clinical Pharmacologist and Hospital Infection Specialists visited the ICU every day. Chest radiography, deep tracheal aspirate, bronchoalveolar lavage (BAL) or mini-broncho-alveolar lavage (mini-BAL) were taken for pathogen identification if VAP was suspected. Blood samples, removed intravascular catheters, urine, urinary and wound catheters were also cultured for microbiological analysis if BSI, UTI or SSI were suspected. Samples were cultured using standard microbiological methods; isolated bacteria were identified by standard microbiological methods and tested for antibiotic susceptibility using Kirby-Bauer disk-diffusion technique according to Clinical and Laboratory Standards Institute (CLCI) specifications [15, 16].

Study ethics

Ethical clearance for this study was obtained from the Ethics committee of the Institutional Review Board of Nazarbayev University. The study was exempt from being classified as human subject research as no personal information related to any of the patients was made available to the Investigators at any time before, during or after the study.

Study population and microbiological culture and analysis

The patients admitted to the NRCOT ICU were from different surgical departments, which included the department of general, oncology, transplant, vascular, orthopedic, and gynecology surgeries. The patients with a diagnosis of HAI received treatment according to the hospital's standard protocol of management of HAI. Samples were taken from all patients admitted to the ICU aged 18 to 90 years of age who developed HAI based on clinical, laboratory and instrumental findings throughout the study duration. For microbiological culture and sensitivity testing, lower respiratory tract secretion, blood and urine samples were taken for diagnosis of VAP, catheter-related BSI, and catheter-associated UTI. Blood culture diagnostics was done for all samples from patients with suspected catheter-related blood stream infections. Data relevant to the diagnosis of HAI were taken by the hospital staff, but only microbiological data regarding etiological agents related to device associated HAI were provided for analysis in this study.

Statistical analysis

The rates of development of each type of HAI (BSI, VAP, UTI and SSI) as well as the total rate per 1000 cases were calculated. Relative risk for these groups was assessed using StataMP 13.0 software, and statistically significant cutoff was determined at a p-value of < 0.05, and highly statistically significant cutoff at a p-value of < 0.001. Prevalence of certain isolated strains of bacteria that caused hospital-acquired infections for each year was determined in percent and compared between the

years 2014 and 2015 using Chi-square analysis in StataMP 13.0 software. Statistically significant level was determined at a p-value < 0.05; and highly statistically significant level at a p-value of < 0.001.

Results
General overview of ICU patients and the proportions with HAI

A total number of 1257 patients were admitted to the ICU from January 2014 to January 2016 of which, 56.6% (711 patients) were admitted in 2014 compared to the remaining 43.4% (546 patients) in 2015. The mean number of ICU stay was 18 days (with a range of 1–330 days) in 2014, while in 2015 the mean ICU stay was 36 days (with a range of 12–62 days); these variations are also a reflection of some changes in perioperative care that took place in between these two time periods. The change we mention here that led to increased mean number of ICU stay in 2015 compared to 2014 was due to the change in patient population. In 2014, the patient population consisted of patients who were transferred to the ICU after emergency surgeries (which were more than 85% of all transfers to ICU) such as patients who underwent appendectomy, cholecystectomy, hernia repair surgeries, etc. In 2015, the ICU patient population consisted of patients who were transferred to the ICU after oncological surgery (50%) and transplant surgery (30%). The period of ICU stay of patients after emergency surgery was generally shorter than the patients who were moved to the ICU after oncological or transplant surgery. Overall, the patients' general health conditions were better for the patients in 2014.

During the study period, 249 out of 1257 patients admitted to the ICU developed HAI; the p-value for the development of HAI between 2014 and 2015 was 0.000127 which is highly statistically significant. A total of 114 microbiological cultures were obtained and identified from patients suspected to have had HAI in 2014 compared to 135 cultures isolated in 2015 (with a p-value of 0.6582 which is not significant).

Device associated infections

The HAIs were classified into four categories: BSI, VAP, UTI and SSI. As evident from the Table 1, in 2014, SSI constituted the highest percentages of all HAIs followed by VAP, BSI and UTI. When compared to 2014, similar profile of device associated HAIs were observed for 2015, whereby SSI was again the most prominent category that caused HAI, followed by VAP. However in 2015, the percent of observed BSI was equal to the percent of UTI as the least frequent types of HAI.

Table 1 Types of Hospital Associated infections in percent for each year

Type of infection	Percent in 2014 (total number)	Percent in 2015 (total number)
BSI	24.6% (28)	18.5% (25)
VAP	25.4% (29)	29.6% (40)
UTI	19.3% (22)	18.5% (25)
SSI	30.7% (35)	33.3% (45)
Total	100% (114)	100% (135)

BSI: Catheter-associated Blood Stream Infections, *VAP*: Ventilator-associated Pneumonia, *UTI*: Catheter-associated Urinary Tract Infections, *SSI*: Surgical Site Infections

Variation in types of infections

Analysis of HAI categories (BSI, VAP, UTI, and SSI) in 2014 compared to 2015 was conducted and revealed significant variation between certain types of HAI (Fig. 1). Specifically, rates of VAP and SSI were found to be statistically different (p-value < 0.05) between the two years of the study period. Rates of VAP infections were higher in 2015 than in 2014. Similar results were obtained for SSI, whereby the rate of infection was again higher in 2015 (p-value < 0.05). On the other hand, no difference in rates of BSI and UTI was observed. The total rate of all types of infections was found to be significantly higher in 2015 when compared to the total infection rate in 2014 (p-value < 0.05). Data was available for the VAP incidence which was determined to be 8.4 per 1000 ventilator days while the incidence of catheter-related blood stream infections was 18 per 1000 line days.

Microbiological etiology of HAI

A total number of 249 microbial pathogens were isolated and identified in 2014 and 2015, and the percent distribution of these etiological agents is represented in Fig. 2a and b. The highest percent in 2014 corresponded to *Pseudomonas aeruginosa* at 23.68%, which was slightly reduced in 2015 to 13.33%. *Klebsiella pneumoniae, Escherichia coli, Staphylococcus aureus, Staphylococcus epidermidis,* and *Acinetobacter baumannii* were isolated and identified from many HAI cases for both 2014 and 2015. Unique and relatively widespread isolate for 2014 was *Enterobacter aerogenes*, representing 17.54% of the cases. Bacterial strains that had an incidence of less than 5% were combined into the subgroup 'Others'. In 2014 *Streptococcus viridans, Citrobacter* spp., *Enterococcus faecium, Achromobacter* spp., *Staphylococcus saprophyticus, Candida albicans and Serratia* spp. were included in this subgroup. In 2015 however, in addition to the above-mentioned *Citrobacter* spp., *S. saprophyticus* and *C. albicans*, unique pathogens such as *Staphylococcus haemolyticus, Enterococcus cloacae, Candida tropicalis, Burkholderia cepacia, Streptococcus mitis* and *Stenotrophomonas maltophilia* were isolated. When comparison analysis was conducted, highly significant difference between two years (p-value < 0.001) was identified. Even though many strains were similar for both years, case-wise analysis revealed important differences that should be taken into account. The types of pathogen described originated from cultures isolated from the different HAI categories as shown in Fig. 3a (VAP), Fig.3b (BSI), Fig. 3c (UTI), and Fig. 3d (SSI), and represented as percent (%) of total number of organisms isolated. We found that

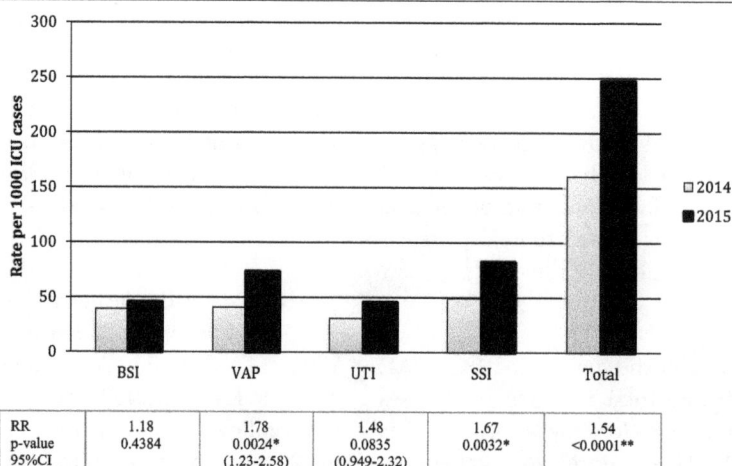

	BSI	VAP	UTI	SSI	Total
RR	1.18	1.78	1.48	1.67	1.54
p-value	0.4384	0.0024*	0.0835	0.0032*	<0.0001**
95%CI		(1.23-2.58)	(0.949-2.32)		

Fig. 1 Samples for microbiological culture and analysis were obtained from patients who presented with HAI symptoms. Blood samples, removed intravascular catheters, urine, urinary and wound catheters were also cultured for microbiological analysis if BSI, UTI or SSI were suspected. Comparison of rates of case-specific infections between 2014 and 2015 were performed. Statistically significant level was determined at a p-value < 0.05; and highly statistically significant level at a p-value of < 0.001. Statistically significant difference is noted for VAP, SSI and combined total between years 2014 and 2015 (statistical significance: *p-value< 0.05; **p-value< 0.001)

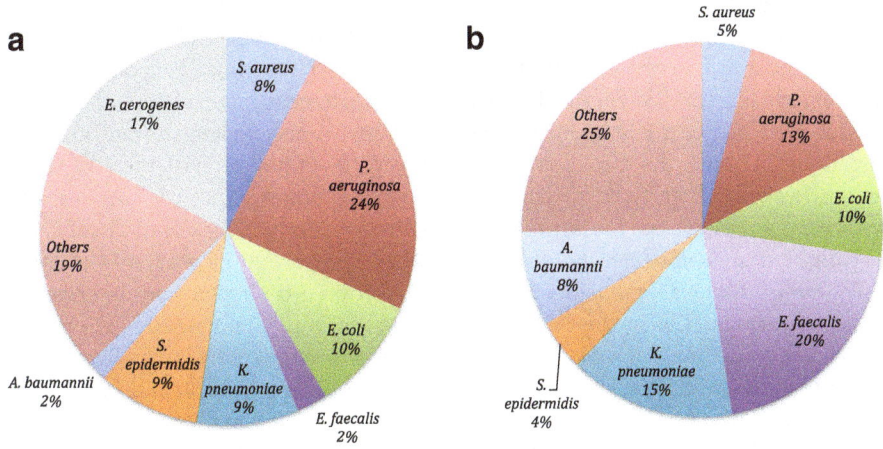

Fig. 2 Samples for bacterial culture and analysis were obtained from patients who presented with HAI symptoms. Samples were cultured using standard microbiological methods; isolated bacteria were identified by standard microbiological methods according to Clinical and Laboratory Standards Institute (CLCI) specifications [12, 13]. For comparison, Chi-square test was conducted with a p-value < 0.001**. The subgroup 'Others' includes rare strains of bacteria (with incidence of < 5%), which were different for each year (comparing 2014 and 2015).

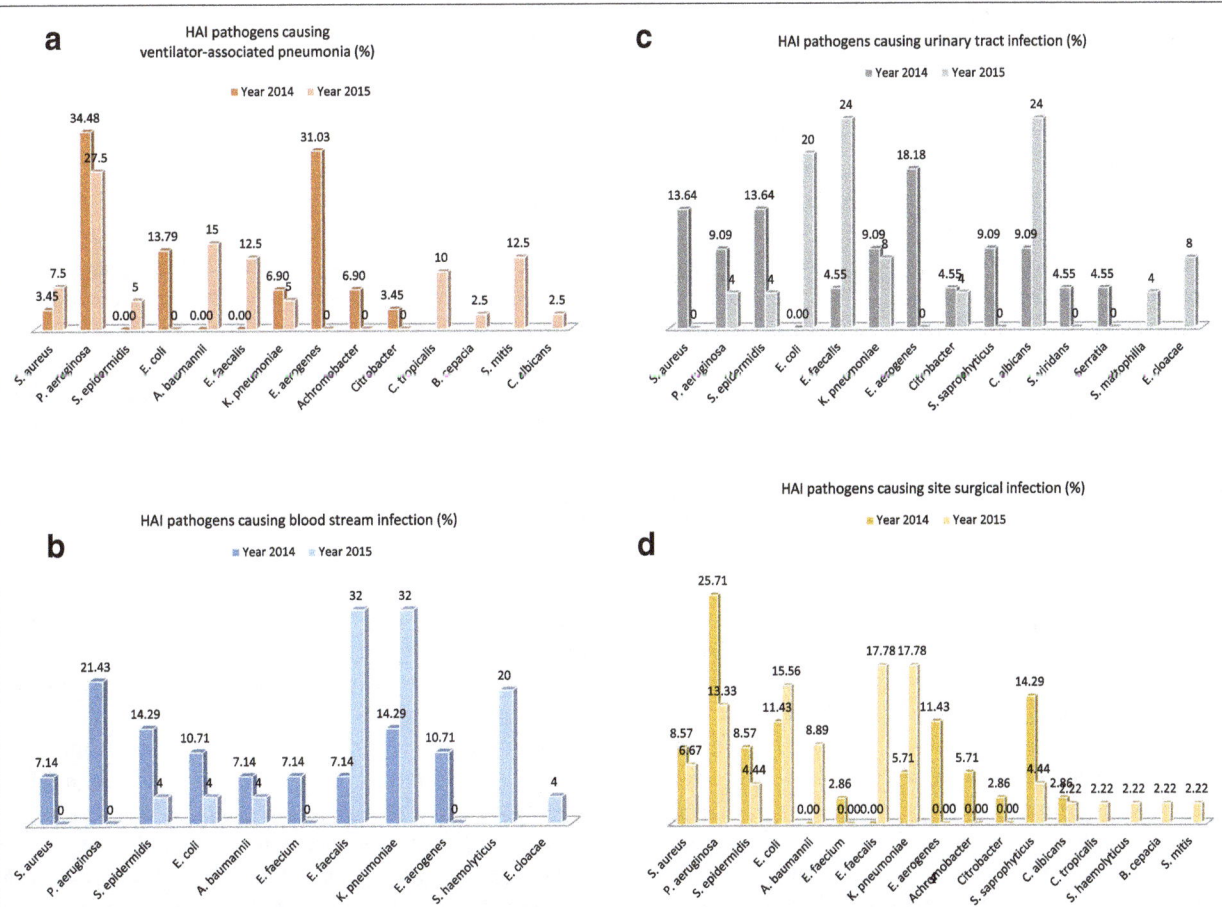

Fig. 3 The types of HAI pathogens shown in Fig. 2 were subdivided into the types of HAI samples they were isolated from; **a** VAP, **b** BSI, **c** UTI, and **d** SSI and represented as percent (%) of total number of bacteria isolated. Samples were cultured using standard microbiological methods; isolated bacteria were identified by standard microbiological methods according to Clinical and Laboratory Standards Institute (CLCI) specifications [12, 13]

HAI were predominantly caused by gram-negative bacterial pathogens, particularly *P. aeruginosa* and *K. pneumoniae*. These strains were most frequently associated with all the HAI types particularly SSI and BSI (as the first two most common types of HAI pathogens isolated) though there are some variations between the two years with these two pathogens as well as other types of bacterial pathogens that predominated, such as *Staphylococcus epidermidis*, *E. faecalis* and *Acinetobacter baumannii*. From our study, *P. aeruginosa* was recognized as a causal agent of the most serious HAI in the ICU. This organism was also causing the majority of VAP and BSIs in two consecutive years. SSI analogously was mainly caused by gram-negative bacteria, of which *P. aeruginosa* prevailed in 2014, while *K. pneumoniae* predominated in 2015.

Discussion

In this study, we have shown that healthcare-associated infections constitute a major healthcare burden in Kazakhstan, which is a rapidly developing nation. Kazakhstan is one of the five Central Asian countries (which also include Kyrgyzstan, Tajikistan, Turkmenistan and Uzbekistan) that achieved independence in 1991 after the collapse of the Soviet Union [17, 18]. At independence, these Central Asian Post-Soviet (CAPS) countries were faced with many problems; progress to build stronger economies varies between countries. Collapse of the Soviet Union led Kazakhstan as well as the other CAPS countries to economic recession. During the Soviet Union era, there were no wide informational, medical and pharmaceutical exchanges with other countries. On the other hand, the dissolution of the Soviet Union mobilized these countries to democracy which initiated important exchanges of products and knowledge with the other countries. Greater successes have been noted for Kazakhstan, Turkmenistan and Uzbekistan, which are the CAPS countries with the richest natural resources [17]. The healthcare systems of these CAPS countries have also gone through many decades of profound revolutions, whereby the rate and quality of progress of the healthcare sectors vary between these countries [19]. Since independence, the CAPS countries have steadily been receiving more attention at the international arena, especially due to the economic and geographical significance of the region. Over the last two decades, Kazakhstan has made significant progress in economy as well as healthcare sector, although there is still much room for improvement.

To our knowledge, this is the only study to be reported in an international journal describing ICU-related HAI situation from the Central Asian region. In our study, HAI represents a significant healthcare problem with ICU related HAI incidence being about 2 to 5 times higher than the incidence in other in-hospital departments [7]. In our study, patients frequently had the following universal host-related risk factors predisposing to HAI which included advanced age, severity of disease, hyperglycemia, neutropenia, immunosuppressive therapy, cancer diagnosis, and malnutrition. Majority of the patients had at least three of these risk factors. The most common type of HAI in our study was SSI whereby the rate increased significantly (p-value < 0.05) when comparing the year 2014 to 2015 (Table 1 and Fig. 1). Between both years, no intervention was introduced in terms of recommendations to improve upon infection control practices which may have been one of the reason there were no observed decrease in device-associated HAI rates. This high incidence of HAI associated with SSI was due to the fact that the Astana NRCOT is a multidisciplinary hospital focusing on multiple types of surgeries. In most cases, patients also had poor nutritional and altered immune status due to devastating diseases, which were either cancer, kidney and liver failure, diabetes, and coexisting infections at the remote body site. Multiple studies stated that the above mentioned medical conditions predispose patients to the development of SSI [20, 21]. Medical procedures in the hospital were typically prolonged, and patients were prone to intraoperative hypothermia, increasing the risk for SSI [22]. In our setting, colorectal surgery was the most frequently performed surgery, which is recognized as a risk factor for SSI worldwide [23].

From our study, VAP was identified as the second most common type of HAI. For patients on mechanical ventilation however, VAP was the leading type of infection, which is consistent with reports from multiple other studies [24, 25]. Majority of the patients who developed VAP had COPD, advanced age, H_2-antagonists and antibiotics use, and Multiple Organ System Failure [26]. Similar to the SSI associated HAI described above, the rates of VAP also increased significantly when comparing 2014 to 2015 (Table 1 and Fig. 1); this may have also been due to absence of intervention that was implemented to reduce the number of VAP cases in the studied ICU. The third most common type of HAI identified in our study was BSI. Almost all patients who developed BSI had the following risk factors; central vein catheterization, malnutrition and surgery, and infection with highly antibiotic resistant pathogens. These findings are supported by evidence from other studies, which report BSI to occur in 5% of all ICU patients [26, 27].

We found that HAI were predominantly caused by gram-negative pathogens, including *P. aeruginosa*, *K. pneumoniae*, and *E. coli*. These strains were most frequently associated with VAP, SSI, BSI and UTI. From our study, *P. aeruginosa* was recognized as a causal agent of the most serious HAI in the ICU [28]. This organism was also causing the majority of VAP and BSI in two consecutive years [9]. SSI analogously was mainly caused by gram-negative bacteria, of which *P. aeruginosa* prevailed in 2014, while *K. pneumoniae* predominated in 2015. Another interesting finding was with regards to the differences between the length of ICU patient stay, the patient population type, rate of HAI as well as the types of pathogens isolated in 2014 when compared to 2015. Since the period of ICU stay of patients after emergency surgeries was much shorter than after oncological or transplant surgeries, the overall period of ICU stay was longer in 2015. Furthermore, ICU patients' general condition was better among patients in 2014. Our results showed that the rate of HAIs was increased and the distribution of pathogen also changed in 2015 compared to 2014. We propose that the difference between patient populations in the ICU partially explained the reason for increased number and rates of HAI in 2015 (Table 1 and Fig. 1), as well as the differences in the types of HAI pathogens that were isolated when these pathogen types were compared between the two years of study. With regards to increased HAI rate, both the oncological and transplant patient populations were immunocompromised due to the surgical procedures, and these patients also received immunosuppressant drugs; this led to further decrease in their immune status. Plus, these patients stayed longer in the ICU thereby had higher risk of acquiring ICU-related HAIs. Interestingly, more HAI pathogens that are more commonly associated with multidrug resistance belonging to the "ESKAPE" pathogen group were identified in 2015. This included *P. aeruginosa, E. faecalis, K. pneumoniae* and *A. baumannii* (Fig. 2); this is not a surprising finding given that these pathogens are associated with many HAI infections within the last few decades [29].

There are limitations to this study, which include the fact that data collected did not include patients' age, sex, and other demographic variables, which might have contributed towards generation of more precise and valuable conclusions. For future studies, the design could include collection of these and other relevant information that would enhance the quality of data and conclusions that can be derived from the study. In this study, some organisms identified were usually not considered common causative agents (such as *Candida, Enterococcus faecalis, Staphylococcus epidermidis* and *Streptococcus mitis* for VAP as in Fig. 3a, and *S. epidermidis* and *S. viridans* for UTI as shown in Fig. 3c). Such unexpected findings further support our conclusion that there is an urgent and definitive need to improve upon HAI prevention practices which include incorporation of surveillance protocols that meet international standards that can more accurately detect and identify the correct etiological agent (which includes incorporation of

quality control measures and established Standard operating procedure) in Kazakhstan and other developing countries within the region. These findings indicate that the surveillance protocols mentioned in the method section were not fully implemented during the study period, which is a major limitation of this study. Therefore the findings from this study demonstrates the need to improve training of infection control personnel regarding the use of and implementation of more stringent practices that meet the international HAI infection control and surveillance guidelines.

HAI is a critical problem for health-care providers worldwide, which should receive appropriate attention for further management. The integrated HAI control program was introduced more than 3 decades ago for the first time, being able to reduce both incidence of infections and related healthcare costs [30]. Unfortunately, many developing countries such as Kazakhstan lack surveillance systems which could effectively decrease incidence of HAIs and healthcare costs for their treatment. Currently, the international guidelines on prevention, diagnosis and treatment of HAI are not actively practiced, and access to newer antibacterial agents is not readily available in Kazakhstan. Within Kazakhstan, there are National and Regional Medical Centers (hospitals). There are no published epidemiological data on HAI from the Regional Medical Centers, therefore, the epidemiological characteristics of HAI from these Centers are unknown. If we compare the National Medical Centers with Regional hospitals, there is an unequal supply of medical equipment and uneven qualification of medical doctors and staff in the latter. For example, several National Medical Centers have internationally educated doctors and staff as well as equipment resembling those that can be found in the best World Class Medical Centers. These medical Centers can be effective in monitoring, diagnosing, treating and preventing the HAI, whereas many Regional (and rural) hospitals do not even follow any guidelines on diagnosis, treatment and preventions of HAIs. The National Medical Centers frequently receive severely ill patients with multiple undiagnosed multi- and pandrug resistant HAI from the Regional Medical Centers.

We propose that the most important recommended measures to prevent HAI at the NRCOT and similar Healthcare Institutions are rational antibacterial therapy, regular infection control audits, and general hygiene measures. Numerous studies in developing countries have shown that the International Nosocomial Infection Control Consortium (INICC) multidimensional infection control strategy with practice bundles can decrease the rate of HAI. Rosenthal et al. found that implementation of a multidimensional infection control strategy can significantly reduce the central line-associated BSI rates in the PICUs of developing countries [31]. In another study, Tao et al. demonstrated that a multidimensional infection control intervention for VAP contributed to a significant cumulative reduction in the VAP rate in their ICUs [32].

This is a first surveillance study on HAI at the NRCOT since its foundation eight years ago. An active surveillance system monitoring incidence and prevalence of HAI as preventative measures is necessary, and this study represents a first step towards this goal.

Conclusions

We conclude that HAI is one of the major problems in healthcare provision in Kazakhstan. SSI, VAP and BSI are the predominant types of HAI. Gram-negative bacteria such as *P. aeruginosa*, *K. pneumoniae* and *E. coli* are the most common causative agents of HAI. The most important risk factors are advanced age, severity of disease, hyperglycemia, neutropenia, immunosuppressive therapy, cancer diagnosis, and malnutrition. For more precise determination of its causality, an ongoing HAI surveillance program is needed to decrease HAI incidence and prevalence at the NRCOT and other healthcare institutions throughout the country. Kazakhstan has made significant effort and progress since independence to establish a healthcare system that is already an improvement over the centralized Semashko health system model inherited from the Soviet Union at independence [19]. One of the ways to continue on the positive trajectory of change for an improved healthcare system is implementation of an efficient active surveillance system for HAI that should be implemented nationwide. The system should include an organized and controlled data collection performed by trained personnel. The data collected should include not only infection-related data, but also patient-related data such as risk factors and history of present illness (such as history of HAI, diagnostic tests, surgeries and invasive methods, as well as the antimicrobial drugs used). A system of monthly HAI analysis and report should also be implemented. Such proactive surveillance system coupled with efficient infection control programs would be highly beneficial to control and reduce the rates of HAI within all Regional and National Medical Centers throughout Kazakhstan.

Acknowledgements

The Authors would like to acknowledge the staff for their contributions including sample retrieval, blinding and randomizing, as well as providing information on sample types available prior to randomizing. The Authors also would like to thank Reviewers for their valuable comments.

Funding

Nazarbayev University School of Medicine.

Author's contribution

DV, AA and YK participated in the study design. ZK and DV participated in the data collection. YK and BC performed the advanced statistical analyses and prepared the associated Figures and Table. YK, DV and AA wrote the manuscript. YK provided technical assistance related to manuscript development. DV and AA conceived of the study, reviewed the data, provided feedback for Figures and Table, and edited the manuscript. AZ and MK provided the technical support to data collection. All authors reviewed and approved the final version of manuscript.

Competing interests

The authors declare that they have no competing interests.

Author details

[1]Nazarbayev University School of Medicine (NUSOM), 5/1 Kerey and Zhanibek Khans Street, Astana, Kazakhstan010000. [2]National Research Center for Oncology and Transplantation, Astana, Kazakhstan. [3]National Research Neurosurgery Center, Astana, Kazakhstan.

References

1. WHO. The burden of health care-associated infection worldwide. 2016. Available at http://www.who.int/gpsc/country_work/burden_hcai/en/. Accessed 22 Apr 2018.
2. Horan TC, Gaynes R. Surveillance of nosocomial infections. In: Mayhall CG, editor. Hospital epidemiology and infection control. Philadelphia: Lippincott Williams & Wilkins; 1999. p. 1285–318.
3. Klevens RM, Edwards JR, Richards CL, et al. Estimating health care-associated infections and deaths in U.S. hospitals, 2002. Public Health Rep. 2007;122(2):160–6.
4. Vincent J. International Study of the Prevalence and Outcomes of Infection in Intensive Care Units. JAMA. 2009;302(21):2323.
5. Magiorakos A, Srinivasan A, Carey R, Carmeli Y, Falagas M, Giske C, et al. Multidrug-resistant, extensively drug-resistant and pandrug-resistant bacteria: an international expert proposal for interim standard definitions for acquired resistance. Clin Microbiol Infect. 2012;18(3):268–81.
6. Arefian H, Vogel M, Kwetkat A, Hartmann M. Economic evaluation of interventions for prevention of hospital acquired infections: a systematic review. PLoS One. 2016;11(1):e0146381.
7. Aly N, Al-Mousa H, Al Asar E. Nosocomial infections in a medical-surgical intensive care unit. Med Princ Pract. 2016;17(5):373–7. https://doi.org/10.1159/000141500
8. Choi J, Kwak Y, Yoo H, Lee S, Kim H, Han S, et al. Trends in the incidence rate of device-associated infections in intensive care units after the establishment of the Korean nosocomial infections surveillance system. J Hosp Infect. 2016;91(1):28–34. https://doi.org/10.1016/j.jhin.2015.06.002
9. Ling M, Apisarnthanarak A, Madriaga G. The burden of healthcare-associated infections in Southeast Asia: a systematic literature review and meta-analysis. Clin Infect Dis. 2016;60(11):1690–9. https://doi.org/10.1093/cid/civ095
10. Dudeck MA, Edwards JR, Allen-Bridson K, Gross C, Malpiedi PJ, Peterson KD, Sievert DM. National Healthcare Safety Network report, data summary for 2013, device-associated module. Am J Infect Control. 2015;43(3):206–21.
11. Al-Mousa HH, Omar AA, Rosenthal VD, Salama MF, Aly NY, Noweir MED, George SM. Device-associated infection rates, bacterial resistance, length of stay, and mortality in Kuwait: international nosocomial infection consortium findings. Am J Infect Control. 2016;44(4):444–9.
12. Yepez ES, Bovera MM, Rosenthal VD, Flores HAG, Pazmiño L, Valencia F, Delgado V. Device-associated infection rates, mortality, length of stay and bacterial resistance in intensive care units in Ecuador: international nosocomial infection control Consortium's findings. World J Biol Chem. 2017;8(1):95.
13. Siegel J, Rhinehart E, Jackson M, Chiarello L. 2007 guideline for isolation precautions: preventing transmission of infectious agents in health care settings.

Am J Infect Control. 2016;35(10):S65–S164. https://doi.org/10.1016/j.ajic.2007.10.007

14. CDC – HICPAC: 2016 Available at http://www.cdc.gov/hicpac/index.html. Accessed 22 Apr 2018.

15. Standards for microbiology investigations - GOV.UK: 2016. Available at https://www.gov.uk/government/collections/standards-for-microbiology-investigations-smi. Accessed 22 Apr 2018.

16. Clinical & Laboratory Standards Institute: CLSI Guidelines: 2016. Available at http://clsi.org/. Accessed 22 Apr 2018.

17. Central Asia after the breakup of the Soviet Union. Jeffrey Hays. Last updated April 2016. http://factsanddetails.com/central-asia/Central_Asian_Topics/sub8_8d/entry-4521.html. Accessed 22 Apr 2018.

18. Central Asia since 1991: The experience of the new independent states. Richard Pomfret. Research programme on: Market Access, Capacity Building and Competitiveness. Working Paper No. 212. OECD Development Centre, 29 July 2003.

19. Ulikpan A, Mirzoev T, Jimenez E, Malik A, Hill PS. Glob Health Action. 2014;7: 24978. https://doi.org/10.3402/gha.v7.24978.

20. Wick E, Vogel J, Church J, Remzi F, Fazio V. Surgical site infections in a "high outlier" institution. Dis Colon rectum. 2009;52(3):374–9.

21. Pedroso-Fernandez Y, Aguirre-Jaime A, Ramos M, Hernández M, Cuervo M, Bravo A, et al. Prediction of SSI after colorectal surgery. Am J Infect Control. 2016;44(4):450–4.

22. Seamon M, Wobb J, Gaughan J, Kulp H, Kamel I, Dempsey D. The effects of intraoperative hypothermia on surgical site infection. Ann Surg. 2012;255(4): 789–95. https://doi.org/10.1097/SLA.0b013e31824b7e35.

23. Kohut A, Liu J, Stein D, Sensenig R, Poggio J. Patient-specific risk factors are predictive for postoperative adverse events in colorectal surgery: an American College of Surgeons National Surgical Quality Improvement Program–based analysis. Am J Surg. 2015;209(2):219–29. https://doi.org/10.1016/j.amjsurg.2014.08.02.

24. Hunter J. Ventilator associated pneumonia. BMJ. 2012;344:e3325. https://doi.org/10.1136/bmj.e3325.

25. Afshari A, Pagani L, Harbarth S. Year in review 2011: critical care - infection. Crit Care. 2012;16(6):242. https://doi.org/10.1186/cc11421.

26. Elatrous S, Boujdaris R, Merghili S, Ouanes L, Boussarsar M, Nouira S, et al. Incidence and risk factors of VAP: a one-year prospective survey. Clin Intensive Care. 1996;7(6):276–81. https://doi.org/10.3109/tcic.7.6.276.281.

27. Vincent J, Rello J, Marshall J, Silva E, Anzueto A, Martin CD, et al. International study of the prevalence and outcomes of infection in ICU. JAMA. 2009;302(21):2323. https://doi.org/10.1001/jama.2009.1754.

28. Neuhauser M, Weinstein R, Rydman R, Danziger L, Karam G, Quinn J. Antibiotic resistance among gram-negative bacilli in US intensive care units. JAMA. 2003;289(7):885.

29. Santajit S, Indrawattana N. Mechanisms of antimicrobial resistance in ESKAPE pathogens. Biomed Res Int. 2016;2016:8. Article ID 2475067. https://doi.org/10.1155/2016/2475067.

30. Higuera F, Rosenthal V, Duarte P, Ruiz J, Franco G, Safdar N. The effect of process control on the incidence of central venous catheter–associated bloodstream infections and mortality in intensive care units in Mexico. Crit Care Med. 2005;33(9):2022–7.

31. Rosenthal VD, Ramachandran B, Villamil-Gomez W, Armas-Ruiz A, Navoa-Ng JA, Matta-Cortes L, Menco A. Impact of a multidimensional infection control strategy on central line-associated bloodstream infection rates in pediatric intensive care units of five developing countries: findings of the international nosocomial infection control consortium (INICC). Infection. 2012;40(4):415–23.

32. Tao L, Hu B, Rosenthal VD, Zhang Y, Gao X, He L. Impact of a multidimensional approach on ventilator-associated pneumonia rates in a hospital of shanghai: findings of the international nosocomial infection control consortium. J Crit Care. 2012;27(5):440–6.

11

Catheter associated urinary tract infections

Lindsay E Nicolle

Abstract

Urinary tract infection attributed to the use of an indwelling urinary catheter is one of the most common infections acquired by patients in health care facilities. As biofilm ultimately develops on all of these devices, the major determinant for development of bacteriuria is duration of catheterization. While the proportion of bacteriuric subjects who develop symptomatic infection is low, the high frequency of use of indwelling urinary catheters means there is a substantial burden attributable to these infections. Catheter-acquired urinary infection is the source for about 20% of episodes of health-care acquired bacteremia in acute care facilities, and over 50% in long term care facilities. The most important interventions to prevent bacteriuria and infection are to limit indwelling catheter use and, when catheter use is necessary, to discontinue the catheter as soon as clinically feasible. Infection control programs in health care facilities must implement and monitor strategies to limit catheter-acquired urinary infection, including surveillance of catheter use, appropriateness of catheter indications, and complications. Ultimately, prevention of these infections will require technical advances in catheter materials which prevent biofilm formation.

Keywords: Urinary catheter, Bacteriuria, Urinary tract infection, Health care acquired infection, Indwelling urethral catheter

Review

Introduction

Catheter acquired urinary tract infection is one of the most common health care acquired infections [1,2]; 70–80% of these infections are attributable to use of an indwelling urethral catheter. Recent prevalence surveys report a urinary catheter is the most common indwelling device, with 17.5% of patients in 66 European hospitals having a catheter [1] and 23.6% in 183 US hospitals [2]. In the NHSN 2011 surveillance report, 45–79% of patients in adult critical care units had an indwelling catheter, 17% of those on medical wards, 23% on surgical wards, and 9% on rehabilitation units [3]. Thus, indwelling urethral catheter use is exceedingly common in health care facilities. Prevention of infections attributable to these devices is an important goal of health-care infection prevention programs.

Indwelling urinary catheters are generally considered to be short term if they are *in situ* for less than 30 days and chronic or long term when *in situ* for 30 days or more [4]. Indwelling catheter use in acute care facilities

Correspondence: lnicolle@exchange.hsc.mb.ca
Departments of Internal Medicine and Medical Microbiology, University of Manitoba, Health Sciences Centre, Room GG443 – 820 Sherbrook Street, Winnipeg, MB R3A 1R9, Canada

is usually short term, while chronic catheters are most common for residents of long term care facilities. Clinical and microbiologic considerations may vary for short and long term catheters. Urinary catheter acquired infection is usually manifested as asymptomatic bacteriuria (CA-ASB). The term catheter associated urinary tract infection (CA-UTI) is used to refer to individuals with symptomatic infection [4]. In early reports, however, asymptomatic and symptomatic catheter-acquired infection were often not differentiated. This review addresses only indwelling urethral catheters, and will not discuss use of intermittent catheters for men or women, or external catheters for men.

Burden of illness

Asymptomatic bacteriuria

Duration of catheterization is the most important determinant of bacteriuria [4]. The daily risk of acquisition of bacteriuria when an indwelling catheter *in situ* is 3–7%. The rate of acquisition is higher for women and older persons [4]. Bacteriuria is universal once a catheter remains in place for several weeks. Patients with chronic indwelling catheters are assumed to be continuously bacteriuric. From 60–80% of hospitalized patients with an indwelling catheter receive antimicrobials, usually for indications other than urinary tract infection [5]. This intense anti-microbial exposure means antimicrobial resistant organisms are frequently isolated from the urine of catheterized individuals. Statewide surveillance of carbapenemase resistant Enterobacteriaceae (CRE) in Michigan reported 61% of isolates were from urine cultures, and a urinary catheter was present in 48% of these patients [6]. Bacteria colonizing the drainage bags of catheterized patients have been reported to be a source for outbreaks of resistant organisms in acute care facilities [4,7]. In the nursing home setting, the urine of residents with chronic indwelling catheters is the most common site of isolation of resistant gram negative organisms [8,9].

Symptomatic urinary tract infection

CA-UTI is the most common adverse event associated with indwelling urinary catheter use (Table 1), although only a small proportion of acute care facility residents with CA-ASB develop symptomatic infection [10]. In the European prevalence survey, 1.3% of patients had urinary infection, representing 17.2% of all healthcare acquired infections, and the third most frequent infection [1]. The presence of any health care acquired infection was independently associated with the number of invasive devices, including indwelling urethral catheters, but the proportion of patients with urinary infections and a catheter was not reported. The recent US point prevalence survey reported urinary tract infection was the fourth most common infection, accounting for 12.9% of health care infections; 67.7% of these patients had a urinary catheter [2]. At one Veteran's Affairs (VA) hospital, 0.3% of all urinary catheter days involved symptomatic UTI [11]. A

comparative British trial evaluating different types of catheters reported rates of CA-UTI of 10.6%-12.6% of catheterized patients, although only 3.2%-5.0% of infections were microbiologically confirmed [12].

CA-UTI rates reported in ICU's in the NHSN hospitals declined by 18.5%-67% among different adult ICU's between 1990 – 2007 [17] (Table 1). In France, a 66% reduction was reported over a 10-year surveillance period [13]. Some of this decrease is attributable to more intense prevention efforts, but modification of definitions to exclude asymptomatic bacteriuria has also contributed.

In US long term care facilities, 3–10% of residents are managed with chronic indwelling catheters [18]. European surveillance reports describe indwelling catheters being present in 12% of residents in 10 nursing homes in the Netherlands [19], 12.3% in 92 homes in Italy [20], and 10.1% in 40 homes in Germany [21]. The prevalence of chronic indwelling catheters was 7% overall among residents of 78 nursing homes in Sweden, but was 16% for men and only 3% for women [22]. Residents with chronic catheters have an increased risk of symptomatic urinary tract infection. CA-UTI rates of 0–7.3/1,000 catheter days (mean 3.2/1,000) were reported in Idaho long term care facilities [23]. The incidence of fever from a presumed urinary source is 0.7–1.1/100 catheter days, which is three times greater than observed for residents with bacteriuria but without a urinary catheter [24,25].

Bacteremia

Less than 3% of subjects with CA-ASB develop bacteremia with the urinary isolate [10] but, given the high frequency of indwelling urinary catheter use, CA-UTI is one of the most common causes of secondary bloodstream infection in acute care facilities. During a 3 year period in Quebec, 21% of health care acquired bloodstream infections were from a urinary source, and 71% of these were device associated. The incidence was 1.4 urinary bloodstream infections/10,000 patient days. All cause 30 day mortality in patients with CA-UTI bacteremia was 15% [26].

CA-UTI is the source of over 50% of episodes of bacteremia in long term care facilities [4,27]. The risk of bacteremia in residents with indwelling catheters in these facilities is 3–36 times that of residents without an indwelling catheter [28].

Other morbidity

Additional infectious complications, usually identified in patients with a chronic indwelling catheter, include urinary catheter obstruction, bladder urolithiasis, purulent urethritis, gland abscesses and, for males, prostatitis [24]. Non-infectious complications attributed to an indwelling urinary catheter include nonbacterial urethral inflammation, urethral strictures, mechanical trauma, and mobility impairment [29,30]. Prospective daily catheter surveillance

Table 1 Recent reports describing incidence of symptomatic catheter-acquired urinary infection

Country (ref)	Population	CA-UTI rate/1,000 catheter days
France [13]	ICU	14.8 (1995);
		8.8 (2004)
Germany [14]	ICU	1.39 (before 2000),
		0.83 (2001, 2002),
		0.68 (2003 or later)
15 developing countries [15]	ICU	7.86 (pre-intervention);
		4.95 (post-intervention)
US NHSN [10]	Critical Care	1.2 – 4.1
	Medical	1.5
	Surgical	3.2
	Burn	4.8
	Postpartum	0.5
	Rehabilitation	3.1
Cyprus [16]	ICU	2.0 – 3.0

in a VA centre identified genitourinary trauma caused by the indwelling catheter on 1.5% of catheter days [11].

Several studies report an association of CA-UTI with increased mortality and prolonged length of stay in acute care facilities. For critical care unit patients, these associations are likely attributable to confounding by unmeasured variables with little, if any, mortality directly attributable to CA-UTI [31]. Long term care facility residents with chronic indwelling catheters have an increased mortality relative to residents without a catheter, but this observation is also attributable to confounding from variable patient characteristics, rather than directly attributable to urinary infection [32].

Pathogenesis of infection
Biofilm
Biofilm formation along the catheter surface is the most important cause of bacteriuria [33]. Biofilm is a complex organic material consisting of micro-organisms growing in colonies within an extra-cellular mucopolysaccharide substance which they produce. Urine components, including Tamm-Horsfall protein and magnesium and calcium ions, are incorporated into this material. Biofilm formation begins immediately after catheter insertion, when organisms adhere to a conditioning film of host proteins which forms along the catheter surface. Both the interior and exterior catheter surfaces are involved. Bacteria usually originate from the periurethral area or ascend the drainage tubing following colonization of the drainage bag. Only about 5% of episodes of CA-ASB follow introduction of periurethral organisms into the bladder at the time of catheter insertion.

Organisms growing in the biofilm are in an environment where they are relatively protected from antimicrobials and host defenses. A single species is usually identified with the initial episode of bacteriuria following insertion of an indwelling catheter. If the catheter remains *in situ* and a mature biofilm develops, polymicrobial bacteriuria becomes the norm. For individuals with long term indwelling catheters, 3–5 organisms are usually isolated [34,35]. The microbiology of biofilm on an indwelling catheter is dynamic with continuing turnover of organisms in the biofilm while the catheter remains *in situ* [36]. Patients continue to acquire new organisms at a rate of about 3–7%/day.

The determinants of CA-UTI are not well described. However, catheter trauma or catheter obstruction are well recognized precipitating events. Risk factors for bloodstream infection from a urinary source in acute care patients are reported to be neutropenia, renal disease and male sex [37]. Bacteremia is not a significant complication of chronic indwelling catheter replacement [28].

Microbiology
The most common infecting organism is *Escherichia coli* [4]. Other Enterobacteriaceae as well as *Enterococci* spp,

coagulase negative *Staphylococcus, Pseudomonas aeruginosa*, other non-fermenters, and *Candida* spp are also frequently isolated [24]. Antimicrobial-resistant organisms are common. The urine of patients with indwelling catheters is the major site of isolation of resistant gram negative organisms in both acute and long term care facilities, including extended spectrum beta-lactamase (ESBL) producing Enterobacteriaceae [8] and CRE [6]. *E. coli* is usually the most frequent species isolated from bacteremic CA-UTI patients in acute care facilities (Table 2). However, *Enterococcus spp* (28.4%) and *Candida spp* (19.7%) were reported to be most common at one US tertiary care academic centre [38].

Proteus mirabilis is an organism of unique importance for patients with chronic indwelling catheters. This species is seldom isolated following initial colonization of the catheterized urinary tract, so it is not common in patients undergoing short term catheterization [42]. The longer a catheter is in place the more likely *P. mirabilis* will be present. This organism is isolated from about 40% of urine samples collected from patients with chronic indwelling catheters [43]. *P. mirabilis* produces more copious biofilm than other bacteria, and these strains also tend to persist for longer periods of time [36].

Bacterial species which produce urease may facilitate the formation of a crystalline biofilm [44,45]. This material is similar to struvite (infection) stones in patients with urolithiasis. Crusts of this material form along the catheter and are the major cause of obstruction of chronic indwelling catheters. About half of patients with chronic indwelling catheters experience catheter blockage at some time, while some patients experience rapid, recurrent obstruction [46,47]. The urease of *P. mirabilis* hydrolyzes urea several times faster than the urease produced by other organisms [48]. This species is isolated from 80% of obstructed catheters [49]. Other urease producing species include *P. aeruginosa, Klebsiella pneumoniae, Morganella morganii*, other Proteus species, some *Providencia* spp and some strains of *Staphylococcus aureus* and coagulase negative staphylococci. Urease production by many of these species, including *M. morganii, K. pneumoniae*, and *P. aeruginosa*, does not generate an alkaline urine, so these strains are seldom associated with appreciable encrustation on catheters [50].

Diagnosis of CA-UTI
Microbiologic diagnosis
Urine specimens for culture should be collected directly from the catheter or tubing, to maintain a closed drainage system. These may be collected either through the catheter collection port or through puncture of the tubing with a needle [4]. CA-ASB is diagnosed when one or more organisms are present at quantitative counts $\geq 10^5$ cful/ml from an appropriately collected urine specimen in a patient with no symptoms attributable to urinary

Table 2 Species isolated from bacteremia attributed to catheter-acquired urinary infection

Population (ref)	US* [38]	UK [39]	Quebec [26]	US [40]**	Europe [40]**	Spain [41]
		% of isolates				
E. coli		43.4%	47%	69.3%	71.3%	42%
Klebsiella spp		7.5%		16.7%	11.2%	15%
Enterococcus spp	28.4%	6%	8%			12%
P. mirabilis		13.3%		6.4%	5.0%	7%
P. aeruginosa		10.8%			4.1%	12%
Candida spp	19.7%		2%			3%

*Tertiary care academic centre.
**Report for gram negative isolates only.

infection [4]. Lower quantitative counts may be isolated from urine specimens prior to ≥10^5 cfu/ml being present, but these lower counts likely reflect the presence of organisms in biofilm forming along the catheter, rather than bladder bacteriuria [5]. A mature biofilm has usually formed once the catheter has been *in situ* for longer than 2 weeks. Urine collected through these catheters are contaminated by organisms present in the biofilm. There is a greater number of species and quantity of organisms isolated than these specimens compared with bladder urine collected simultaneously. Thus, it is recommended that the catheter be removed and a new catheter inserted, with specimen collection from the freshly placed catheter, before antimicrobial therapy is initiated for symptomatic infection [4]. Organisms isolated with quantitative counts <10^5 cfu/ml from the replacement catheter tend not to persist [51].

Clinical diagnosis

The diagnosis of symptomatic CA-UTI is often a diagnosis of exclusion [4,24]. Fever without localizing findings is the usual presentation of CA-UTI. Localizing signs or symptoms such as catheter obstruction, acute hematuria, recent trauma, suprapubic pain, or costovertebral angle pain or tenderness are helpful to identify a urinary source of fever, but are present in only a minority of episodes of presumed symptomatic infection. If localizing genitourinary findings are not present, fever in bacteriuric patients should be attributed to urinary infection only when there are no other potential sources. When the same organism is isolated from both the urine and a simultaneous blood culture, a diagnosis of CA-UTI is presumed in the absence of an alternate source for the bacteremia.

Pyuria

Bacteriuric patients usually have pyuria, irrespective of symptoms. Patients with an indwelling catheter may also have pyuria without bacteriuria, as the catheter itself may cause bladder inflammation [10]. Other potential non-infectious causes of pyuria include renal disease, such as interstitial nephritis. Thus, the presence of pyuria in urine

specimens obtained from a patient with an indwelling urinary catheter does not identify symptomatic infection in a bacteriuric subject, nor is it an indication for antimicrobial therapy [4,28].

Prevention of catheter acquired urinary tract infections
Guidelines

Several evidence-based guidelines provide recommendations for the development and maintenance of prevention programs for CA-UTI [4,7,52-54]. Approaches to prevention include avoidance of catheter use, policies for catheter insertion and maintenance, catheter selection, surveillance of CA-UTI and catheter use, and recommendations for quality indicators.

Program implementation

The facility infection prevention and control program should incorporate measures to limit CA-UTI. Improved outcomes following implementation of these programs have been reported [15,55-57]. The program for a given institution should be individualized to be relevant to local experience, population characteristics, and resources. An essential element of any program is leadership at the senior management level [58].

Infrastructure to support an effective program includes development of policies for catheter indications, catheter selection, and catheter insertion and maintenance [4,7,52]. There must be sufficient staffing and staff education, together with access to adequate and appropriate supplies. A means for documentation of urinary catheter use, including indications and dates of insertion and removal, should be established. Where an electronic patient record is used, documentation of catheter use and automatic reminders for removal should be incorporated into this record. The development and implementation of "bundles" for prevention of catheter acquired urinary tract infections has been described. Introduction of a urinary catheter bundle which included education, catheter insertion and management guidelines, and CA-UTI surveillance, in intensive care units in 15 developing countries was followed by a 37% reduction in CA-UTI rate [15]. A state wide initiative in Michigan introduced a CA-UTI bundle with specific practical recommendations addressing implementation under the concepts of "engage and educate", "execute" and "evaluate" [59].

Avoidance of catheter use

The single most important intervention to prevent CA-UTI is to avoid use of an indwelling urinary catheter. There are only a limited number of accepted indications for catheter use [46]:

- Monitoring of hourly urine output in acutely ill patients.
- Perioperative use for selected surgical procedures
    Urologic surgery
    Surgery on contiguous structures of the genitourinary tract
    Large volume infusions or diuretics during surgery
    Requirement for intraoperative monitoring of urine output
- Management of acute urinary retention and urinary obstruction.
- To facilitate healing of open pressure ulcers or skin grafts in selected patients with urinary incontinence.
- In exceptional circumstances (e.g. end-of-life care), at patient request to improve comfort.

Alternate voiding management strategies such as intermittent catheterization or, for men, external condom catheters, should be used when possible. Institutional policies should also minimize perioperative catheter use by promoting early post-procedure catheter removal and monitoring of bladder volume with ultrasound bladder scanners, where available, to limit catheter reinsertion for potential urinary retention. When a catheter is indicated, it should be removed promptly once it is no longer required. Patients with indwelling catheters should be identified and reviewed on a continuing basis, preferably at daily rounds, and the catheter removed when no longer indicated. Catheters have been reported to frequently remain *in situ* beyond necessary, sometimes because health-care personnel are not aware the catheter is present [7,52]. A systematic review of catheter discontinuation strategies for hospitalized patients reported that the intervention of a "stop order" to facilitate prompt removal of unnecessary catheters reduced the duration of catheter use by 1.06 days, and use of either catheter reminders or stop orders decreased the CA-UTI rate by 53% [60].

Selection of urinary catheter

The smallest gauge catheter possible should be used, to minimize urethral trauma [4,52]. Infection risks are similar with latex or silicone catheters, and whether or not there is hydrogel coating of the catheter. Residents with

chronic catheters have a decreased frequency of obstruction with silicone catheters, but this observation is attributed to the larger bore size of the catheter, rather than the catheter material. The use of silver alloy coated catheters does not decrease the frequency of CA-UTI [12,61-63]. Nitrofurazone coated catheters have been reported to be associated with a small decrease in CA-UTI [12], but are accompanied by more frequent catheter removal and increased catheter discomfort. Thus, current evidence does not support the routine use of antimicrobial coated catheters [52].

Catheter insertion and maintenance

Recommended practices for catheter insertion and maintenance include [4,7,52].

- Catheter insertion:
    Appropriate hand hygiene
    Choice of catheter
    Aseptic techniques/sterile equipment
    Barrier precautions
    Antiseptic meatal cleaning
- Catheter maintenance
    Appropriate hand hygiene
    Secure catheter
    Closed drainage system
    Obtain urine samples aseptically
    Replace system if breaks in asepsis
    Avoid irrigation for purpose of prevention of infection

These recommendations are primarily based on consensus, but there is strong evidence supporting a decreased rate of acquisition of bacteriuria by maintaining a closed drainage system. There are no benefits with routine daily periurethral cleaning using normal saline, soap, or an antiseptic [52,64], or with the addition of antiseptics to the drainage bag [52].

Monitoring of infection

The surveillance of catheter use and complications is important to document the facility CA-UTI rate, the effectiveness of interventions, and to allow comparison with benchmark rates [7,52]. Surveillance with benchmarking was reported, by itself, to decrease infection rates in German intensive care units, although the impact for CA-UTI was not as great as observed for ventilator-associated pneumonia or primary blood stream infections [14]. Standardized surveillance definitions for infection should be used [52]. Core data elements which must be collected to support effective surveillance include recording of catheter indication, catheter insertion and removal dates, urine culture results, and monitoring of bacteremia. Relevant quality indicators are CA-UTI incidence, CA-

UTI bacteremia incidence, and the proportion of indwelling catheter use meeting accepted indications.

The outcomes of CA-UTI and bacteremic infection are described using a denominator of device days [52]. However, an effective infection prevention program will minimize catheter use, potentially leading to overall higher device day infection rates as fewer low-risk patients will have catheters [65,66]. Thus, an outcome based on total patient days, the standardized infection ratio, should also be reported [7]. Surveillance data should be reviewed by appropriate individuals and committees, and observations reported back to caregivers on patient wards [7,52].

Prevention of CA-UTI in long term care facilities

The prevention of CA-UTI in long term care facilities addresses primarily residents with a chronic indwelling catheter [4,24,28]. There should be frequent, systematic review of any resident with a chronic indwelling catheter to determine whether the catheter remains necessary. Bacteriuria in these residents is not avoidable. Interventions should focus on removing the catheter, whenever feasible, minimizing catheter trauma, and early identification of catheter obstruction. Chronic indwelling catheters should not be changed routinely. They should be replaced only if there is obstruction or other malfunction, or prior to initiating antimicrobial therapy when symptomatic urinary infection is treated [52]. Residents with chronic catheters may use a leg bag for drainage to facilitate mobility. Facility policies should address reuse and cleaning or replacement of the leg bags [67]. Antimicrobial therapy for the treatment of bacteriuria in long term care residents with chronic indwelling catheters does not decrease CA-UTI, but there is an increased isolation of resistant organisms with the antimicrobial therapy. Thus, treatment of asymptomatic bacteriuria should be avoided [24].

Conclusions

CA-UTI is an important device-associated health care acquired infection. The use of an indwelling urethral catheter is associated with an increased frequency of symptomatic urinary tract infection and bacteremia, and additional morbidity from non-infectious complications. Infection control programs must develop, implement, and monitor policies and practices to minimize infections associated with use of these devices. A major focus of these programs should be to limit the use of indwelling urethral catheters, and to remove catheters promptly when no longer required. Ultimately, however, the avoidance of CA-ASB will likely require development of biofilm resistant catheter materials.

Competing interests
The author declares that she has no competing interests.

References

1. Zarb P, Coignard B, Griskevicienne J, Muller A, Vankerckho ven Weist K, Goossens MM, Vaerenberg S, Hopkins S, Catry B, Monnet DL, Goosens H, Suetens C: **The European Centre for Disease Prevention and Control (ECDC) pilot point prevalence survey of healthcare-associated infections and antimicrobial use.** *Euro Surveill* 2012, **17**(46):pii=20316.

2. Magill SS, Edwards JR, Bamberg W, Beldaus ZG, Dumyati G, Kainer MA, Lynfield R, Maloney M, McAllister-Hollod L, Nadle J, Ray SM, Thompson D, Wilson LE, Fridkin SK: **Multistate point-prevalence survey of health care-associated infections.** *N Engl J Med* 2014, **370**:1198–1208.

3. Centers for Disease Control and Prevention (CDC): **National Healthcare Safety Network (NHSN) Report, Data Summary for 2011, Device-Associated Module, Atlanta: CDC.** 2013, http://www.cdc.gov/nhsn/PDFs/dataStat/NHSN-Report-2011-Data-Summary.pdf.

4. Hooton TM, Bradley SF, Cardenas DD, Colgan R, Geerlings SE, Rice JC, Saint S, Schaeffer AJ, Tambyah PA, Tenke P, Nicolle LE: **Diagnosis, prevention and treatment of catheter-associated urinary tract infection in adults; 2009 international clinical practice guidelines from the Infectious Diseases Society of America.** *Clin Infect Dis* 2010, **50**:625–663.

5. Stark RP, Maki DG: **Bacteriuria in the catheterized patient. What quantitative level of bacteriuria is relevant?** *N Engl J Med* 1984, **311**:560–564.

6. Brennan BM, Coyle JR, Marchaim D, Pogue JM, Boehme M, Finks J, Malani AN, Verhec KE, Buckley BO, Mollon N, SUrdin DR, Washer LL, Kaye KS: **Statewide surveillance of carbapenem-resistant Enterobacteriaceae in Michigan.** *Infection Control Hosp Epidemiol* 2014, **35**:342–349.

7. Lo E, Nicolle LE, Coffin SE, Gould C, Maragakis L, Meddings J, Pegues DA, Pettis AM, Saint S, Yokoe DS: **Strategies to prevent catheter-associated urinary tract infections in acute care hospitals: 2014 update.** *Infect Control Hosp Epidemiol* 2014, **35**:464–479.

8. Arnoldo L, Migliavasca R, Regastin L, Raglio A, Pagani L, Nucleo E, Spalla M, Vailati F, Agodi A, Mosea A, Zoth C, Tardivo S, Bianco I, Rulli A, Gualdi P, Panetta P, Pasini C, Pedroni M, Brusaferro S: **Prevalence of urinary colonization by extended spectrum-beta-lactamase Enterobacteriaceae among catheterized inpatients in Italian long term care facilities.** *BMC Infect Dis* 2013, **13**:124.

9. Mody L, Matieshwari S, Galecki A, Kauffman CA, Bradley SF: **Indwelling device use and antibiotic resistance in nursing homes: identifying a high-risk group.** *J Am Geriatr Soc* 2007, **55**:1921–1926.

10. Tambyah PA, Maki DG: **Catheter-associated urinary tract infection is rarely symptomatic.** *Arch Intern Med* 2000, **160**:678–687.

11. Leuck A-M, Wright D, Ellingson L, Kraemer L, Kuskowski MA, Johnson JR: **Complications of Foley catheters – is infection the greatest risk?** *J Urol* 2012, **187**:1662–1666.

12. Pickard R, Lam T, MacLennan G, Starr K, Kilonzo M, McPherson G, Gillies K, McDonald A, Walton K, Buckley B, Glazener C, Boachie C, Burr J, Norrie J, Vale L, Grant A, Nidow J: **Types of urethral catheter for reducing symptomatic urinary tact infections in hospitalized adults requiring short-term catheterization: multicenter randomized controlled trial and economic evaluation of antimicrobial- and antiseptic-impregnated urethral catheters (the CATHETER trial).** *Health Technol Assess* 2012, **16**(47). doi:10.3310/hta16470.

13. Venhems P, Baratin D, Voirin N, Savey A, Caillat-Vallet E, Metzger M-H, Lepape A: **Reduction of urinary tract infections acquired in an intensive care unit during a 10-year surveillance program.** *Eur J Epidemiol* 2008, **23**:641–645.

14. Gastmeier P, Behnke M, Schwab F, Geffers C: **Benchmarking of urinary tract infection rates, experiences from the intensive care unit component of the German national nosocomial infections surveillance system.** *J Hosp Infect* 2011, **78**:41–44.

15. Rosenthal VD, Todi SK, Alvarez-Moreno C, Pawar M, Karlekar A, Zeggwagh AA, Mitrev Z, Udwadia FE, Navoa-Ng JA, Chakravarthy M, Salomao R, Sahu S, Dilek A, Kanj SS, Guanche-Garcell H, Cuellar LE, Ersoz G, Nevzat-Yolein A, Jagg N, Madeiros EA, Ye G, Akan DA, Mapp T, Castenada-Sabogal A, Matta-Cortes L, Sirmate IF, Olark N, Torres-Hernandes H, Barahona-Guzman N, Fernandez-Hidalgo R, *et al*: **Impact of a multidimensional infection control strategy on catheter-associated urinary tract infection rates in the adult intensive care units of 15 developing countries: findings of the**

International Nosocomial Infection Control Consortium. *Infection* 2012, **40:**517–526.

16. Giks A, Roumbelaki M, Bagatzoumi-Pieridou D, Alexandrou M, Zinseri V, Dimitradis I, Krixtsotaks EI: **Device-associated infections in the intensive care units of Cyprus: results of the first national incidence study.** *Infection* 2010, **38:**165–171.

17. Burton DC, Edwards JR, Srinivasion A, Fredkin SK, Gould CV: **Trends in catheter-associated urinary tract infections in adult intensive care units – United States, 1990–2007.** *Infect Control Hosp Epidemiol* 2011, **32:**748–756.

18. Crnich CJ, Drinka P: **Medical device-associated infections in the long-term care setting.** *Infect Dis Clin North Am* 2012, **26:**143–164.

19. Eilers R, Veldman-Ariesen MJ, Van Bentham BH: **Prevalence and determinants associated with healthcare-associated infections in long-term care facilities in the Netherlands, May to June 2010.** *Euro Surveill* 2012, **17**(34):pil=20252.

20. Moro ML, Ricchizzi E, Morsillo F, Marchi M, Purs V, Zotti CM, Prato R, Privitera G, Poli A, Mora I, Fedeli U: **Infections and antimicrobial resistance in long term care facilities: a national prevalence study.** *Ann Ig* 2013, **25:**109–118.

21. Heudorf L, Boehicke K, Schade M: **Healthcare-associated infections in long-term care facilities in Frankfurt am Main, Germany, January to March 2011.** *Euro Surveill* 2012, **17**(35):pil=20256.

22. Jonsson K, Loft A-L E, Nasic S, Hedelin H: **A prospective registration of catheter life and catheter interventions in patients with long-term indwelling catheters.** *Scand J Urol Nephrol* 2011, **45:**401–403.

23. Stevenson KB, Moore J, Colwell H, Sleeper B: **Standardized infection surveillance in long-term care: interfacility comparisons from a regional cohort of facilities.** *Infect Control Hosp Epidemiol* 2004, **25:**985–994.

24. Nicolle LE: **Urinary catheter associated infections.** *Infect Dis Clin North Am* 2012, **26:**13.28.

25. Warren JW, Damron D, Tenney JH, Hoopes JM, Deforge B, Muncie HL Jr: **Fever, bacteremia and death as complications of bacteriuria in women with long-term urethral catheters.** *J Infect Dis* 1987, **155:**1151–1158.

26. Fortin E, Rocher I, Frenette C, Temblay C, Quach C: **Healthcare-associated bloodstream infections secondary to a urinary focus: the Quebec Provincial Surveillance results.** *Infect Control Hosp Epidemiol* 2012, **33:**456–462.

27. Mylotte JM: **Nursing home acquired bloodstream infection.** *Infect Control Hosp Epidemiol* 2005, **26:**838–837.

28. Nicolle LE: **Urinary tract infections in the elderly.** *Clin Geriatr Med* 2009, **25:**423–436.

29. Hollingsworth JM, Rogers MA, Krein SL, Hickner A, Kuhn L, Cheng A, Chang R, Saint S: **Determining the noninfectious complications of indwelling urethral catheters: a systematic review and meta-analysis.** *Ann Intern Med* 2013, **159:**401–410.

30. Saint S, Baker PD, McDonald LL, Ossenkop K: **Urinary catheters: what type do men and their nurses prefer?** *J Am Geriatr Soc* 1999, **47:**1453–1457.

31. Chant C, Smith DM, Marshall JC, Friedrich JO: **Relationship of catheter associated urinary tract infection to mortality and length of stay in critically ill patients: a systematic review and meta-analysis of observational studies.** *Crit Care Med* 2011, **39:**1167–1173.

32. Kunin CM, Chin QF, Chambers S: **Morbidity and mortality associated with indwelling urinary catheters in elderly patients in a nursing home – confounding due to the presence of associated diseases.** *J Am Geriatr Soc* 1987, **35:**1001–1006.

33. Stickler DJ: **Bacterial biofilms in patients with indwelling urinary catheters.** *Nat Clin Pract Urol* 2008, **5**(11):598–608.

34. Nicolle LE: **The chronic indwelling catheter and urinary infection in long term care facility residents.** *Infect Control Hosp Epidemiol* 2001, **22:**316–321.

35. Warren JW: **The catheter and urinary tract infection.** *Med Clin North Am* 1991, **75:**481–493.

36. Warren JW, Tenney JH, Hoopes JM, Muncie HL, Anthony WC: **A prospective microbiologic study of bacteriuria in patients with chronic indwelling urethral catheters.** *J Infect Dis* 1982, **146:**719–723.

37. Greene MT, Chang R, Kuhn L, Rogers MA, Chenoweth CE, Shuman E, Saint S: **Predictors of hospital-acquired urinary tract-related bloodstream infection.** *Infect Control Hosp Epidemiol* 2012, **33:**1001–1007.

38. Chang R, Greene MT, Chenoweth CE, Kuhn L, Shuman E, Rogers NAM, Saint S: **Epidemiology of hospital-acquired urinary-tract related blood stream infection at a university hospital.** *Infect Control Hosp Epidemiol* 2011, **32:**1127–1129.

39. Melzer M, Welch C: **Outcomes in UK patients with hospital-acquired bacteremia and the risk of catheter-associated urinary tract infections.** *Postgrad Med J* 2013, **89:**329–334.

40. Sader HS, Flamm RK, Jones RN: **Frequency of occurrence and antimicrobial susceptibility of Gram-negative bacteremia isolates in patients with urinary tract infection: results from United States and European hospitals (2009–2011).** *J Chemother* 2014, **26:**133–138.

41. Ortega M, Marco F, Soriano A, Almela M, Martinez JA, Pitart C, Mensa J: **Epidemiology and proynostic determinants of bacteremic catheter acquired urinary tract infection in a single institution from 1991–2010.** *J Infect* 2013, **67:**282–287.

42. Matsukawa M, Kunishima Y, Takahashi S, Takeyama K, Tsukamoto T: **Bacterial colonization on intraluminal surface of urethral catheter.** *Urology* 2005, **65:**440–444.

43. Mobley HT: **Virulence of *Proteus mirabilis*.** In *Urinary tract infections: molecular pathogenesis and clinical management*. Edited by Mobley HL, Warren JW. Washington DC: ASM Press; 1996:245–270.

44. Getliffe KA, Mulhall AB: **The encrustation of indwelling catheters.** *Br J Urol* 1991, **67:**337–341.

45. Stickler DJ, Zimakoff J: **Complications of urinary tract infections associated with devices used for long-term bladder management.** *J Hosp Infect* 1994, **28:**177–194.

46. Getliffe KA: **The characteristics and management of patients with recurrent blockage of long-term urinary catheters.** *J Adv Nurs* 1994, **20:**140–149.

47. Kohler-Ockmore J, Feneley RC: **Longterm catheterization of the bladder: prevalence and morbidity.** *Br J Urol* 1996, **77:**347–351.

48. Jones BD, Mobley HL: **Genetic and biochemical diversity of ureases of *Proteus*, *Providencia*, and *Morganella* species isolated from urinary tract infection.** *Infect Immun* 1987, **55:**2198–2203.

49. Jacobsen SM, Stickler DJ, Mobley HL, Shirtliff ME: **Complicated catheter-associated urinary tract infections due to *Escherichia coli* and *Proteus mirabilis*.** *Clin Microbiol Rev* 2008, **21:**26–59.

50. Stickler D, Morris N, Moreno MC, Sabbaba N: **Studies on the formation of crystalline bacterial biofilms on urethral catheters.** *Eur J Clin Microbiol Infect Dis* 1998, **17:**649–652.

51. Tenney JH, Warren JW: **Bacteriuria in women with long term catheters: paired comparison of indwelling and replacement catheters.** *J Infect Dis* 1988, **157:**199–207.

52. Gould CV, Umscheid CA, Agarwal RK, Kuntz G, Pegues DA: **Healthcare Infection Control Practices Advisory Committee (HICPAC): guideline for prevention of catheter-associated urinary tract infections.** 2009, http://www.cdc.gov/hicpac/cauti/011_cauti.html.

53. Pratt RJ, Pellowe C, Loveday HP, Robinson N, Smith GW, Epic Guideline Development Team: **Guidelines for preventing infections associated with the insertion and maintenance of short-term indwelling urethral catheters in acute care.** *J Hosp Infect* 2001, **47**(suppl):S39–S46.

54. Pratt RJ, Pellowe CM, Wilson JA, Loveday HP, Harper PJ, Jones SR, McDougall C, Wilcox MH: **Epic 2: national evidence-based guidelines for preventing healthcare-associated infections in NHS hospitals in England.** *J Hosp Infect* 2007, **65**(suppl):S1–S64.

55. Fakih MG, Watson SR, Green MT, Kennedy EH, Olmsted RN, Krein SL, Saint S: **Reducing inappropriate urinary catheter use: a statewide effort.** *Arch Intern Med* 2012, **172:**255–260.

56. Marigliano A, Barbadoro P, Pennacchietti L, D'Errico MM, Prospero E: **Active training and surveillance: two good friends to reduce urinary catheterization rate.** *Am J Infect Control* 2012, **40:**692–695.

57. Titsworth WL, Hester J, Correia T, Reed R, Williams M, Guin P, Layon AJ, Archibald LK, Mocco J: **Reduction of catheter-associated urinary tract infections among patients in a neurological intensive care unit: a single institution's success.** *J Neurosurg* 2012, **116:**911–920.

58. Saint S, Kowalski CP, Forman J, Damschroder L, Hofer TP, Kaufman SR, Creswell JW, Krein SL: **A multicenter qualitative study on preventing hospital-acquired urinary tract infection in US hospitals.** *Infect Control Hosp Epidemiol* 2008, **29:**333–341.

59. Saint S, Olmsted RN, Fakih MG, Kowalski CP, Watson SR, Sales AE, Krein SL: **Translating health care-associated urinary tract infection prevention research into practice via the bladder bundle.** *Jt Comm J Qual Patient Saf* 2009, **35:**449–455.

60. Meddings J, Rogers MA, Krein SL, Fakih MG, Olmsted RN, Saint S: **Reducing unnecessary urinary catheter use and other strategies to prevent**

catheter-associated urinary tract infection: an integrative review. *BMJ Qual Saf* 2013, Electronically published ahead of print. doi:10.1136/bmjqs-2012-001774.

61. Johnson JR, Roberts PL, Olsen RJ, Moyer KA, Stamm WE: Prevention of catheter-associated urinary tract infection with a silver-oxide-coated urinary catheter: clinical and microbiologic correlation. *J Infect Dis* 1990, **162**:1145–1150.

62. Srinivasan A, Karchmer T, Richards A, Song X, Perl T: A prospective trial of a novel, silicone-based, silver-coated Foley catheter for the prevention of nosocomial urinary tract infection. *Infect Control Hosp Epidemiol* 2006, **27**:38–43.

63. Riley DK, Classen DC, Stevens LE, Burke JP: A large, randomized clinical trial of a silver-impregnated urinary catheter: lack of efficacy and staphylococcal superinfection. *Am J Med* 1995, **98**:349–356.

64. Huth TS, Burke JP, Larsen RA, Classen DC, Stevens LE: Randomized trial of meatal care with silver sulfadiazine cream for the prevention of catheter-associated bacteriuria. *J Infect Dis* 1992, **165**:14–18.

65. Fakih MG, Greene MT, Kennedy EH, Meddings JA, Krein SL, Olmsted RN, Saint S: Introducing a population-based outcome measure to evaluate the effect of interventions to reduce catheter-associated urinary tract infection. *Am J Infect Control* 2012, **40**:359–364.

66. Burns AC, Petersen NJ, Garza A, Arya M, Patterson JE, Naik AD, Trautner BW: Accuracy of a urinary catheter surveillance protocol. *Am J Infect Control* 2012, **40**:55–58.

67. Smith P, Bennett G, Bradley S, Drinka P, Lautenbach E, Marx J, Mody L, Nicolle L, Stevenson K: SHEA/APIC Guideline: infection prevention and control in the long-term care facility. *Infect Control Hosp Epidemiol* 2008, **29**:785–814.

12

Molecular characterization of extended spectrum β -lactamases enterobacteriaceae causing lower urinary tract infection among pediatric population

Nahla O. Eltai[1]* , Asmaa A. Al Thani[1,4], Khalid Al-Ansari[2], Anand S. Deshmukh[3], Eman Wehedy[1], Sara H. Al-Hadidi[1] and Hadi M. Yassine[1,4]*

Abstract

Background: The β-lactam antibiotics have traditionally been the main treatment of Enterobacteriaceae infections, nonetheless, the emergence of species producing β- Lactamases has rendered this class of antibiotics largely ineffective. There are no published data on etiology of urinary tract infections (UTI) and antimicrobial resistance profile of uropathogens among children in Qatar. The aim of this study is to determine the phenotypic and genotypic profiles of antimicrobial resistant Enterobacteriaceae among children with UTI in Qatar.

Methods: Bacteria were isolated from 727 urine positive cultures, collected from children with UTI between February and June 2017 at the Pediatric Emergency Center, Doha, Qatar. Isolated bacteria were tested for antibiotic susceptibility against sixteen clinically relevant antibiotics using phoenix and Double Disc Synergy Test (DDST) for confirmation of extended-spectrum beta-lactamase (ESBL) production. Existence of genes encoding ESBL production were identified using polymerase chain reaction (PCR). Statistical analysis was done using non-parametric Kappa statistics, Pearson chi-square test and Jacquard's coefficient.

Results: 201 (31.7%) of samples were confirmed as Extended Spectrum β -Lactamases (ESBL) Producing Enterobacteriaceae. The most dominant pathogen was *E. coli* 166 (83%) followed by *K. pneumoniae* 22 (11%). Resistance was mostly encoded by *bla* CTX-M (59%) genes, primarily *bla* CTX-MG1 (89.2%) followed by *bla* CTX-MG9 (7.7%). 37% of isolated bacteria were harboring multiple *bla* genes (2 genes or more). *E. coli* isolates were categorized into 11 clusters, while *K. pneoumoniae* were grouped into five clonal clusters according to the presence and absence of seven genes namely *bla* TEM, *bla* SHV, *bla* CTX-MG1, *bla* CTX-MG2, *bla* CTX-MG8 *bla* CTX-MG9, *bla* CTX-MG25.

Conclusions: Our data indicates an escalated problem of ESBL in pediatrics with UTI, which mandates implementation of regulatory programs to reduce the spread of ESBL producing Enterobacteriaceae in the community. The use of cephalosporins, aminoglycosides (gentamicin) and trimethoprim/sulfamethoxazole is compromised in Qatar among pediatric population with UTI, leaving carbapenems and amikacin as the therapeutic option for severe infections caused by ESBL producers.

Keywords: Urinary tract infection (UTI), Enterobacteriaceae, Antibiotic resistance, Children, ESBL, Qatar

* Correspondence: nahla.eltai@qu.edu.qa; hyassine@qu.edu.qa
[1]Biomedical Research Center, Qatar University, P.O. Box 2713, Doha, Qatar
Full list of author information is available at the end of the article

Background

Enterobacteriaceae carrying extended-spectrum β-lactamases (ESBLs) is a global concern that demands global attention due to the limited available treatment options [1–4]. Over the past two decades, there has been an exponential increase in β-lactamase resistance worldwide accompanied with a significant escalation in the prevalence of ESBL-producing Enterobacteriaceae [5]. Unfortunately, ESBL-producing bacteria in children have come to the forefront of emerging antibiotic-resistant bacteria worldwide [6]. β-lactamases are divided into four functional groups: penicillinases, ESBLs, carbapenemases, and AmpC-type cephalosporinases [7]. Specifically, ESBLs is a group of plasmid-encoded enzymes that confer resistance to third generation cephalosporins [8–10]. ESBLs are divided into three groups according the encoding of TEM, SHV and CTX-M genes [11, 12]. CTX-M enzymes are the most common and are further classified into five major phylogenetic groups based on gene sequences namely, CTX-M -1, CTX-M-2, CTX-M-8, CTX-M-9, and CTX-M-25 [11]. ESBL-producing *Escherichia coli (E. coli)* and *Klebsiella pneumoniae (K. pneumoniae)* are the predominant organisms in childhood infections, and they pose significant threat to human health [13]. These organisms are listed among the pathogens for which there are few potentially effective drugs [1]. About 57% of bloodstream infections are caused by ESBL-producing Enterobacteriaceae, which are more likely to result in death compared to the infections caused by a non ESBL-producing strains [14].

Urinary Tract Infections (UTIs) continue to be one of the most common cause of illness in young children worldwide [9]. It distresses the child, concern the parent, and may cause permanent renal sequelae. The β-lactam antibiotics have traditionally been the main antibiotics for treatment of infections caused by Enterobacteriaceae, but the emergence of ESBL has rendered this class of antibiotics largely ineffective. It is therefore important to run epidemiological studies to define the epidemiology and profiles of these resistant bacteria for its impact on the development and implementation of stewardship programs.

High prevalence of extended-spectrum-β-lactamase (ESBL) and carbapenemase producing gram negative bacteria (GNB) has been reported in the Arabian Peninsula [15]. Nonetheless, little is known about the prevalence and profile of these bacteria in pediatric population [16] in the region. Prevalence of ESBL in urine among pediatric population has been gradually increasing in Qatar (HMC annual antibiogram). For example, the percentage of *E.coli* ESBL producers have gradually increased from 18% in 2010 to 24% in 2014, and reached 31.7% in 2017 (January–June) as reported in this study.

This is the first study that describes at the molecular level the genotypic profile of ESBL producing bacteria among children with UTIs in Qatar. Our data indicates rapid increase in ESBL resistance among Enterobacteriaceae in pediatrics with UTI, which mandates rapid regulatory and monitoring reforms at the State level.

Methods
Clinical isolates and controls strains

Ethical approval for this study was obtained from the Medical Research Centre (MRC), Hamad Medical Corporation (HMC), Doha, Qatar, protocol no. 16434/16. A total of 727 urine Samples were collected between February and June of 2107 from children (0–15 years of age) hospitalized with lower UTI at the Pediatric Emergency Center-HMC. All urine analysis were performed on patients presented with symptoms, mainly fever and dysuria. Urinary catheter was applied for all patients less than or equal 2 years of age, cerebral palsy (CP) patients and patients under intermittent catheterization. Otherwise, urine was obtained from mid-stream catch. Samples that did not yield significant bacterial growth, those that had multiple organisms and samples with suspected contamination as per lab report, were excluded from the study, and no duplicate samples were collected. All of the reported cases had UTI as their primary diagnosis. For each patient, demographic data such as age, nationality, and gender were collected. Out of the above samples, 635 (87.3%) were positive for Enterobacteriaceae species which were then isolated using readymade Cystine Lactose Electrolyte-Deficient media (IMES, Doha, Qatar). Isolated bacteria were identified by MALDI-TOF (Bruker Daltonik GmbH, Leipzig, Germany) and initial antimicrobial susceptibility testing was performed by Phoenix using the NMIC/ID-5 panel (BD Biosciences, Heidelberg, Germany) according to the manufacturer's recommendations. Both automated tests were performed at Hamad General Hospital Microbiology laboratory. All intermediate resistant isolates were considered as susceptible. Initial testing with Phoenix revealed 201 (31.7%) isolates as Extended Spectrum β -Lactamases (ESBL) producer Enterobacteriaceae. Susceptibility testing was done for 16 clinically relevant antibiotics. 110 of these samples were randomly selected for further genotypic analysis.

Standard strains, *E. coli* ATCC® 25,922 and *E. coli* ATCC® 35,218, were used as controls for antimicrobial drug susceptibility testing. *E. coli* NCTC® 13,461™, *E. coli* NCTC® 13,462™, *E. coli* NCTC ®13,463™, *Enterobacter cloacae* NCTC ®13,464™ and *K. pneumonia* NCTC® 13,465™, *E. coli* ATCC® 35,218™ and *E. coli* NCTC ®13,368™ were used as positive controls, for CTX-M G1, CTX-M G 2, CTX-M G 8, CTX-M G 9, CTX-M G25

25, [bla] TEM and [bla] SHV, polymerase chain reaction (PCR) assays, respectively.

ESBL phenotype confirmation

Isolates that were tested positive for ESBL by Phoenix were consequently confirmed by Double Disc Synergy Test (DDST) as previously described [17, 18]. Briefly, synergy was determined between a 20/10 µg disc of amoxicillin-clavulanate (BD- Sensi Disc™) and 30-µg disc of ceftazidime and ceftriaxone (BD- Sensi Disc™), placed onto Mueller–Hinton agar (Oxoid Ltd., Basingstoke, Hampshire, England) inoculated with a microbial suspension of 0.5 McFarland turbidity, at a distance of 15 mm apart from the edge of the amoxicillin-clavulanate disc. The cefoxitin (30 µg, BD- Sensi Disc™) disc was placed in any available space remaining on the plate. Extension of the edge of the exhibition zone by > 5 mm towards the disc of amoxicillin-clavulanate disc, together with susceptibility to cefoxitin was interpreted as positive for the ESBL production [18].

Molecular genotyping of ESBL genes

DNA was extracted from bacterial cultures using QIAamp® UCP pathogen mini Kit (Qiagen, Germany) following manufacturer's instructions. Extracted DNA was then used to run PCR for seven genes and using previously published primers [19, 20] . The conditions used for [bla]TEM and [bla]SHV reactions were as follows: PCR mixture was made in volume of 20 µl containing 0.5 µM of each primer, 50 ng DNA, 1× master mix (Hot star *Taq* plus master mix (Qiagene, Germany)) and DPEC H2O up to 20 µl. The reaction was amplified in GeneAmp® PCR system 9700 thermocycler under the following conditions: 1. Initial denaturation at 96 °C for 5 min.; 2. 32 cycles consisting of denaturation at 96 °C for 30 s., annealing at 44 °C ([bla] TEM) and at 58 °C ([bla] SHV) for 45 s, and extension for 60 s. at 72 °C; and 3. A final extension cycles at 72 °C for 10 min. Multiplex PCR (MPCR) was performed in a final volume of 30 µl containing 0.23 µM of each primer ([bla] CTX-M-G$_{(1,2,8,9 \&25)}$), 50 ng DNA, 1× master mix (Hot star *Taq* plus master mix (Qiagene, Germany) [19]) and DPEC H2O up to 30 µl to screen for [bla] CTX-M- G (1,2,8,9 & 25) genes. Amplified products were subjected to electrophoresis in 1.2% agarose (Agarose- LE, Ambion®, USA), stained with ethidium bromide (Promega, Madison, USA) and visualized using Bio-Rad gel doc system (Bio - rad, Gel Doc ᵗᵐ XR System 170–8170, Canada).

Clustering of ESBL-positive isolates

An agglomerative hierarchical algorithm was used to derive a cluster analysis dendrogram to establish the relationship between individual *E. coli* (*n* = 95) and *Klebsiella pneumoniae* (*n* = 13) isolates based on the

presence and absence of 7 genes ([bla]TEM, [bla]SHV, [bla] CTXM -G 1, [bla] CTXM -G2, [bla] CTXM -G8, [bla] CTXM -G9 & [bla] CTXM –G25), whichare reported in the literature to encode for ESBL. The scores '1' and '0' were given for the presence and absence of bands respectively [21–23]. The data obtained by scoring of the genetic profiles of different ESBL genes were subjected to cluster analysis, and hierarchical cluster dendrogram was created using Past software version 1.91 [24]. A similarity matrix values were used for cluster analysis.

Data analysis

Data were introduced into Microsoft Excel 2010 (Microsoft Corporation, New York, USA) to generate figures and run initial analysis and further statistical analysis were done using SPSS statistics 24 (Statistical Package for the Social Science; SPSS Inc., Chicago, IL, USA). Relation between gene type and resistance of each antibiotic was cross-tabulated using non-parametric Kappa statistics; on the other hand, relation between gene type, nationality and age grouping was calculated using Pearson chi-square test. Probability value (*P* value) less than 0.05 was considered statistically significant. Past software, version 1.91, was used to construct hierarchical clustering dendrogram and Jacquard's coefficient was applied to generate the similarity values for generation of the cluster analysis [24].

Results
Demography of the study population

The demographic profile of the studied population is summarized in Table 1. Sixteen percent (*n* = 34) of samples were collected from males compared to 83.% (*n* = 167) from females (0–15 years of age), with Male to female ratio of approximately 1:5. ESBL producing Enterobacteriaceae were more prevalent among Qataris 46 (22.8%), Egyptians 37 (18.4%), Indians 27 (13.4%), and to lesser extent in Pakistani 21(10.4%). Most of the ESBL

Table 1 Demographic profile of the study population (*n* = 201) with ESBL UTI in the State of Qatar

Gender	Total number/ percentage	Nationality	
		Qatari	Non Qatari (*n*ª=24)
Male	34 (16.9%)	5 (2.5%)	29 (14.42%)
Female	167(83%)	41 (20.4%)	126 (62.7%)
Total no./percentage	201 (100%)	46 (22.9%)	155 (77.11%)
Age group (years)			
< 2	60 (29.9%)	7 (36.8%)	53 (26.4%)
2–5	82 (40.8%)	18 (9%)	64 (31.8%)
6–15	59 (29.4%)	20 (10%)	39 (19.4)

ªRepresent the number of nationalities tested

was detected among children between 0 and 5 years of age, $n = 142$ (70.6%).

Etiology of ESBL-associated UTI infections

Out of 635 Enterobacteriaceae positive urine cultures, 201 (31.7%) were found to be ESBL producing bacteria. *E. coli* species was the most prominent with prevalence rate of 83% ($n = 166$), followed by *Klebsiella pneumoniae* 11% ($n = 22$) and the rest 6% included *Citrobacter koseri, Enterobacter cloacae, Serratia marcescens, Citrobacter amalonaticus*.

Phenotypic resistance profile of ESBL isolates

Antibiotics resistance profile of ESBL-producing pathogens is depicted in Fig. 1. All ESBL-producing isolates showed 100% resistance to ampicillin, and to all cephalosporins including cephalothin, cefazolin, ceftriaxone and cefepime. Low resistance was recorded to carbapenems. Resistance ranged between 2.5% to meropenem, ertapenem and 10% to imipenem. Among the β-lactam/β-lactamase inhibitor combinations, 9% were resistant to piperacillin/tazobactam, whereas 99% were resistant to amoxicillin/clavulanic acid. Regarding aminoglycosides, all the isolates were susceptible to amikacin, and 24.4% of which were resistant to gentamicin. The resistance prevalence to other classes of antibiotics namely, cefoxitin, nitrofurantoin, trimethoprim/sulfamethoxazole and ciprofloxacin was 19.4, 13, 59.7 and 36%, respectively.

Molecular genotyping profile of ESBL isolates

110 ESBL producing bacterial isolates representing 95 *E. coli*, 13 *K. Pneumonia*, one *Citrobacter koseri* and one *Enterobacter cloacae* were randomly selected and characterized with PCR for genes encoding resistance (Fig. 2). Of these, the highest resistance ($n = 65$, 59%) was

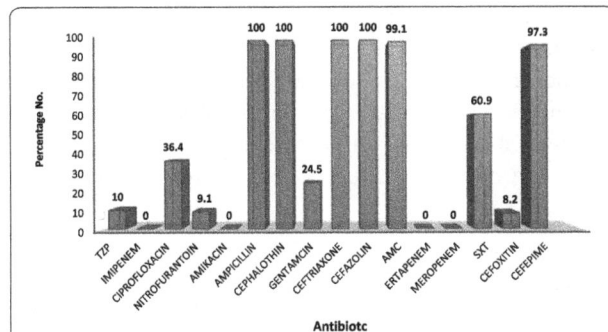

Fig. 2 Detection of ^{bla}SHV, blaTEM and ^{bla}CTX-M-G (1,2,8,9, &25) antibiotic resistance genes in 110 ESBL Enterobacteriaceae pathogens isolated from children with UTIs. Representative samples are shown. Multiplex PCR was performed for detection of CTX-M groups while monoplex PCR was used for detection of TEM and SHV. The amplification products of each isolate were run on the same lane for detection of bla genes. Lane 1: ^{bla}TEM, blaSHV& ^{bla}CTX-MG1; Lane 2: ^{bla}TEM, ^{bla}SHV & bla CTX-M-G1: Lane 3: ^{bla}CTXM-G9; Lane 4: ^{bla}SHV & ^{bla}CTXM-G1; Lane 5: ^{bla}SHV; Lane6: ^{bla}CTX-MG1; Lane 7: ^{bla}CTXM-G2; Lane 8; ^{bla}CTXM-G8, Lane 9: ^{bla}TEM &^{bla}CTXM-G8; Lane 10, ^{bla} TEM, ^{bla}SHV &^{bla}CTXM-G8; Lane 11: ^{bla}SHV & ^{bla}CTXM-G1; Lane 12: ^{bla}NCTC 13,351 *E. coli* Positive control for ^{bla}TEM, NCTC 13368 *K. pneumonia* positive control for ^{bla}SHV, NCTC 13461 *E. coli* positive control for ^{bla}CTX-MG1: Lane 13: ATCC 25922 *E. coli* negative control

encoded by ^{bla} CTX-M genes: ^{bla} CTX-MG1 (89.2%), ^{bla} CTX-MG9 (7.7%), and ^{bla} CTX-MG2 (0.9%) and ^{bla} CTX-MG8 (1.5%). ^{bla} TEM and ^{bla} SHV genes were detected in 2.7 and 0.9% of the isolates, respectively. 37.3% of bacteria harbored multiple *bla* genes ($\geq$ two genes). Two *bla* genes were detected in 20 (18.2%) *E. coli* and 3 (3.2%) of *K. pneoumoniae* isolates. 77% of *K. pneoumoniae* and 6.3% of *E. coli* isolates were harboring three *bla* genes. While majority of the ESBL *E. coli* resistance was encoded by one gene, ^{bla}CTX-M-G1 58 (61.1%), resistance in *k. pneoumoniae* isolates was encoded by ^{bla}SHV, ^{bla}TEM and ^{bla}CTX-MG1 genes (46.2%) concurrently (Fig. 3). ^{bla}CTX-M-G25 was not detected in any isolate.

Correlation between phenotypic and genotypic profiles

The antibiotic resistance outcomes (resistance or susceptible [i.e., binary]) were cross- tabulated with the six detected ESBL genes using kappa statistics (Table 2). A significant association ($p < 0.05$) were found between the presence of TEM, nitrofurantoin and trimethoprim/ sulfamethoxazole; SHV and nitrofurantoin; CTXM-G2 and piperacillin/tazobactam. The presence of individual ESBL genes was not significantly different ($P > 0.05$, Pearson Chi- square test) by nationality or age.

Clustering and similarity of ESBL-positive isolates

Cluster analysis was used to study similarity among individual *E.coli* ($n = 94$) and *K. pneumoniae* ($n = 13$) isolates

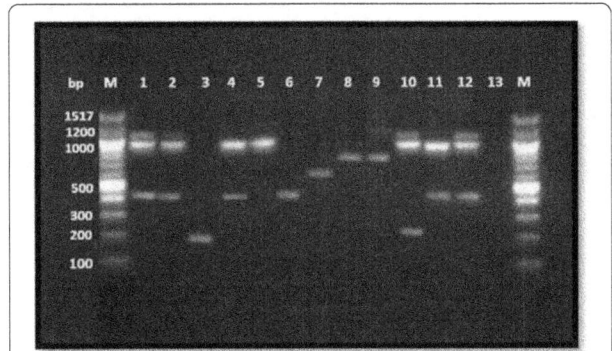

Fig. 1 Antimicrobial resistance profile of 201 ESBL producing bacteria isolated from children (age 0 to 15 years) with UTI. Isolates were tested for antibiotics resistance against 16 clinically relevant antibiotics using phoenix NMIC/ID-5 panel (BD Biosciences, Heidelberg, Germany). The figure depicts the percentage of isolates with resistance to each of the antibiotics. TZP: piperacillin/ tazobactam; SXT: trimethoprim/sulfamethoxazole; AMC: Amoxicillin/clavulanic acid

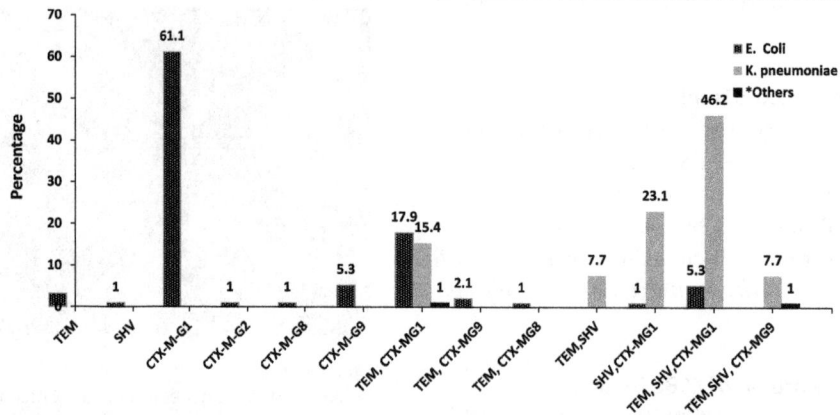

Fig. 3 Distribution of bla genes among ESBL Enterobacteriaceae obtained from urine samples of children with lower urinary tract infection

according to presence and absence of 7 genes ([bla] TEM, [bla] SHV, [bla] CTXM -G 1, [bla] CTXM- G2, [bla] CTXM G8, [bla] CTXM G9 & [bla] CTXM G25). The *E. coli* positive isolates were distributed into one of the three main branches A, B and C (Fig. 4a), then sub grouped into 11 clusters (A1, A2, A3, A4 A5, B1, B2, B3, B4, B5 and C1). Most of the *E. coli* isolates clustered in A2 (61.7%) which includes only CTXM-G1 enzyme.Around 20.2% clustered in A5 (which includes a combination of TEM and CTXM-G1 enzymes. On the other hand, *K. pneoumoniae* were distributed into one of the two main branches A and B (Fig. 4b), then sub grouped into five clusters (A1, A2, B1, B2 and B3), with the main cluster being B2 (46.2%) which represent combination of TEM, SHV and CTXM-G1 type enzymes.

Discussion

Out of a 635 Enterobacteriaceae isolated from urine samples obtained from a cohort of children with UTI, 201 (31.7%) were found to be ESBL. *E. coli* species was the most prevalent representing 83% (*n* = 166) of the isolates, followed by *K. pneumoniae* which represented 11% (*n* = 22). This is in agreement with other studies including a recent one from Sri Lanka [25] in which *E. coli* and *Klebsiella* species represented 86.8 and 13.1% of UTI infections among adult patients. Expectedly, ESBL was more predominant among females than males with a ratio of 4.9 to 1. It has been frequently reported thatU-TIs occur far more frequently in girls than in boys during the first few months of life, presumably due to the shorter length of the female urethra [26, 27]. The most affected group of our study were the children ranging in

Table 2 Measure of agreement between resistance of antibiotics and presence of ESBL genes by cross tabulation Kappa statistics

Antibiotic	Number of resistance / Kappa significant value					
	TEM	SHV	CTXM-G1	CTXM-G2	CTXM-G8	CTXM-G9
Piperacillin/Tazobactam	11/0.186	11/0.253	11/0.5	11/0.003	11/0.634	11/0.328
Ciprofloxacin	40/0.06	40/0.654	40/0.401	40/0.2	40/0.9	40/0.9
Nitrofurantoin	12/0.021	12/0.000	12/0.825	12/0.7	12/0.074	12/0.3
Gentamicin	28/0.2	28/0.843	28/0.08	28/0.4	12/404	12/0.9
Trimethoprim/Sulfamethoxazole	67/0.02	67/0.727	67/0.2	67/0.08	67/0.75	67/0.396
Cefoxitin	11/0.180	11/0.538	11/0.7	11/0.057	11/0.057	11/0.8

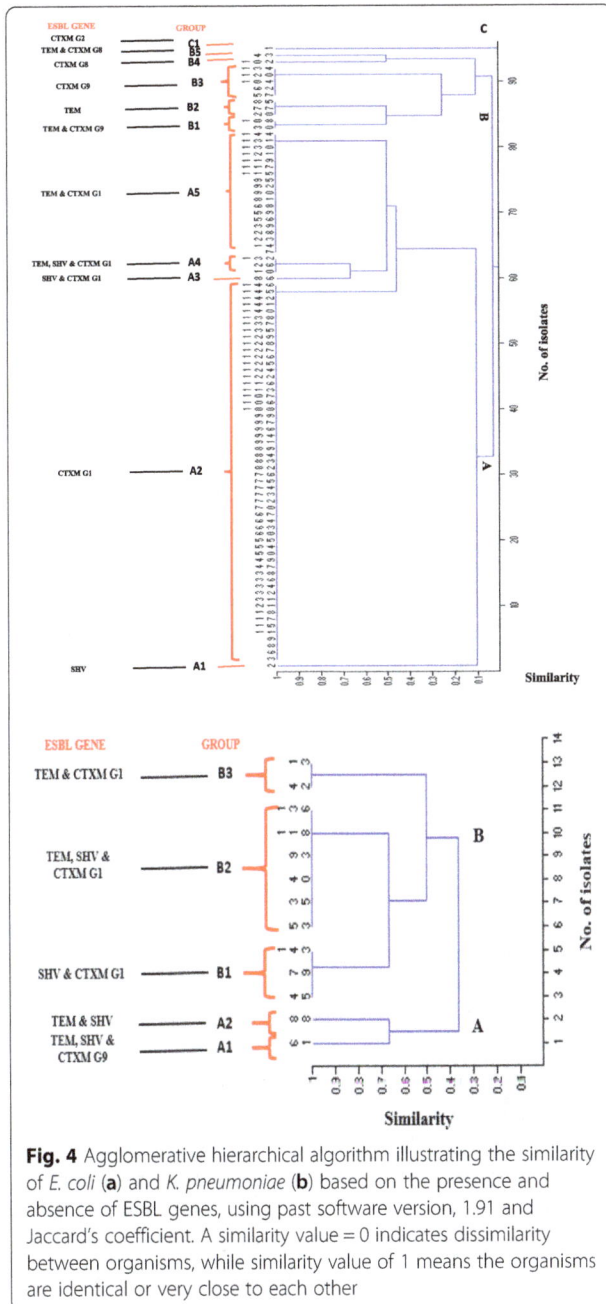

Fig. 4 Agglomerative hierarchical algorithm illustrating the similarity of *E. coli* (**a**) and *K. pneumoniae* (**b**) based on the presence and absence of ESBL genes, using past software version, 1.91 and Jaccard's coefficient. A similarity value = 0 indicates dissimilarity between organisms, while similarity value of 1 means the organisms are identical or very close to each other

gene, that contributes to the dissemination of CTX-M enzymes to the community and could cause extra horizontal transmission in healthcare facilities [32]. In busy health care facilities, especially in developing countries, the rapid turnover of patients to accommodate multiple patients' treatment could lead to breaching of infection control measures, such as compliance with hand hygiene, which could lead to this horizontal transmission of resistant bacteria from one patient to another. Unfortunately, we could not compare our findings to others from the region due to the scarcity of published data. However, it has been globally reported that the predominant genotype of ESBL-producing *E. coli* and *K. pneumonia* has changed from TEM and/or SHV to CTX-M-1 since 2006 [33, 34], which seems to be the trend in Qatar. Interestingly, our results indicated that three [bla] genes ([bla]SHV, [bla]TEM and [bla]CTX-MG1/[bla]CTX-MG9) were concurrently detected in 77% of *K. pneoumoniae isolates*, whereas only 6.3% of the *E. coli* isolates had combinations of the three genes (Fig. 3). On the other hand, two out of seven [bla] genes were simultaneously detected in 18.2 and 3.2% of *E. coli* and *K. pneumonia*, respectively. These results indicate different genotypic profile of ESBL resistance between *E. coli* and *K. pneumoniae* in urine samples which might indicate a high transfer of genes among *K. pneumoniae* than *E. coli*. Concerning the cephalosporins, all ESBL-producing isolates showed 100% resistance to ampicillin, cephalothin, cefazolin, ceftriaxone and 97.3% resistance to cefepime. This finding coincided with a study carried in intensive care unit (ICU) among adult patients at HMC, Qatar, on respiratory tract and blood samples [35]. No resistance in ESBL-producing isolates were observed against amikacin, ertapenem, meropenem and imipenem. Among the β-lactam/β-lactamase inhibitor combinations, 10% were resistant to piperacillin/tazobactam, whereas 99.1% were resistant to amoxicillin/clavulanic acid. The clinical isolates presented 24.5% resistance to gentamicin compared with 100% susceptibility to amikacin among aminoglycosides. Similarly, these findings concur with the findings from the aforementioned study in ICU patients, [35] with an exception of piperacillin/tazobactam resistance which was reported at 22% in ICU adult patients compared to 10% in pediatrics with UTI. Resistance to piperacillin/tazobactam and ciprofloxacin were significantly lower in our study (10 and 36.4% respectively) compared with another one from Kingdom Saud Arabia (KSA) in a hospital at Dammam-Eastern province, where resistance reached63.2 and 84.6%, respectively [30]. Authors attributed high resistance to these antibiotics due to the misuse of ciprofloxacin and restriction of aminoglycosides among adult in Dammam hospital. Whereas, ciprofloxacin is restricted for use among adult patients at HMC

age from 0 to 5 years (70.7%), wherecolonization with *E. coli* and enterococci is known to diminish after 5 years of age [26].

Molecular genotyping of ESBL-positive isolates showed that the highest resistance was due to the presence of [bla] CTX-M genes (59%), particularly [bla] CTX-MG1 (89.2%). [bla] TEM and [bla] SHV genes contributed to only 2.7 and 0.9% of ESBL resistance, which is consistent with previous reports from the region and around the globe [15, 28–31]. The high occurrence of [bla] CTX-MG1 gene among pediatric population suggests high dynamic transmission-ability of the plasmid-carried

and very rarely used in pediatric population (personal communication, 2017).

The resistance to oral antibiotics namely, nitrofurantoin, trimethoprim/sulfamethoxazole and ciprofloxacin was found to be 9.1, 60.9 and 36.4%, respectively. Obtained results were comparable to those observed in the Middle East region [27], which indicate rapid dissemination of multidrug resistance bacteria in the communities [15, 36]. Worldwide, previous studies have reported higher prevalence of ESBL resistance in Europe compared to United States (US), but lower than South America and Asia [37]. Our results indicate that the patterns of ESBL resistance in Qatar, at least in pediatric population, is more similar to Asia. It is worth noting that 80% of population in Qatar is expatriates; arriving mostly from countries in South East Asia. This could partially explain our findings. Cumulatively, our findings mandates the establishment of the antimicrobial stewardship program and formulation of guidelines for empirical use of prescription of antibiotics for UTI infections among pediatric population.

We found that the majority of ESBL (156, 77.6%) producers were multidrug resistant (resistant to 3 or more different classes of antibiotics), with the most common resistance pattern being to amoxicillin-clavulanate, ampicillin, ciprofloxacin, Sulfamethoxazole/trimethoprim in addition to cephalosporines. Plasmids encoding ESBL resistance often carry multiple genes conferring multiple resistance, thus simultaneous resistance to fluoroquinolones, aminoglycosides, tetracyclines, and trimethoprim sulfamethoxazole [12]. Our study revealed a significant association ($p < 0.05$) between the presence of TEM, nitrofurantoin and trimethoprim/sulfamethoxazole; SHV and nitrofurantoin; CTXM-G2 and piperacillin/tazobactam resistance. Thus, in our study, the use of extended-spectrum cephalosporins, ciprofloxacin, aminoglycosides (gentamicin) and trimethoprim/sulfamethoxazole is compromised, leaving carbapenems as the therapeutic option for severe infections caused by ESBL producers. In agreement with our findings, [38] found that plasmid-mediated quinolone resistance has been associated with [bla] CTX-M genes, where genes conferring resistance to aminoglycosides and tetracycline and other [bla] genes have been found on the same plasmids as the [bla] CTXM [39]. Isolates in this study were all from pediatric patients in the community who attended emergency setting This highlights the therapeutic challenges posed by ESBL producers, particularly in the UTI treatment of community-onset [40].

Using seven genes to run agglomerative hierarchical algorithm analysis [21–24] our study revealed eleven clonal clusters among the 94 tested E. coli isolates. Clonally related strains of cluster A2 were responsible for the predominant UTI in pediatrics population 67.1% (58/

94), which produce only CTXM-G1 type enzyme, followed by A5 (20.2%), which produce a combination of TEM and CTXM-G1type enzymes. Five clonal clusters were detected among K. pneumoniae with the main cluster B2 producing concurrently a combination of three enzyme types SHV, TEM and CTXM-G1. Whole plasmid sequencing for representative isolates from each cluster can be very helpful to better understand the relatedness and typing differences between the clusters and elucidating further information on the mechanism of resistance in these isolates. Unfortunately, similar molecular analysis of ESBL bacteria are lacking in the surrounding country. This limit our understanding of the trends and distribution of the strains, noting that more than 80% of Qatari population are expats that arrive from MENA region and South East Asia.

Conclusions

Although ESBL-producing members of Enterobacteriaceae have been reported in all Arabian Gulf region, very limited data is available about the genetic makeup encoding for such resistance. This is the first study among pediatric population in the state of Qatar that demonstrate the correlation between genetic and phenotypic profile of ESBL producing Enterobacteriaceae. The study highlights an escalated problem of ESBL resistance in Enterobacteriaceae causing UTI in pediatric population in Qatar. Resistance was predominantly mediated by CTX-MG1-type enzymes. The use of cephalosporins, aminoglycosides (gentamicin) and trimethoprim/sulfamethoxazole is compromised in Qatar among pediatric population with UTI, leaving carbapenems and amikacin as the therapeutic option for severe infections caused by ESBL producers. The negative impact of extensive use of carpabenemes could lead to carbapenamase resistant Enterobacteriaceae. This mandates further epidemiological studies and implementation of regulatory programs to reduce spread of ESBL producing Enterobacteriaceae in the community. Further next generation sequencing (NGS) studies are necessary for a more comprehensive analysis of ESBL variants.

Abbreviations

CP: Cerebral palsy; DDST: Double disc synergy test; ESBL: Extended-spectrum beta-lactamase; GCC: Gulf cooperation council; GNB: Negative bacteria; HMC: Hamad medical corporation; MRC: Medical research centre; NGS: Next generation sequencing; UTI: Urinary tract infection

Acknowledgements

This work was funded by Qatar University Grant No. QUUG-BRC-2017-2 to Dr. Nahla Omer Ahmed Eltai.

Authors' contributions

NOE, HMY, AAA, KA, and AD designed the study and drafted the manuscript. NOE, EW, SH and AD performed the experimental work. NO and HMY analyzed the data. All authors read and approved the final manuscript.

Competing interests

The authors declare that they have no competing interests.

Author details

[1]Biomedical Research Center, Qatar University, P.O. Box 2713, Doha, Qatar. [2]Pediatrics Department, Hamad Medical Corporation, Doha, Qatar. [3]Department of Laboratory Medicine and Pathology, Hamad Medical Corporation, Doha, Qatar. [4]College of Health Sciences, Qatar University, Doha, Qatar.

References

1. Talbot GH, Bradley J, Edwards Jr JE, Gilbert D, Scheld M, Bartlett JG: Bad bugs need drugs: an update on the development pipeline from the antimicrobial availability task force of the Infectious Diseases Society of America. Clin Infect Dis 2006, 42(5):657–668.
2. Goyal A, Prasad K, Prasad A, Gupta S, Ghoshal U, Ayyagari A: Extended spectrum beta-lactamases in Escherichia coli & Klebsiella pneumoniae & associated risk factors. 2009.
3. Sharma M, Pathak S, SrivaStava P. Prevalence and antibiogram of extended Spectrum β-lactamase (ESBL) producing gram negative bacilli and further molecular characterization of ESBL producing Escherichia coli and Klebsiella spp. J Clin Diagn Res. 2013;7(10):2173.
4. Nakamura T, Komatsu M, Yamasaki K, Fukuda S, Miyamoto Y, Higuchi T, Ono T, Nishio H, Sueyoshi N, Kida K. Epidemiology of Escherichia coli, Klebsiella species, and Proteus mirabilis strains producing extended-spectrum β-lactamases from clinical samples in the Kinki region of Japan. Am J Clin Pathol. 2012;137(4):620–6.
5. Birgy A, Mariani-Kurkdjian P, Bidet P, Doit C, Genel N, Courroux C, Arlet G, Bingen E. Characterization of extended-spectrum-beta-lactamase-producing Escherichia coli strains involved in maternal-fetal colonization: prevalence of E. Coli ST131. J Clin Microbiol. 2013;51(6):1727–32.
6. Lukac PJ, Bonomo RA, Logan LK. Extended-Spectrum β-lactamase–producing Enterobacteriaceae in children: old foe, emerging threat. Clin Infect Dis: Offic Public Infect Dis Soc Am. 2015;60(9):1389–97.
7. Bush K. Alarming β-lactamase-mediated resistance in multidrug-resistant Enterobacteriaceae. Curr Opin Microbiol. 2010;13(5):558–64.
8. Paterson DL, Bonomo RA. Extended-spectrum β-lactamases: a clinical update. Clin Microbiol Rev. 2005;18(4):657–86.
9. Pitout JD, Laupland KB. Extended-spectrum β-lactamase-producing Enterobacteriaceae: an emerging public-health concern. Lancet Infect Dis. 2008;8(3):159–66.
10. Stedt J, Bonnedahl J, Hernandez J, Waldenström J, McMahon BJ, Tolf C, Olsen B, Drobni M. Carriage of CTX-M type extended spectrum β-lactamases (ESBLs) in gulls across Europe. Acta Vet Scand. 2015;57(1):74.
11. Lahlaoui H, Khalifa A, Haj B, Moussa MB. Epidemiology of Enterobacteriaceae producing CTX-M type extended spectrum β-lactamase (ESBL). Medecine et maladies infectieuses. 2014;44(9):400–4.
12. Malloy AM, Campos JM. Extended-spectrum beta-lactamases: a brief clinical update. Pediatr Infect Dis J. 2011;30(12):1092–3.
13. Bakshi R, Walia G, Shikha J. Prevalence of extended spectrum β-lactamases in multidrug resistant strains of gram negative bacilli. J Acad Indus Res. 2013;1:558–60.
14. CDC. Antibiotic resistance threats in the United States, 2013. In: Centers for disease control and prevention USA; 2013.
15. Zowawi HM, Balkhy HH, Walsh TR, Paterson DL. β-Lactamase production in key gram-negative pathogen isolates from the Arabian peninsula. Clin Microbiol Rev. 2013;26(3):361–80.
16. Chandramohan L, Revell PA. Prevalence and molecular characterization of extended-spectrum-β-lactamase-producing Enterobacteriaceae in a

pediatric patient population. Antimicrob Agents Chemother. 2012;56(9): 4765–70.
17. Eltai NO, Abdfarag EA, Al-Romaihi H, Wehedy E, Mahmoud MH, Alawad OK, Al-Hajri MM, Al Thani AA, Yassine HM. Antibiotic resistance profile of commensal Escherichia coli isolated from broiler chickens in Qatar. J Food Prot. 2017;81(2):302–7.
18. CLSI. Clinical and laboratory standards institute. Performance standards for antimicrobial susceptibility testing. M100S. 2016;26:1–129.
19. Woodford N, Fagan EJ, Ellington MJ. Multiplex PCR for rapid detection of genes encoding CTX-M extended-spectrum β-lactamases. J Antimicrob Chemother. 2005;57(1):154–5.
20. Bora A, Hazarika NK, Shukla SK, Prasad KN, Sarma JB, Ahmed G. Prevalence of blaTEM, blaSHV and blaCTX-M genes in clinical isolates of Escherichia coli and Klebsiella pneumoniae from Northeast India. Indian J Pathol Microbiol. 2014;57(2):249.
21. Ahmed SF, Ali MMM, Mohamed ZK, Moussa TA, Klena JD. Fecal carriage of extended-spectrum β-lactamases and AmpC-producing Escherichia coli in a Libyan community. Ann Clin Microbiol Antimicrob. 2014;13(1):22.
22. Kamatchi C, Magesh H, Sekhar U, Vaidyanathan R. Identification of clonal clusters of Klebsiella pneumoniae isolates from Chennai by extended spectrum beta lactamase genotyping and antibiotic resistance phenotyping analysis. Am J Infect Dis. 2009;5(2):74–82.
23. Chapman TA, Wu X-Y, Barchia I, Bettelheim KA, Driesen S, Trott D, Wilson M, Chin JJ-C. Comparison of virulence gene profiles of Escherichia coli strains isolated from healthy and diarrheic swine. Appl Environ Microbiol. 2006; 72(7):4782–95.
24. Hammer Ø, Harper D, Ryan P. Paleontological Statistics Software Package for Education and Data Analysis. Palaeontol Electron. 2001;4:9.
25. Fernando M, Luke W, Miththinda J, Wickramasinghe R, Sebastiampillai B, Gunathilake M, Silva F, Premaratna R. Extended spectrum beta lactamase producing organisms causing urinary tract infections in Sri Lanka and their antibiotic susceptibility pattern–a hospital based cross sectional study. BMC Infect Dis. 2017;17(1):138.
26. Hellerstein S. Urinary tract infections in children: why they occur and how to prevent them. Am Fam Physician. 1998;57(10):2440–6. 2452-2444
27. Zeyaullah M, Kaul V. Prevalence of urinary tract infection and antibiotic resistance pattern in Saudi Arabia population. Global J Biol, Agricult Health Sci. 2015;4(1):206–14.
28. Zhao W-H, Hu Z-Q. Epidemiology and genetics of CTX-M extended-spectrum β-lactamases in gram-negative bacteria. Crit Rev Microbiol. 2013; 39(1):79–101.
29. Potz NA, Hope R, Warner M, Johnson AP, Livermore DM. Prevalence and mechanisms of cephalosporin resistance in Enterobacteriaceae in London and south-East England. J Antimicrob Chemother. 2006;58(2):320–6.
30. Hassan H, Abdalhamid B. Molecular characterization of extended-spectrum beta-lactamase producing Enterobacteriaceae in a Saudi Arabian tertiary hospital. J Infect Dev Countries. 2014;8(03):282–8.
31. Bindayna K, Khanfar HS, Senok AC, Botta GA. Predominance of CTX-M genotype among extended spectrum beta lactamase isolates in a tertiary hospital in Saudi Arabia. Saudi Med J. 2010;31(8):859–63.
32. Mendonça N, Leitão J, Manageiro V, Ferreira E, Caniça M. Portugal ARSPi: spread of extended-spectrum β-lactamase CTX-M-producing Escherichia coli clinical isolates in community and nosocomial environments in Portugal. Antimicrob Agents Chemother. 2007;51(6):1946–55.
33. Cantón R, Coque TM. The CTX-M β-lactamase pandemic. Curr Opin Microbiol. 2006;9(5):466–75.
34. Livermore DM, Canton R, Gniadkowski M, Nordmann P, Rossolini GM, Arlet G, Ayala J, Coque TM, Kern-Zdanowicz I, Luzzaro F. CTX-M: changing the face of ESBLs in Europe. J Antimicrob Chemother. 2007;59(2):165–74.
35. Ahmed AMS, Sultan AA, Deshmukh A, Acharya A, Elmi AA, Bansal D, Ibrahim E, Hamid JM, Ahmed MAS, Bilal NE. Antimicrobial susceptibility and molecular epidemiology of extended-spectrum beta-lactamase-producing Enterobacteriaceae from intensive care units at Hamad Medical Corporation, Qatar. Antimicrob Resist Infect Control. 2016;5(1):4.
36. Balkhy HH, Assiri AM, Al Mousa H, Al-Abri SS, Al-Katheeri H, Alansari H, Abdulrazzaq NM, Aidara-Kane A, Pittet D, Erlacher-Vindel E. The strategic plan for combating antimicrobial resistance in gulf cooperation council states. J Infect Public Health. 2016;9(4):375–85.
37. Giamarellou H. Multidrug resistance in gram-negative bacteria that produce extended-spectrum β-lactamases (ESBLs). Clin Microbiol Infect. 2005;11(s4):1–16.

38. Jacoby GA, Walsh KE, Mills DM, Walker VJ, Oh H, Robicsek A, Hooper DC.
     qnrB, another plasmid-mediated gene for quinolone resistance. Antimicrob
     Agents Chemother. 2006;50(4):1178–82.
39. Boyd DA, Tyler S, Christianson S, McGeer A, Muller MP, Willey BM, Bryce E,
     Gardam M, Nordmann P, Mulvey MR. Complete nucleotide sequence of a
     92-kilobase plasmid harboring the CTX-M-15 extended-spectrum beta-
     lactamase involved in an outbreak in long-term-care facilities in Toronto,
     Canada. Antimicrob Agents Chemother. 2004;48(10):3758–64.
40. Heffernan H, Dyet K, Woodhouse R, Williamson D: Antimicrobial
     susceptibility and molecular epidemiology of extended-spectrum β-
     lactamase producing Enterobacteriaceae in New Zealand, 2013. 2014.

13

Implementing an infection control and prevention program decreases the incidence of healthcare-associated infections and antibiotic resistance in a Russian neuro-ICU

Ksenia Ershova[1]*[iD], Ivan Savin[2], Nataliya Kurdyumova[2], Darren Wong[3], Gleb Danilov[4], Michael Shifrin[5], Irina Alexandrova[6], Ekaterina Sokolova[2], Nadezhda Fursova[7], Vladimir Zelman[1,8] and Olga Ershova[9]

Abstract

Background: The impact of infection prevention and control (IPC) programs in limited resource countries such as Russia are largely unknown due to a lack of reliable data. The aim of this study is to evaluate the effect of an IPC program with respect to healthcare associated infection (HAI) prevention and to define the incidence of HAIs in a Russian ICU.

Methods: A pioneering IPC program was implemented in a neuro-ICU at Burdenko Neurosurgery Institute in 2010 and included hand hygiene, surveillance, contact precautions, patient isolation, and environmental cleaning measures. This prospective observational cohort study lasted from 2011 to 2016, included high-risk ICU patients, and evaluated the dynamics of incidence, etiological spectrum, and resistance profile of four types of HAIs, including subgroup analysis of device-associated infections. Survival analysis compared patients with and without HAIs.

Results: We included 2038 high-risk patients. By 2016, HAI cumulative incidence decreased significantly for respiratory HAIs (36.1% vs. 24.5%, *p*-value = 0.0003), urinary-tract HAIs (29.1% vs. 21.3%, p-value = 0.0006), and healthcare-associated ventriculitis and meningitis (HAVM) (16% vs. 7.8%, p-value = 0.004). The incidence rate of EVD-related HAVM dropped from 22.2 to 13.5 cases per 1000 EVD-days. The proportion of invasive isolates of *Klebsiella pneumoniae* and *Acinetobacter baumannii* resistant to carbapenems decreased 1.7 and 2 fold, respectively. HAVM significantly impaired survival and independently increasing the probability of death by 1.43.

Conclusions: The implementation of an evidence-based IPC program in a middle-income country (Russia) was highly effective in HAI prevention with meaningful reductions in antibiotic resistance.

Keywords: Cross infection, Intensive care unit, Infection control, Drug resistance, Survival analysis

* Correspondence: ksenia.ershova@skolkovotech.ru
[1]Center for Data-Intensive Biotechnology and Biomedicine, Skolkovo Institute
of Science and Technology, Moscow, Russia
Full list of author information is available at the end of the article

Background

Infection prevention and control (IPC) programs have been repeatedly shown to be effective at decreasing the incidence of healthcare-associated infections (HAIs). A landmark paper on this topic in 1985 showed a 32% decrease in the hospital infection rate after 5 years of an ongoing IPC program [1]. In 1999 the CDC identified seven key evidence-based elements of an effective IPC strategy including voluntary participation of all hospitals, standardized case definitions and protocols, targeted interventions for high risk patient populations, risk adjusted comparisons of infection rates across hospitals, education and adequacy of resources, and feedback to healthcare providers [2]. The elements of an IPC program have since been significantly updated, forming the concept of "multimodal strategy" [3].

To prevent HAIs, the WHO recommends implementing an IPC program in every acute healthcare facility [4]. However, according to the most-recent survey, only 29% of 133 countries surveyed have IPC programs in all tertiary hospitals [3]. In Russia, IPC programs are also not widely used. The rate of HAIs in Russia has been heavily underestimated for decades. In 2016 it was reported to be approximately 0.08% (24,771 [5] cases per 31.3 million hospitalized patients [6]) yet a concurrent meta-analysis which included Russia reported the prevalence of HAIs at 15.5% [7]. According to the latest World Bank report, Russia has a gross national income per capita of US $9720, corresponding to a middle-income country [8].

Besides significant underreporting of HAIs, Russia faces other challenges in establishing IPC programs, such as lack of commitment, punishment-based HAI reporting systems, lack of expertise, and inadequate allocation of resources [9]. Since the dissolution of the Soviet Union, Russia has made some progress in adopting the IPC programs [10]. A pioneering Russian hospital where an evidence-based IPC program was implemented in 2010 is Burdenko National Medical Research Center of Neurosurgery (NSI) in Moscow. Herein we report the results of our study which aimed to evaluate the impact of this program on HAI prevention in the ICU.

Methods

Study design and healthcare facility

This study was a prospective observational cohort study with annual interim data analyses. The study was done in the neuro-ICU department at NSI in Moscow, Russia. NSI is a specialized neurosurgical hospital with 300 beds that cares for approximately 8000 patients per year, 95% of whom undergo surgery. The NSI ICU has 38 single-bed rooms with a flow of approximately 3000 patients per year.

Infection prevention and control program

In September 2010, an IPC program was first set up in the neuro-ICU, inspired by the results of the European HELICS-ICU program [11]. The protocols for our IPC program were adopted from the 2007 CDC guidelines [12] and included three key components: education, infection prevention measures, and surveillance (Fig. 1). The surveillance software was designed in-house and integrated in the NSI electronic health record system [13]. At the time of initiation of this program, an antibiotic stewardship program was in existence at our facility. However, during the study period there were refinements to this program and coordination of antibiotic stewardship initiatives with the infection control program.

Patients

We studied a high-risk patient population, which we defined as patients who required > 48 h of care in the neurosurgical ICU. All of these patients were qualified to participate in the study until discharge or death. Enrollment period was between January 1st, 2011 and December 31st, 2016. Following ICU discharge, the parameters of total length of stay and outcome were collected.

To identify cases of HAIs, we used the 2008 CDC definition [14]. Four types of HAIs were surveilled: bloodstream, respiratory and urinary-tract infections, and healthcare-associated ventriculitis and meningitis (HAVM). We specifically focused on the subgroup of device-related infections, such as central line-associated bloodstream infections (CLABSI), ventilator-associated pneumonia (VAP), catheter-associated urinary-tract infections (CAUTI), and external ventricular drain (EVD)-associated HAVM. In accordance with the CDC case definitions, an infection was considered device-related if the patient had a device in place for > 48 h prior to developing the HAI [12].

In addition to HAIs, we monitored superficial surgical-site infections (SSSI) after neurosurgery, and ICU-acquired intestinal dysfunction. The latter was clinically defined by the presence of one or more of the following gastrointestinal symptoms, as delineated in the literature [15]: vomiting, diarrhea, absence or abnormality of bowel sounds, bowel dilation, gastrointestinal bleeding, or increased nasogastric aspirate volume (> 500 ml/day).

Data collection and preprocessing

Data was collected prospectively on a daily basis and incorporated 54 different characteristics (Additional file 1: Table S1). The spectrum and susceptibility profile of identified organisms causing the HAIs was built for each infection type. In January of each year, interim analysis was performed, and the results were then disseminated to NSI staff to encourage compliance with IPC measures.

Microbiological analysis

Clinical samples were collected form patients with HAIs and delivered to the microbiological laboratory without

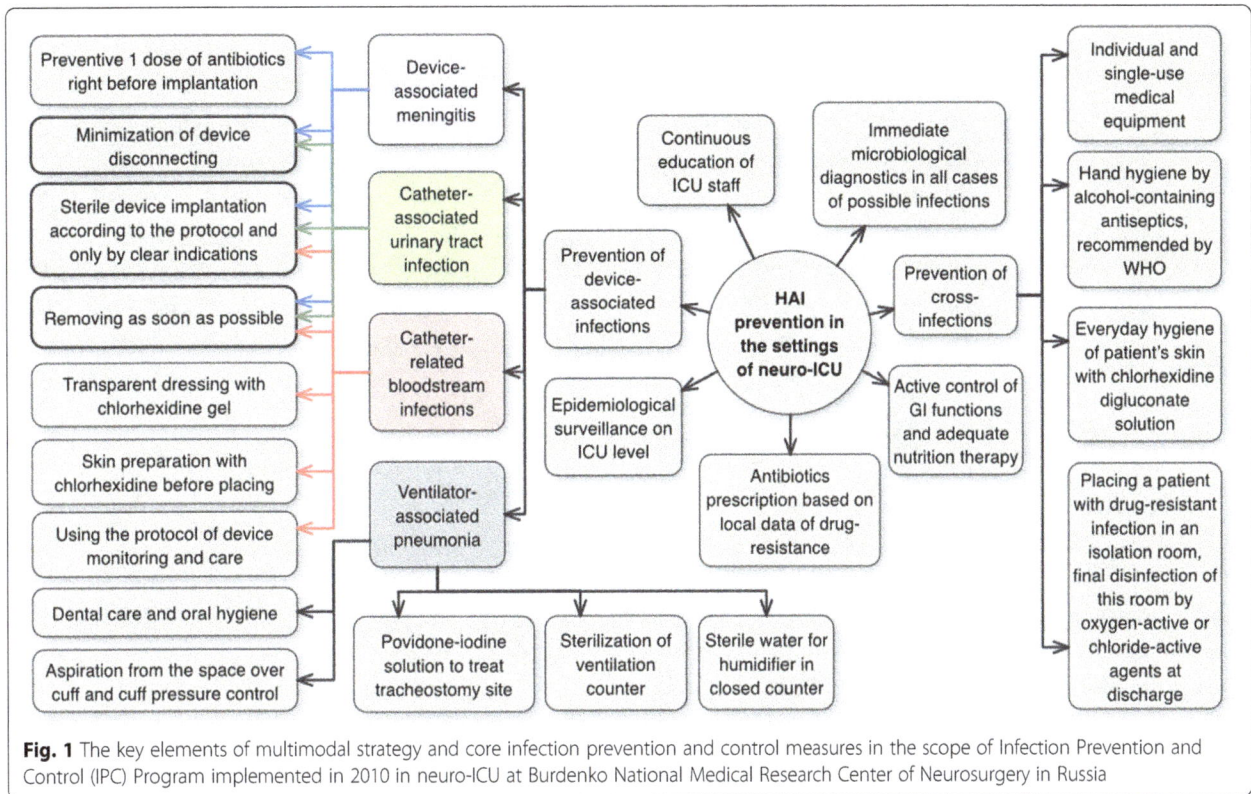

Fig. 1 The key elements of multimodal strategy and core infection prevention and control measures in the scope of Infection Prevention and Control (IPC) Program implemented in 2010 in neuro-ICU at Burdenko National Medical Research Center of Neurosurgery in Russia

delay. Blood and CSF samples were processed using BD BACTEC (Becton, Dickinson and Company, USA). All samples of pure bacterial cultures underwent automated identification by VITEK®2 (Biomerieux, France) with standard AST Cards. Selected samples of pure bacterial cultures were subsequently identified by MALDI-TOF MS, MALDI Biotyper® (Bruker Daltonik GmbH, Germany). Minimal inhibitory concentrations obtained from VITEK®2 were interpreted in accordance with the current CLSI guidelines [16]. A profile of antibiotic resistance for each strain was built using the WHONET software [17].

Statistical analysis

Statistical analysis was performed in Python3.6 using StatsModels [18] and Scipy [19]. Categorical variables for dichotomous events were reported as number of events of one category with percentage and 95% confidence interval (CI) for binomial distribution. Continuous variables were reported as a median value with first and third quartiles (Q1; Q3). Incidence of HAIs was calculated as a number of cases per 100 high-risk patients or as a number of cases per 1000 patient-days. DA-HAIs were measured as cases per 1000 device-days. Device utilization ratio (DUR) was calculated as proportion of device-days to patient-days. We used Chi-square test to compare binary and categorical variables and linear regression analysis to compare continuous variables over years. In survival analysis we

used Cox regression, including HAIs, diagnosis, surgeries, and preexisting characteristics. Log-rank test was used to compare survival curves. *P*-values below 0.05 were considered statistically significant.

Results

A total of 2038 patients of all ages and both genders were included in the study during 6 years (the study data set is available at https://doi.org/10.5281/zenodo.1021503). The code for data analysis is available at https://github.com/KseniaErshova/IPC_paper.git.

Study population included 50% males, 16.9% children under 18 years, and a patient median age of 46 [Q1;Q3: 26.0; 59.0] years. The patients were uniformly distributed across the years by disease types, surgery types, and patient features. However, the number of lethal outcomes and the length of stay in the ICU decreased from 2011 to 2016. The baseline characteristics of the study population for each year and averaged over the 6 years are shown in Table 1.

HAIs and patients' stay in the ICU

A median number of 344 [Q1;Q3: 330; 349] patients per year accounted for a median 6998 [Q1;Q3: 6678; 7399] patient-days per year (Additional file 1: Table S2). Since the number of patients increased from 2011 to 2016 by an average of 2.3% annually and the number of patient-days gradually decreased simultaneously by 2.7%

Table 1 Baseline characteristics of the study population by years

	Parameters	Total	2011	2012	2013	2014	2015	2016	p-value
			No of pts. (%)	No of pts. (%)	No of pts. (%)	No of pts. (%)	No of pts. (%)	No of pts. (%)	
	Patients, total	2038	313 (100%)	350 (100%)	361 (100%)	341 (100%)	326 (100%)	347 (100%)	1.000
	Children	345 (16.9%)	52 (16.6%)	57 (16.3%)	58 (16.1%)	65 (19.1%)	42 (12.9%)	71 (20.5%)	0.315
	Male gender	1020 (50%)	154 (49.2%)	184 (52.6%)	186 (51.5%)	168 (49.3%)	164 (50.3%)	164 (47.3%)	0.976
Diagnosis	Brain trauma	255 (12.5%)	43 (13.7%)	54 (15.4%)	51 (14.1%)	41 (12.0%)	28 (8.6%)	38 (11.0%)	0.192
	Brain tumor	1271 (62.4%)	185 (59.1%)	221 (63.1%)	240 (66.5%)	200 (58.7%)	209 (64.1%)	216 (62.2%)	0.911
	Congenital disorders	23 (1.1%)	4 (1.3%)	5 (1.4%)	3 (0.8%)	7 (2.1%)	2 (0.6%)	2 (0.6%)	0.436
	Vascular brain diseases	454 (22.3%)	77 (24.6%)	60 (17.1%)	63 (17.5%)	89 (26.1%)	80 (24.5%)	85 (24.5%)	0.066
	Other diseases	29 (1.4%)	3 (1.0%)	10 (2.9%)	4 (1.1%)	4 (1.2%)	4 (1.2%)	4 (1.2%)	0.302
Surgeries	Craniotomy	1537 (75.4%)	230 (73.5%)	261 (74.6%)	279 (77.3%)	262 (76.8%)	245 (75.2%)	260 (74.9%)	0.998
	INSD	650 (31.9%)	101 (32.3%)	130 (37.1%)	124 (34.3%)	112 (32.8%)	94 (28.8%)	89 (25.6%)	0.227
	Endovascular surgery	194 (9.5%)	31 (9.9%)	37 (10.6%)	26 (7.2%)	40 (11.7%)	25 (7.7%)	35 (10.1%)	0.407
	EETS	87 (4.3%)	13 (4.2%)	15 (4.3%)	15 (4.2%)	14 (4.1%)	15 (4.6%)	15 (4.3%)	1.000
	Spinal surgery	4 (0.2%)	1 (0.3%)	0 (0.0%)	0 (0.0%)	0 (0.0%)	2 (0.6%)	1 (0.3%)	0.377
	Other surgeries	873 (42.8%)	151 (48.2%)	161 (46.0%)	156 (43.2%)	146 (42.8%)	127 (39.0%)	132 (38.0%)	0.523
Outcomes	Recovery	80 (3.9%)	15 (4.8%)	14 (4.0%)	14 (3.9%)	19 (5.6%)	9 (2.8%)	9 (2.6%)	0.365
	Positive dynamics	934 (45.8%)	133 (42.5%)	153 (43.7%)	170 (47.1%)	159 (46.6%)	150 (46.0%)	169 (48.7%)	0.934
	No dynamics	210 (10.3%)	34 (10.9%)	41 (11.7%)	37 (10.2%)	30 (8.8%)	29 (8.9%)	39 (11.2%)	0.818
	Negative dynamics	505 (24.8%)	81 (25.9%)	67 (19.1%)	78 (21.6%)	92 (27.0%)	96 (29.4%)	91 (26.2%)	0.153
	Death	307 (15%)	50 (16.0%)	75 (21.4%)	62 (17.2%)	41 (12.0%)	41 (12.6%)	38 (11.0%)	0.009
		Median [Q1;Q3]	Median [Q1;Q3]	Median [Q1;Q3]	Median [Q1;Q3]	Median [Q1;Q3]	Median [Q1;Q3]	Median [Q1;Q3]	p-value
	Age, years	46 [26.0; 59.0]	44 [25.0; 57.0]	44 [25.0; 58.0]	47 [26.0; 60.0]	44 [25.0; 57.0]	50 [30.0; 59.75]	48 [24.5; 60.5]	0.099
	CCI score	3 [2.0; 5.0]	3 [2.0; 4.0]	3 [2.0; 5.0]	3 [2.0; 5.0]	3 [2.0; 4.0]	3 [2.0; 5.0]	3 [2.0; 4.0]	1.000
	Length of stay in ICU, days	10 [6.0; 22.0]	13 [7.0; 27.0]	12 [6.0; 25.0]	10 [6.0; 24.0]	8 [6.0; 22.0]	9 [6.0; 22.0]	8 [5.0; 17.0]	0.010

Abbreviations: *INSD* Implantation of neurosurgical devices, *EETS* Endoscopic endonasal transsphenoidal surgery, *CCI* Charlson comorbidity index

per year (from 6778 to 5809), an average patient spent less time in the ICU, from the median of 13 days [Q1;Q3: 7.0; 27.0] in 2011 to 8 days [Q1;Q3: 5.0; 17.0] in 2016, p-value = 0.01 (Table 1). We found that over the six-year study, the lowest percentage of DA-HAIs was in the HAVM group: 40.4% [95% CI 33.6–47.1]. The highest percentage of DA-HAIs was in healthcare-associated bloodstream infections: 86.6% [95% CI 80.4–92.7]. Thus, most healthcare-associated bloodstream infections were CLABSI, whereas less than half of HAVM cases were EVD-associated (Additional file 1: Table S3, Fig. 2).

DUR was relatively high for mechanical ventilation (0.65 [Q1;Q3: 0.65; 0.69]), central line (0.70 [Q1;Q3: 0.66; 0.76]), and urinary catheter (0.70 [Q1;Q3: 0.67; 0.72]), but low for EVD (0.12 [Q1;Q3: 0.12; 0.13]) (Additional file 1: Table S2, Fig. 2). Although, DURs varied slightly over time, we observed a significant decrease in the number of days with respiratory HAIs: from 1643 days in 2011 to 690 in 2016 (mean annual reduction rate 11.9%, p-value = 0.038), while the number of

days with VAP remained unchanged (Fig. 2a). The number of patients with HAVM and with DA-HAVM decreased significantly from 2011 to 2016 (Fig. 2d).

Incidence of healthcare-associated infections

The incidence of all-cause HAIs and DA-HAIs was analyzed. The cumulative incidence of all-cause HAIs decreased significantly for respiratory infections (from 36.1% [95% CI 30.8–41.4] in 2011 to 24.5% [95% CI 20.0–29.0] in 2016, p-value = 0.0003), urinary tract infections (from 29.07% [95% CI 24.0–34.1] in 2011 to 21.33% [95% CI 17.0–25.6], p-value = 0.0006), and HAVM (from 15.97% [95% CI 11.9–20.0] in 2011 to 7.78% [95% CI 5.0–10.6] in 2016, p-value = 0.004) (Fig. 3a, Additional file 1: Table S4). Time-adjusted incidence rate of all-cause HAIs identified a declining trend for all four types of HAIs (Fig. 3c). In the group of DA-HAIs, only the cumulative incidence of CAUTI decreased significantly, from 28.04 [95% CI 22.7–33.4] per

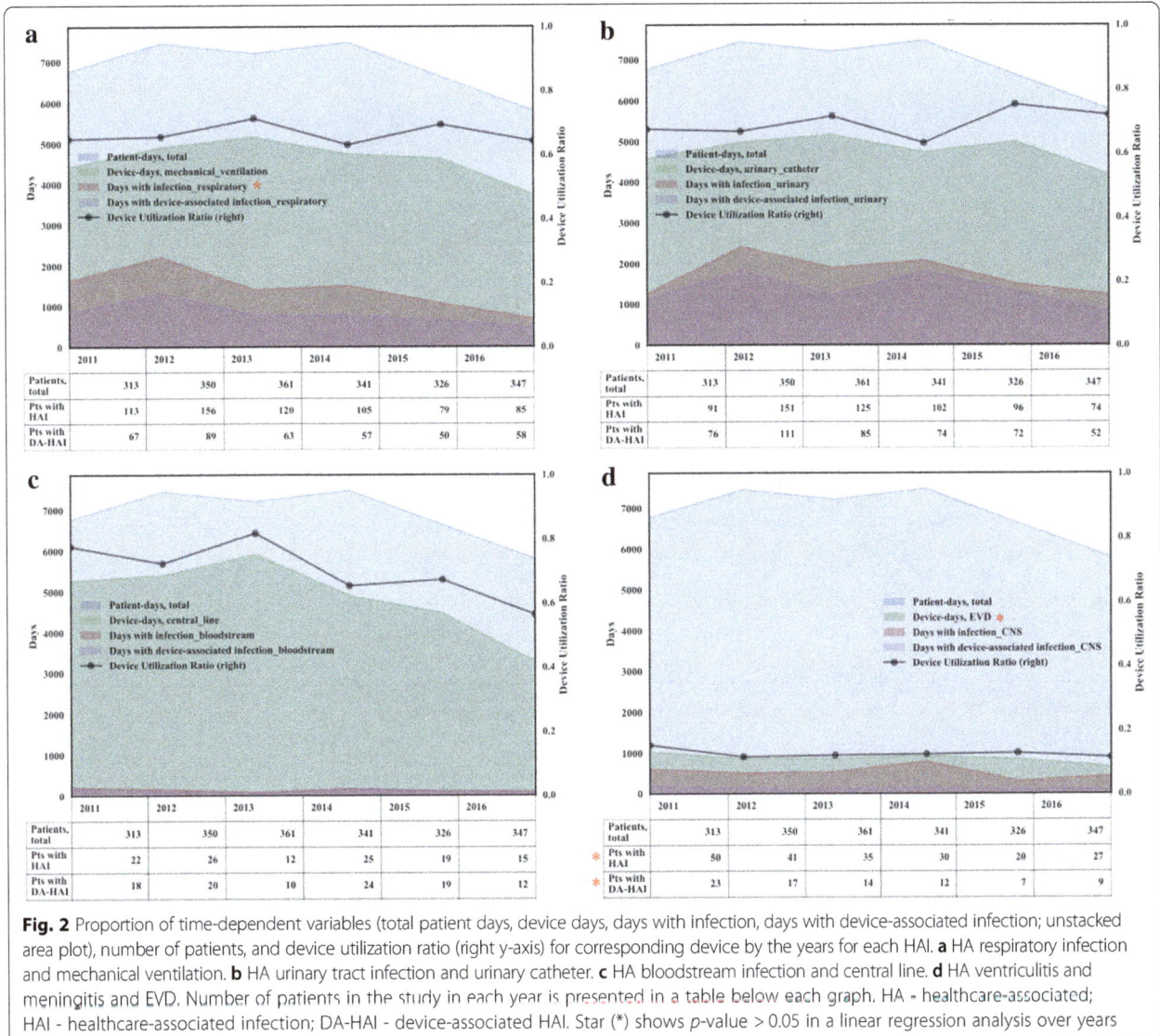

Fig. 2 Proportion of time-dependent variables (total patient days, device days, days with infection, days with device-associated infection; unstacked area plot), number of patients, and device utilization ratio (right y-axis) for corresponding device by the years for each HAI. **a** HA respiratory infection and mechanical ventilation. **b** HA urinary tract infection and urinary catheter. **c** HA bloodstream infection and central line. **d** HA ventriculitis and meningitis and EVD. Number of patients in the study in each year is presented in a table below each graph. HA - healthcare-associated; HAI - healthcare-associated infection; DA-HAI - device-associated HAI. Star (*) shows p-value > 0.05 in a linear regression analysis over years

100 patients with a urinary catheter in 2011 to 18.31 [95% CI 13.8–22.8] in 2016, p-value = 0.026 (Fig. 3b, Additional file 1: Table S4). However, once we adjusted incidence to the device-days at risk, EVD-associated HAVM demonstrated a significant drop from 2011 to 2016 (22.2 vs. 13.5 cases per 1000 EVD-days, respectively) (Fig. 3d, Additional file 1: Table S2). Risk-adjusted incidence of VAP and CAUTI also trended toward a decrease. The incidence rate of CLABSI did not change and remained at the median level of 3.7 [Q1;Q3: 3.5; 4.1] per 1000 central line-days (Fig. 3d, Additional file 1: Table S2). Of note, in 2012 the rates of respiratory and urinary HAIs as well as VAP and CAUTI spiked increasing 4–14% compare to 2011 (Additional file 1: Table S4). Therefore, the reduction in infection rate at the end of the study period in 2016 was more pronounced when compared to peak rates seen in 2012.

Microbiological profile of HAIs

We observed that in 2011–2012 approximately half of bloodstream HAIs were caused by *Klebsiella pneumoniae* and *Acinetobacter baumannii*. However, in 2016 the proportion of *K. pneumoniae* decreased to 14% from a high of 47% in 2012 and *A. baumannii* did not appear on the profile for the first time (Fig. 4a). There was a tendency for Gram-negative species to be replaced by Gram-positive species (Fig. 4a). For other HAIs, the etiological spectrum remained relatively stable over time (Additional file 1: Figures S1–S3).

By 2016 *K. pneumoniae* became more susceptible to the most-tested antibiotics: there were significantly fewer isolates resistant to cephalosporins, ciprofloxacin, and imipenem as compared to 2011 (Additional file 1: Figure S4). The proportion of imipenem-resistant *K. pneumoniae* decreased from 34.5% [95% CI 29.9–39.1] in 2011 to 20.2% [95% CI 15.6–24.8], p-value < 0.001 (Fig. 4b).

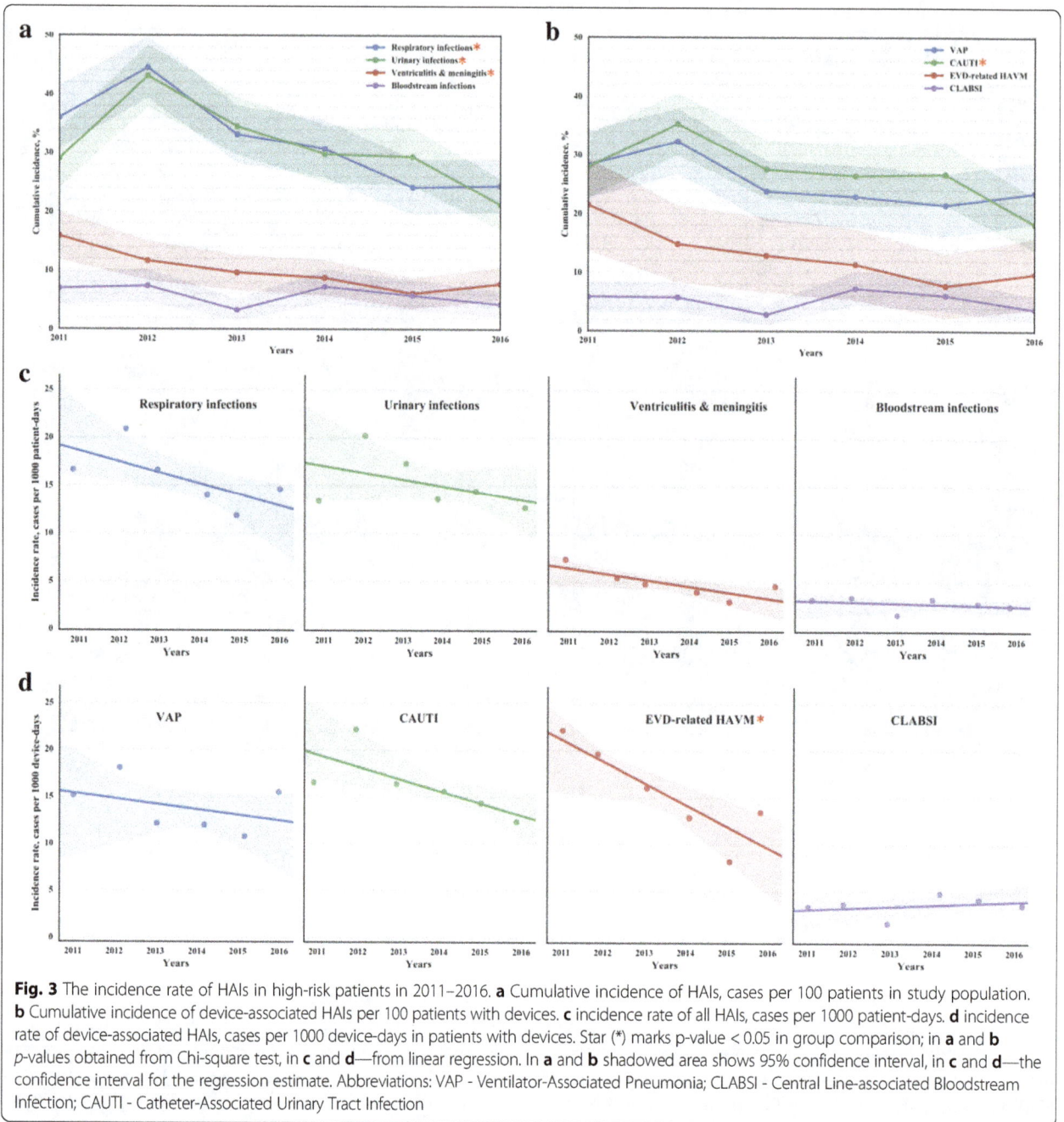

Fig. 3 The incidence rate of HAIs in high-risk patients in 2011–2016. **a** Cumulative incidence of HAIs, cases per 100 patients in study population. **b** Cumulative incidence of device-associated HAIs per 100 patients with devices. **c** incidence rate of all HAIs, cases per 1000 patient-days. **d** incidence rate of device-associated HAIs, cases per 1000 device-days in patients with devices. Star (*) marks p-value < 0.05 in group comparison; in **a** and **b** p-values obtained from Chi-square test, in **c** and **d**—from linear regression. In **a** and **b** shadowed area shows 95% confidence interval, in **c** and **d**—the confidence interval for the regression estimate. Abbreviations: VAP - Ventilator-Associated Pneumonia; CLABSI - Central Line-associated Bloodstream Infection; CAUTI - Catheter-Associated Urinary Tract Infection

Dramatic changes were found in cephalosporin resistance, e.g. in 2011 there were 90.3% isolates resistant to cefepime [95% CI 87.4–93.1] vs. 45.6% [95% CI 39.9–51.4] in 2016, p-value < 0.001 (Additional file 1: Figure S4).

The number of imipenem-resistant isolates of *A. baumannii* decreased from 77.7% [95% CI 72.3–83.0] in 2011 to 38% [95% CI 30.9–45.1] in 2016, p-value < 0.001 (Fig. 4b). While the proportion of ampicillin/sulbactam-resistant isolates increased from 48.1% [95% CI 34.8–61.5] in 2011 to 82% [95% CI 76.2–87.9] in 2016, p-value < 0.001, the resistance to the rest of tested antibiotics

remained virtually unchanged (Additional file 1: Figure S5). These changes in resistance occurred with a concurrent reduction in antibiotic utilization over the study period. Antibiotic use was measured as antibiotic-days per 1000 patient-days. The rate of antibiotic utilization was initially 1066 antibiotic days per 1000 patient-days in 2011. This highlights that multiple antibiotics were administered in many patients and a high overall usage rate was in effect. Over the six-year study period the utilization rate consistently declined. In 2016 the utilization rate was 807 antibiotic days per 1000 patient-days.

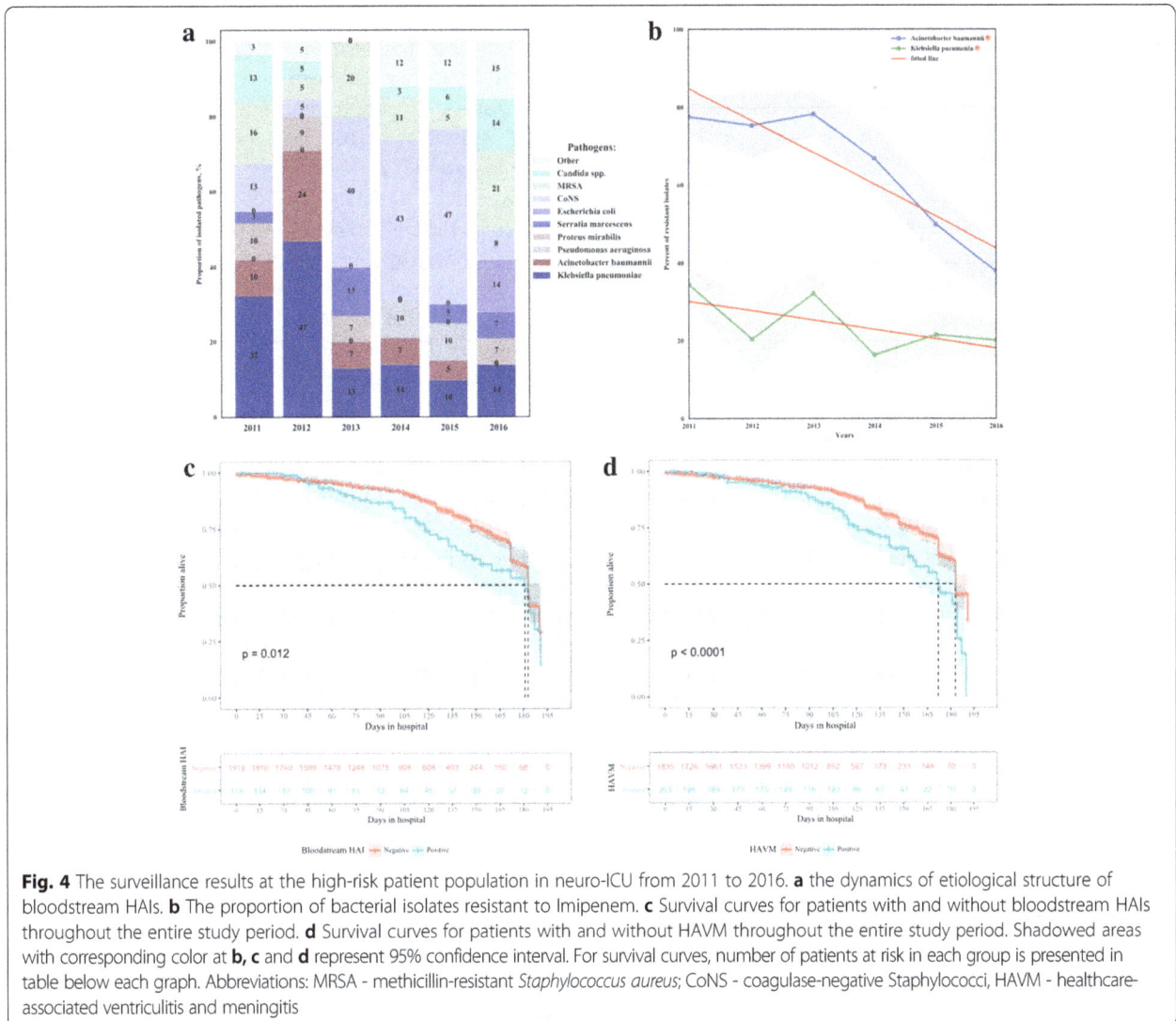

Fig. 4 The surveillance results at the high-risk patient population in neuro-ICU from 2011 to 2016. **a** the dynamics of etiological structure of bloodstream HAIs. **b** The proportion of bacterial isolates resistant to Imipenem. **c** Survival curves for patients with and without bloodstream HAIs throughout the entire study period. **d** Survival curves for patients with and without HAVM throughout the entire study period. Shadowed areas with corresponding color at **b**, **c** and **d** represent 95% confidence interval. For survival curves, number of patients at risk in each group is presented in table below each graph. Abbreviations: MRSA - methicillin-resistant *Staphylococcus aureus*; CoNS - coagulase-negative Staphylococci, HAVM - healthcare-associated ventriculitis and meningitis

Survival analysis in patients with HAIs

Bloodstream HAIs and HAVM significantly impair survival (log-rank p-values = 0.012 and < 0.0001, respectively), Fig. 4c and 4d. In order to confirm their influence on mortality, multifactorial survival analyses were done by Cox regression (Additional file 1: Table S5). We confirmed that only HAVM affected survival independently from other factors, increasing the probability of death 1.43 times (95% CI 1.03–1.98, p-value = 0.034). Other types of HAIs did not influence survival (Additional file 1: Figure S6). Besides HAIs, other factors were shown to independently affect survival. While brain tumor (HR = 1.57 [95% CI 1.1–2.24], p-value = 0.012) and implantation of neurosurgical devices (HR = 1.59 [95% CI 1.24–2.03], p-value = 0.0002) enhanced mortality, craniotomy decreased mortality: HR = 0.64 [95% CI 0.48–0.87], p-value = 0.0037 (Additional file 1: Figure S7).

ICU-acquired intestinal dysfunction

The cumulative incidence of overall intestinal dysfunctions dropped from 54.9% [95% CI 49.4–60.5] in 2011 to 23.9% [95% CI 19.4–28.4] in 2016, p-value < 0.001 (Additional file 1: Figure S8A, Additional file 1: Table S6). Intestinal dysfunction impaired survival independently increasing the probability of death 1.46 times [95% CI 1.11–1.93], p-value = 0.0069; log-rank test p-value = 0.019 (Additional file 1: Figure S8D).

Discussion

A comprehensive IPC program with a focus on hand hygiene and patient isolation was started in NSI's ICU in 2010 (Fig. 1a). By that time, the use of our IPC program to prevent HAIs in the ICU became a paradigm-shifting solution across Russia as HAI prevention strategies had previously remained unchanged for years and had become outdated [20].

The importance of HAI prevention programs is clearly indicated by the observation that HAIs directly deteriorate patient survival. It was found that HAIs increased the probability of death by 1.4–1.5 [21] and odds of mortality increased 1.5 to 1.9-fold [22]. In our study, we found that HAVM decreased the probability of survival by 1.43, while other HAIs did not significantly influence survival. It has been previously reported that HAVM increased mortality rate approximately three times [23]. Although the exact mechanism is not yet understood, prospective studies have found that in ICU patients, gastrointestinal dysfunction is also an independent risk factor for increased mortality [15]. We can postulate that the intestinal microbiome serves an important role in immune function and consequently, is a well described reservoir for antibiotic resistance [24]. Additionally, in critically ill patients intestinal dysbiosis could be postulated as a potential contributor to gut translocation of pathogens and may play a role in enteric absorption. In our study, ICU-acquired intestinal dysfunction decreased the probability of survival by 1.46, which is consistent with earlier studies. The implementation of IPC initiatives and the accompanying reduction in the incidence of infections, thereby reducing the requirement for antibiotics, can be assumed to at least in part account for reduction in gastrointestinal dysbiosis. This finding further highlights the potential unseen morbidity impact of IPC beyond simple measures of antibiotic utilization and resistance rates.

The implementation of the IPC program was followed by significant reduction of HAIs in the ICU. In fact, the impact of this program may actually be under-estimated. Our IPC program was implemented in 9/2010 whereas study data collection began 1/2011. Therefore, although adherence to IPC protocols would be expected to improve with greater time and familiarity, the totality of impact of this program may be under-estimated. Key initiatives, such as early removal of indwelling catheters, would be expected to have an immediate impact in the reduction of nosocomial infections. Even discounting the IPC impact in the initial months after implementation, the fact that a sustained and continued reduction in HAI rate occurred is both meaningful and serves as a reinforcement of overall utility. In high-risk ICU patients we observed a substantial decrease in HAI incidence: cumulative incidence of respiratory HAIs declined by 1.47 (from 36.1 to 24.5%), urinary tract HAIs by 1.4-fold (from 29.1 to 21.3%), HAVM by twofold (from 16 to 7.8%), CAUTI by 1.93 (from 35.4 to 18.3%) (Fig. 3), and ICU-acquired intestinal dysfunction by 2.3 fold. These results are consistent with previously reported evidence, demonstrating a reduction of HAI prevalence by approximately 1.7 fold (from 11.7 to 6.8%) [25].

We also found that the risk-adjusted incidence of EVD-related HAVM reduced 1.64 fold (from 22.2 to 13.5 cases per 1000 EVD-days) over the six-year study period. The impact of an IPC program on decreasing DA-HAI incidence has been previously reported. For example, one publication reported a 2.7-fold decrease in CAUTI episodes per 100 patients within a year after IPC implementation [26]. However, for some HAIs, like HAVM, such statistics are absent. In addition, the changes in the incidence of intestinal dysfunction could be confounded by the implementation of an advanced nutritional protocol in 2012 at the ICU.

We did find that in 2012 the rates of several infection subcategories did increase in comparison to 2011. The rate of respiratory and urinary HAIs had increases ranging from 4 to 14% compared to 2011. The reason for this increase is unclear, but we postulate that this may be related to several factors. One contributor may be that staff were educated on the appropriate identification of HAIs and utilized clear standardized case definitions. As staff became more familiar with these definitions, they may have been able to better identify cases leading to an apparent increase in infection rates. Additionally, during initial implementation of IPC protocols, staff underwent in-service training and consequently there was a specific focus on the strict adherence to protocols. However, adherence to infection control practices may wane with time, and that probably what happened in 2012. Therefore, continued reinforcement of best practices along with feedback to healthcare teams is necessary for sustained adherence to IPC initiatives. Following the re-education of staff, a renewed attention to IPC may have contributed to reductions seen in 2013 HAI rate.

Additionally, both the length of patients' stays in the ICU and the incidence of patient mortality did decrease over the study period. Although a direct causality cannot be determined, it would be fair to postulate that the associated decrease in HAI incidence may at least have been a partial contributor for this reduction. Thus, a reduction in the rate of HAIs may result in a meaningful reduction in healthcare cost, and potential benefit in overall mortality. However, we did not monitor all other parameters that could have influenced the mortality and the length of stay, thus other explanations should be investigated. Additionally, we admit that the overall approach in patient treatment did not change much, and the DUR did not change for any of the devices we monitored.

The prevention of the spread of carbapenem-resistant, Gram-negative bacteria was named the first priority of IPC efforts by the latest WHO guidelines because these strains pose significant threat to global health [27]. We found firstly that the proportion of such Gram-negatives as *K. pneumoniae* and *A. baumannii* in the spectrum of bloodstream HAIs decreased and secondly that the resistance of both pathogens to carbapenems was significantly reduced. In our study the initial percentage of isolates resistant to imipenem was 34.5% for *K. pneumonia* and 77.7% for *A. baumannii.* By the end of the study, the percentage decreased 1.7- and 2-fold, respectively (Fig. 4b). The initial prevalence of carbapenem-resistant isolates in the NSI neuro-ICU was shown to be higher than the mean prevalence in Europe (8.1% for *K. pneumoniae* and 50% for *A. baumannii*), and in the U.S. (7.9% for *K. pneumoniae* and 49.5% for *A. baumannii*) [27]. This finding could partly be explained by the study population because we analyzed only intensive care unit patients which may be a higher risk population. However, we postulate these initial rates of carbapenem resistance were at least in part due to nosocomial cross-infection of patients.

Our hypothesis is that the implementation of IPC protocols acted in a two-fold manner with an initial reduction in nosocomial patient-to-patient transmission which consequently lead to a reduction in nosocomial infection rate. Our most critical interventions involved implementation of contact precautions utilizing gloves, gown, and mask, isolation of patients identified with carbapenemase resistance genes, and cohorting of patients with *Acinetobacter* or *Klebsiella* (Fig. 1). These efforts were paired with intensive environmental disinfection measures, skin antisepsis for indwelling devices, as well as initiates focused on hand hygiene as a multi-modal strategy (Fig. 1).

Of note, hand hygiene compliance was particularly difficult to implement with a compliance rate of 27% in 2011. Compliance with hand hygiene in the subsequent years 2012 through 2016 were 40, 69, 63, 68, and 81% respectively. The reduction in infection rate over time could reasonably be postulated to result in a secondary reduction in the necessity of broad spectrum antibiotic therapy. This reduction in antibiotic utilization is underscored by the dramatic decline in the rate of antibiotic utilization over the study period. It must be noted that an antibiotic stewardship program was in existence prior to IPC implementation. Antibiotic stewardship involved institutional protocols for perioperative antibiotic prophylaxis and for empiric antibiotic therapy. However, integration of IPC protocols, including surveillance measures may have enhanced the effectiveness of antibiotic stewardship interventions. The ultimate result was that within the study period, our observed resistance rates decreased to the level of global and regional estimations.

This improvement in susceptibility rates, is in contrast to the global trend of increasing carbapenem resistance over the past decade [27], indicating that in limited-resource settings IPC programs can be highly effective. The programs may be especially significant in healthcare settings with high levels of resistance where they can serve as a cost-effective intervention leading to a substantial clinical impact. The substantial diminution in carbapenem resistance supports the notion that

implemented IPC strategies contain effective measures to prevent and control the resistance to carbapenems (Fig. 1). Moreover, this is supported by the recent WHO guidelines which affirmed that the core components of multimodal IPC strategy can help to prevent carbapenem resistance.

This paper reports a prospective study of the impact of an infection control program in a high acuity limited resource setting with regard to the reduction in HAI risk. Such studies are limited to date but have been identified by the WHO as particularly needed [27]. Thus, this study can help to fill this research gap providing insight regarding an approach to implantation of these programs and highlighting the most essential IPC components. Our results suggest that a focus on robust surveillance paired with isolation/infection control measures can promote a sustainable and meaningful reduction in HAI incidence and antibiotic resistance.

The current study has certain limitations. It is a single-center study in a highly specialized ICU facility. Thus, one should be careful when generalizing these results to other hospitals and other wards. In addition, we only studied a cohort of high-risk patients, those staying in the dedicated neuro-ICU for > 48 h—not the entire ICU population. Thus, reported HAI incidences are higher than those calculated for the entire ICU population. However, the underlying principles of our IPC program leading to the reduction of CAUTI, CLABSI, and VAP would be expected to be generalizable to other hospitalized settings with a similar expected impact.

One aspect that was not able to be fully evaluated were *Clostridium difficile* infections (CDI). The prevalence of CDI, identified by a positive PCR stool assay and compatible symptoms, was measured quarterly. However, the quarterly rate included all patients in the ICU at the time of a positive diagnosis and included patients that did not meet the defined criteria for high-risk population that were studied. Additionally, the incidence rate was low throughout the six-year period with a peak rate of 1.5% in 2011 and a nadir of 0.9% in 2015. Notably, patients who were transferred out of the ICU and subsequently developed CDI would not have been identified. Therefore, we can postulate that IPC initiatives may result in a reduction in CDI as the rate did decline from 2011; however, the low overall incidence of CDI and aforementioned limitations do not allow for definitive conclusions.

By design, the study did not include a control group (i.e. a group treated in the ICU before the IPC program had been implemented), because HAI rates without surveillance are unknown. Moreover, the decrease of HAI incidence and length of stay in the ICU could be explained by modification of clinical practices and by regression to the mean. It should be mentioned that survival analysis in our study suffers from immortal time bias. Patients in the HAI group are "immortal" until they get the infection, that favors the HAI group by lowering mortality rate in this group. Thus, HAIs have a stronger influence on survival, posing a higher risk of death in patients once they get HAIs.

Conclusion

Implementation of an evidence-based IPC program was strongly associated with a significant reduction in HAIs in the neuro-ICU. Over a six-year period, there was a decreasing HAI incidence, reduction in the prevalence of carbapenem-resistant invasive bacterial isolates, and consequently improved patient outcomes. Our study supports the finding that an IPC program can be highly effective in a middle-income country (Russia) despite the lack of a national surveillance system and limited resources. Expansion of IPC initiatives, potentially paired with a robust antimicrobial stewardship program, should be considered in resource limited settings as a feasible cost-effective opportunity to achieve meaningful reductions in antibiotic resistance and HAI incidence.

Additional file

Additional file 1: Supplementary materials for the research study report "Implementing an infection control and prevention program decreases the incidence of healthcare-associated infections and antibiotic resistance in a Russian neuro-ICU". (PDF 35444 kb)

Abbreviations

CAUTI: Catheter-associated urinary tract infection; CDC: Centers for Disease Control and Prevention; CI: Confidence interval; CLABSI: Central line-associated bloodstream infections; DA-HAI: Device-associated HAI; DUR: Device utilization ratio; EVD: External ventricular drain; HAI: Healthcare-associated infection; HAVM: Healthcare-associated ventriculitis and meningitis; HR: Hazard ratio; ICU: Intensive care unit; IPC: Infection prevention and control; NSI: Burdenko National Medical Research Center of Neurosurgery; Q1; Q3: First and third quartiles; SSSI: Superficial surgical site infection; VAP: Ventilator-associated pneumonia; WHO: World Health Organization

Acknowledgements

The authors gratefully acknowledge the contributions of many people who helped to develop, support, implement, and guide this study. Special thanks to all NSI clinicians, nurses, and administrators who patiently accepted and complied with the IPC program, and helped to collect data. We'd like to acknowledge the contribution of Dr. Yulia Savochkina and Dr. Svetlana Sazykina who helped with the microbiological assay. We are grateful for the help with data analysis to Dr. Anton Barchuk (Saint Petersburg Cancer Center), Dr. Rashied Amini (NASA-JPL), and Oleg Khomenko (Skoltech). We thank for providing language help and proofreading to Michael Saint-Onge (Los Angeles Public Library), also Travis Nielsen (University of Southern California).

Authors' contributions

KE and DW analyzed data and wrote the manuscript; OE and IS developed, implemented and maintained IPC program in the ICU; NK, GD, and ES collected data, evaluated and treated study subjects; MS developed and supported electronic surveillance protocol; NF and IA performed microbiological testing; VZ consulted with study design and promoted the IPC program implementation. All authors read and approved the final manuscript.

Competing interests

The authors declare that they have no competing interests.

Author details

[1]Center for Data-Intensive Biotechnology and Biomedicine, Skolkovo Institute of Science and Technology, Moscow, Russia. [2]Department of Intensive Care, Burdenko National Medical Research Center of Neurosurgery, Moscow, Russia. [3]Division of Infectious Diseases, Keck School of Medicine, University of Southern California, Los Angeles, USA. [4]Laboratory of Biomedical Informatics, Burdenko National Medical Research Center of Neurosurgery, Moscow, Russia. [5]IT Department, Burdenko National Medical Research Center of Neurosurgery, Moscow, Russia. [6]Department of Microbiology, Burdenko National Medical Research Center of Neurosurgery, Moscow, Russia. [7]Federal Budget Institution of Science "State Research Center for Applied Microbiology & Biotechnology" (SRCAMB), Moscow, Russia. [8]Department of Anesthesiology, Keck School of Medicine, University of Southern California, Los Angeles, USA. [9]Department of Epidemiology and Infection Control, Burdenko National Medical Research Center of Neurosurgery, Moscow, Russia.

References

1. Haley R, Culver D, White J, Morgan W, Emori T, Munn V, Hooton T. The efficacy of infection surveillance and control programs in preventing nosocomial infections in US hospitals. Am J Epidemiol. 1985;121(2):182–205. https://www.ncbi.nlm.nih.gov/pubmed/4014115.
2. Centers for Disease Control and Prevention (CDC). Monitoring hospital-acquired infections to promote patient safety, United States, 1990-1999. MMWR Morb Mortal Wkly Rep. 2000;49(8):149–53. https://www.ncbi.nlm.nih.gov/pubmed/10737441.
3. Storr J, Twyman A, Zingg W, Damani N, Kilpatrick C, Reilly J, Price L, et al. Core components for effective infection prevention and control Programmes: new WHO evidence-based recommendations. Antimicrob Resist Infect Control. 2017;6(January):6. https://doi.org/10.1186/s13756-016-0149-9.
4. Guidelines on core components of infection prevention and control programmes at the national and acute health care facility level. Geneva: World Health Organization; 2016. https://www.ncbi.nlm.nih.gov/pubmed/27977095.
5. State report "On the state of sanitary and epidemiological well-being of the population in Russian federation in 2016". Moscow: Federal Service for Surveillance on Consumer Rights Protection and Human Well-being; 2017 128–131. Accessed 16 Aug 2017. http://www.rospotrebnadzor.ru/upload/iblock/0b3/gosudarstvennyy-doklad-2016.pdf.
6. Official report "Health care in Russia in 2015". Moscow: Federal State Statistics Service; 2016. Accessed 16 Sept 2017. http://www.gks.ru/wps/wcm/connect/rosstat_main/rosstat/ru/statistics/publications/catalog/doc_1139919134734. Pages 18 and 97.
7. Allegranzi B, Bagheri Nejad S, Combescure C, Graafmans W, Attar H, Donaldson L, Pittet D. Burden of endemic health-care-associated infection in developing countries: systematic review and meta-analysis. Lancet. 2011; 377(9761):228–41. https://doi.org/10.1016/S0140-6736(10)61458-4.
8. "World Development Indicators." World development indicators data. Accessed 22 Nov 2017. https://data.worldbank.org/data-catalog/world-development-indicators.
9. Ider B-E, Adams J, Morton A, Whitby M, Clements A. Infection control Systems in Transition: the challenges for post-soviet bloc countries. J Hosp Infect. 2012;80(4):277–87. https://doi.org/10.1016/j.jhin.2012.01.012.
10. Stratchounski L, Dekhnitch A, Kozlov R. Infection control system in Russia. J Hosp Infect. 2001;49(3):163–6. https://doi.org/10.1053/jhin.2001.1042.
11. Suetens C, Morales I, Savey A, Palomar M, Hiesmayr M, Lepape A, Gastmeier P, Schmit JC, Valinteliene R, Fabry J. European surveillance of ICU-acquired infections (HELICS-ICU): methods and main results. J Hosp Infect. 2007; 65(Suppl 2):171–3. https://doi.org/10.1016/S0195-6701(07)60038-3.
12. Siegel J, Rhinehart E, Cic R, Jackson M, Chiarello L, Ms RN. Guideline for isolation precautions: preventing transmission of infectious agents in healthcare settings. HICPAC. 2007; https://stacks.cdc.gov/view/cdc/6878.
13. Shifrin M, Kurdumova N, Danilov G, Ershova O, Savin I, Alexandrova I, Sokolova E, Tabasaranskiy T. Electronic patient records system as a monitoring tool. Stud Health Technol Inform. 2015;210:236–8. https://www.ncbi.nlm.nih.gov/pubmed/25991140.

14. Horan T, Andrus M, Dudeck M. CDC/NHSN surveillance definition of health care-associated infection and criteria for specific types of infections in the acute care setting. Am J Infect Control. 2008;36(5):309–32. https://doi.org/10.1016/j.ajic.2008.03.002.

15. Reintam A, Parm P, Kitus R, Kern H, Starkopf J. Gastrointestinal symptoms in intensive care patients. Acta Anaesthesiol Scand. 2009;53(3):318–24. https://doi.org/10.1111/j.1399-6576.2008.01860.x.

16. Clinical and Laboratory Standard Institute. M100: performance standards for antimicrobial susceptibility testing. 26th ed; 2016. 1–56238–804-5.

17. Agarwal A, Kapila K, Kumar S. WHONET software for the surveillance of antimicrobial susceptibility. Med J Armed Forces India. 2009;65(3):264–6. https://doi.org/10.1016/S0377-1237(09)80020-8.

18. Seabold S, Perktold J. Statsmodels: econometric and statistical modeling with python. In: Proceedings of the 9th python in science conference; 2010.

19. E. Jones, T. Oliphant, and P. Peterson. 2001. "SciPy: open source scientific tools for python." http://www.scipy.org.

20. Shestopalov N, Akimkin V, Panteleeva L, Fedorova L, Abramova I. Measures for disinfection and sterilization as the most significant concept in health care infection control system in Russia. Antimicrob Resist Infect Control. 2015;4(1):P47. https://doi.org/10.1186/2047-2994-4-S1-P47.

21. Koch A, Nilsen R, Eriksen H, Cox R, Harthug S. Mortality related to hospital-associated infections in a tertiary hospital; repeated cross-sectional studies between 2004-2011. Antimicrob Resist Infect Control. 2015;4:57. https://doi.org/10.1186/s13756-015-0097-9.

22. Glance L, Stone P, Mukamel D, Dick A. Increases in mortality, length of stay, and cost associated with hospital-acquired infections in trauma patients. Arch Surg. 2011;146(7):794–801. https://doi.org/10.1001/archsurg.2011.41.

23. Korinek A-M, Baugnon T, Golmard J-L, van Effenterre R, Coriat P, Puybasset L. Risk factors for adult nosocomial meningitis after craniotomy: role of antibiotic prophylaxis. Neurosurgery. 2008;62(Suppl 2):532–9. https://doi.org/10.1227/01.neu.0000316256.44349.b1.

24. O'Fallon E, Gautam S, D'Agata E. Colonization with multidrug-resistant gram-negative bacteria: prolonged duration and frequent cocolonization. Clin Infect Dis. 2009;48(10):1375–81. Oxford University Press. https://doi.org/10.1086/598194.

25. Ebnöther C, Tanner B, Schmid F, La Rocca V, Heinzer I, Bregenzer T. Impact of an infection control program on the prevalence of nosocomial infections at a tertiary Care Center in Switzerland. Infect Control Hosp Epidemiol. 2008;29(1):38–43. https://doi.org/10.1086/524330.

26. Stéphan F, Sax H, Wachsmuth M, Hoffmeyer P, Clergue F, Pittet D. Reduction of urinary tract infection and antibiotic use after surgery: a controlled, prospective, before-after intervention study. Clin Infect Dis. 2006; 42(11):1544–51. https://doi.org/10.1086/503837.

27. World Health Organization. "Guidelines for the prevention and control of carbapenem-resistant Enterobacteriaceae, Acinetobacter baumannii and Pseudomonas aeruginosa in health care facilities." Geneva: World Health Organization; 2017. http://www.who.int/infection-prevention/publications/guidelines-cre/en/.

14

Risk for subsequent infection and mortality after hospitalization among patients with multidrug-resistant gram-negative bacteria colonization or infection

Wen-Pin Tseng[1], Yee-Chun Chen[2,3], Shang-Yu Chen[1], Shey-Ying Chen[1*] and Shan-Chwen Chang[2]

Abstract

Background: Risks for subsequent multidrug-resistant gram-negative bacteria (MDRGNB) infection and long-term outcome after hospitalization among patients with MDRGNB colonization remain unknown.

Methods: This observational study enrolled 817 patients who were hospitalized in the study hospital in 2009. We defined MDRGNB as a GNB resistant to at least three different antimicrobial classes. Patients were classified into MDRGNB culture-positive (MDRGNB-CP; 125 patients) and culture-negative (MDRGNB-CN; 692 patients) groups based on the presence or absence of any MDRGNB identified from either active surveillance or clinical cultures during index hospitalization. Subsequent MDRGNB infection and mortality within 12 months after index hospitalization were recorded. We determined the frequency and risk factors for subsequent MDRGNB infection and mortality associated with previous MDRGNB culture status.

Results: In total, 129 patients had at least one subsequent MDRGNB infection (MDRGNB-CP, 48.0%; MDRGNB-CN, 10.0%), and 148 patients died (MDRGNB-CP, 31.2%; MDRGNB-CN, 15.9%) during the follow-up period. MDR *Escherichia coli* and *Acinetobacter baumannii* were the predominant colonization microorganisms; patients with *Proteus mirabilis* and *Pseudomonas aeruginosa* had the highest hazard risk for developing subsequent infection. After controlling for other confounders, MDRGNB-CP during hospitalization independently predicted subsequent MDRGNB infection (hazard ratio [HR], 5.35; 95% confidence interval [CI], 3.72–7.71), all-cause mortality (HR, 2.42; 95% CI, 1.67–3.50), and subsequent MDRGNB infection-associated mortality (HR, 4.88; 95% CI, 2.79–8.52) after hospitalization.

Conclusions: Harboring MDRGNB significantly increases patients' risk for subsequent MDRGNB infection and mortality after hospitalization, justifying the urgent need for developing effective strategies to prevent and eradicate MDRGNB colonization.

Keywords: Multidrug resistance, Gram-negative bacteria, Colonization, Subsequent infection, Mortality

* Correspondence: erdrcsy@ntu.edu.tw
[1]Department of Emergency Medicine, National Taiwan University Hospital, College of Medicine, National Taiwan University, No. 7, Zhongshan S. Rd., Zhongzheng Dist., Taipei 100, Taiwan
Full list of author information is available at the end of the article

Key points

Harboring multidrug-resistant gram-negative bacteria (MDRGNB) significantly increases patients' risk for subsequent infection after hospital discharge. The association between MDRGNB colonization and increased long-term mortality further justifies the need for effective, collaborative strategies to prevent and eradicate MDRGNB colonization.

Background

The emergence and spread of multidrug-resistant gram-negative bacteria (MDRGNB) have become a major public health threat globally [1, 2]. Infections with MDRGNB are associated with higher hospital cost, prolonged hospitalization, and mortality [3–7]. Acquisition and infection of MDRGNB are common among hospitalized patients, especially for critically ill patients who were vulnerable to high MDRGNB selection pressure following extensive antimicrobial therapy [8–12]. The risk for subsequent infection was significantly higher for hospitalized patients with initial antimicrobial-resistant GNB colonization than patients without colonization [8, 13–15]. Approximately 9.1–39% of inpatients who were initially colonized with various antimicrobial-resistant GNB developed subsequent infection during the same hospital stay [8, 10, 12–14]. Therefore, the effect of initial MDRGNB colonization on the risk for subsequent infection and clinical outcomes among hospitalized patients is well documented, and it significantly influences the recommendations for controlling and treating MDRGNB infections in hospital settings.

In contrast to in-hospital settings, decreased risk for MDRGNB colonization and infection over time following hospital discharge was usually deemed as a matter of course. Although the clearance of MDRGNB colonization of a patient after being away from nosocomial, high-antibiotic pressure environment has been demonstrated [16], prolonged effect from persistent MDRGNB colonization remains a potential contributing factor for subsequent MDRGNB infections and threats on the treatment outcomes of community patients with recent hospitalization history. However, the effects of MDRGNB colonization on subsequent infection and long-term outcome of patients after hospitalization have not been comprehensively explored.

In this study, we used any positive culture for MDRGNB, either from active surveillance cultures on index hospitalization admission or decision-driven clinical cultures during index hospitalization, to identify patients with potential MDRGNB colonization, irrespective of the antibiotic treatment history. Then, we hypothesized that MDRGNB colonization along with certain patient characteristics synergistically affects the risk for subsequent MDRGNB associated infection and long-term mortality after hospital discharge. We also hypothesized that there exists different species-specific and isolation site-specific colonization effects that contribute to the different risk for subsequent MDRGNB infection. Therefore, this study aimed to provide data on the characteristics of subsequent infection pattern and outcome effects associated with prior MDRGNB colonization or infection to help first-line physicians in making treatment decisions for patients with community-onset infection.

Methods
Study design, setting, and patients
The National Taiwan University Hospital is a 2200-bed teaching hospital that provides both primary and tertiary care in northern Taiwan. This retrospective study used an adult patient cohort of one prospective study that recruited 995 patients in the emergency department who received active microbiological surveillance cultures for the development a MDRGNB prediction model on patients' hospital admission (index hospitalization) [17]. The results of active surveillance cultures, which included anterior nares swab, posterior pharyngeal wall (throat) swab, urine, and areas of skin breakdown if presented, and all clinical cultures during index hospitalization of the 995 patients were recorded to determine the MDRGNB colonization status on admission and before hospital discharge. Among the 995 patients, 118 (11.6%) died during hospitalization and 60 (6.0%) did not have any outpatient department (OPD) follow-up record after hospital discharge; hence, they were excluded from this study. Therefore, only 817 patients who survived the index hospitalization discharge and had at least one OPD follow-up record were finally enrolled. We then conducted this observational study to investigate the risk for subsequent MDRGNB infections and mortality in these patients during 12 months after discharge from the index hospitalization (Appendix).

Definition of MDRGNB and determination of colonization status
We defined MDRGNB as the presence of *Enterobacteriaceae* or glucose non-fermentative gram-negative bacilli (NFGNB) that are resistant to at least three different antimicrobial classes. For *Enterobacteriaceae*, MDR was defined as resistance to at least three classes of the following agents: third- or fourth-generation cephalosporins, aminoglycosides, fluoroquinolones, and ampicillin/sulbactam. For NFGNB, MDR was defined as resistance to at least three classes of the following agents: antipseudomonal cephalosporins (ceftazidime or cefepime), aminoglycosides, fluoroquinolones (levofloxacin or

ciprofloxacin), antipseudomonal penicillins (ticarcillin-clavulanic acid or piperacillin-tazobactam), and carbapenem (imipenem or meropenem) [1, 18]. Patients with and without any positive culture for MDRGNB from either active surveillance cultures on admission or decision-driven clinical cultures during index hospitalization were classified as MDRGNB culture-positive (MDRGNB-CP) and MDRGNB culture-negative (MDRGNB-CN) groups, respectively.

Data collection and information on variables
For all study patients, clinical data, including age, sex, preexisting comorbidities, antibiotic exposure, intensive care unit (ICU) admission, receiving of tracheal intubation, length of hospital stay (LOS), clinical cultures within 1 year prior to index hospitalization, active surveillance cultures on admission, and decision-driven clinical cultures obtained during index hospitalization were prospectively obtained from medical records [17]. Follow-up data 12 months after index hospitalization were retrospectively collected from the hospital and OPD electronic medical records, including repeated hospitalization, subsequent clinical culture results, occurrence of culture-confirmed MDRGNB infection, and mortality.

Several comorbid medical conditions were investigated. Malignancy included either an active malignant solid tumor or hematological disease. Severity of preexisting comorbidities was assessed using a modified Charlson comorbidity score [19, 20]. The diagnosis of MDRGNB infection of a study patient was independently evaluated by two investigators based on clinical, radiographic, and microbiological findings and National Nosocomial Infections Surveillance criteria [21, 22]. A third investigator confirmed and finalized the decision if the two investigators did not agree on the diagnosis of MDRGNB infection. All subsequent MDRGNB infections were described according to the number of days between the onset of infection and the index hospitalization discharge date, source of infection, and causative microorganism. For patients with multiple episodes of subsequent MDRGNB infection during the 12 months follow-up period, only the first episode was analyzed, because the causative microorganism of later episodes of MDRGNB infection could be a new colonization acquired during subsequent hospitalization for the first episode of MDRGNB infection treatment. MDRGNB-associated mortality was defined as MDRGNB bacteremia occurring within 7 days of death or active MDRGNB infection at the time of death [23].

Statistical analyses
Means (±SD) were calculated for continuous variables, and percentages were used for categorical variables.

Independent Student's t-test or Mann–Whitney U test was used to compare continuous variables, and Chi-square or Fisher's exact test was used to analyze categorical variables. Kaplan–Meier method and log-rank tests were used to compare the cumulative probability of the first episode of subsequent MDRGNB infection and survival after index hospitalization of both the study groups. We screened for variables with P values of ≤0.2 using univariate analysis and included these as candidate variables in the multivariate Cox regression model. We then used stepwise selection of these variables to investigate independent risk factors associated with subsequent MDRGNB infection and 1-year survival. The risks for subsequent infection due to the same MDRGNB species or isolation site were presented as hazard risk between patients with positive culture for the indicated MDRGNB species or isolation site and those without any MDRGNB culture during index hospitalization. Data were analyzed using SAS 9.4 (SAS Institute, Cary NC). All P values are two sided, and findings with P values of < 0.05 were considered statistically significant.

Results
In total, 817 patients were enrolled in this study, including 125 patients with at least one positive MDRGNB from surveillance (71 patients), clinical (93 patients), or both (39 patients) cultures. The microbiological distribution of MDRGNB species is detailed in Table 1. *Escherichia coli* was the most predominant MDRGNB isolate (37.6% [47/125]), followed by *Acinetobacter baumannii* (25.6% [32/125]), *Pseudomonas aeruginosa* (17.6% [22/125]), and *Klebsiella pneumoniae* (16.8% [21/125]) during the index hospitalization. Demographic and clinical characteristics of the 817 study patients with and without positive MDRGNB culture during index hospitalization are summarized in Table 2. MDRGNB-CP patients were older, had longer index hospitalization LOS, and had higher percentage of prior healthcare-associated exposure or MDRGNB culture before index hospitalization. MDRGNB-CP patients also had a higher percentage of having cardiovascular diseases and a bed-ridden status, presence of a pressure sore or indwelling urinary catheter, receiving ICU care and tracheal intubation, and antibiotic exposure during index hospitalization.

After discharge from index hospitalization, 129 patients (60 MDRGNB-CP and 69 MDRGNB-CN) had at least one episode of subsequent MDRGNB infection during the 12-month follow-up period. The median duration from index hospitalization discharge to the first subsequent MDRGNB infection episode was 74 (range, 2–354) days for all the 129 patients with subsequent infection episodes, 44.5 (range, 2–

Table 1 Bacteriology and Culture Site of Multidrug-resistant Gram-negative Bacteria (MDRGNB) Isolates Identified during Index Hospitalization and Within 1 year after Index Hospitalization Discharge

Bacterial species	MDRGNB culture positive group[a] (n = 125)										MDRGNB culture negative group[b] (n = 692)									
	Overall		Isolation site								Overall		Isolation site							
			Respiratory[c]		Urine		Blood		Others[d]				Respiratory[c]		Urine		Blood		Others[d]	
Index hospitalization[e,f]																				
Escherichia coli	47	(37.6)	17	(13.6)	26	(20.8)	4	(3.2)	7	(5.6)	–	–	–	–	–	–	–	–	–	–
Acinetobacter species	32	(25.6)	25	(20.0)	7	(5.6)	2	(1.6)	4	(3.2)	–	–	–	–	–	–	–	–	–	–
Pseudomonas aeruginosa	22	(17.6)	17	(13.6)	5	(4.0)	0	(0.0)	0	(0.0)	–	–	–	–	–	–	–	–	–	–
Klebsiella pneumoniae	21	(16.8)	15	(12.0)	6	(4.8)	1	(0.8)	1	(0.8)	–	–	–	–	–	–	–	–	–	–
Enterobacter species	17	(13.6)	11	(8.8)	5	(4.0)	1	(0.8)	3	(2.4)	–	–	–	–	–	–	–	–	–	–
Proteus mirabilis	4	(3.2)	3	(2.4)	1	(0.8)	0	(0.0)	0	(0.0)	–	–	–	–	–	–	–	–	–	–
Other bacteria[g]	20	(16.0)	13	(10.4)	2	(1.6)	3	(2.4)	2	(1.6)	–	–	–	–	–	–	–	–	–	–
Subsequent infection[f,h,i]																				
Escherichia coli	24	(40.0)	9	(15.0)	13	(21.7)	3	(5.0)	1	(1.7)	13	(18.8)	2	(2.9)	8	(11.6)	3	(4.3)	2	(2.9)
Acinetobacter species	15	(25.0)	12	(20.0)	2	(3.3)	1	(1.7)	2	(3.3)	23	(33.3)	22	(31.9)	1	(1.4)	3	(4.3)	0	(0.0)
Pseudomonas aeruginosa	12	(20.0)	10	(16.7)	2	(3.3)	0	(0.0)	0	(0.0)	8	(11.6)	6	(8.7)	1	(1.4)	1	(1.4)	0	(0.0)
Klebsiella pneumoniae	10	(16.7)	6	(10.0)	4	(6.7)	0	(0.0)	0	(0.0)	14	(20.3)	9	(13.0)	2	(2.9)	3	(4.3)	1	(1.4)
Enterobacter species	1	(1.7)	0	(0.0)	0	(0.0)	1	(1.7)	0	(0.0)	7	(11.7)	7	(10.1)	0	(0.0)	0	(0.0)	0	(0.0)
Proteus mirabilis	5	(8.3)	3	(5.0)	0	(0.0)	0	(0.0)	2	(3.3)	3	(4.3)	1	(1.4)	0	(0.0)	0	(0.0)	1	(1.4)
Other bacteria	2	(3.3)[j]	0	(0.0)	2	(3.3)	0	(0.0)	0	(0.0)	5	(7.2)[k]	1	(1.4)	1	(1.4)	1	(1.4)	0	(0.0)

[a]Indicates patients with at least 1 positive MDRGNB culture during index hospitalization
[b]Indicates patients without any positive MDRGNB culture during index hospitalization
[c]Including nasal swab, throat swab, and sputum culture
[d]Including axillary or inguinal skin, wound, soft tissue pus, drainage, bile, pleural fluid, ascites, and catheter tip culture
[e]Including surveillance and clinical culture during index hospitalization
[f]One MDR-GNB species could be isolated from different anatomical sites
[g]Including *Serratia marcescens* (4), *Morganella morganii* (2), *Achromobacter xylosoxidans* (2), *Burkholderia cepacia* complex (1), *Citrobacter freundii* (3), *Aeromonas hydrophila* (1), *Aeromonas sobria* (1), *Providencia stuartii* (1), *Sphingomonas paucimobilis* (1), *Klebsiella oxytoca* (1), and unidentified nonfermentative gram-negative bacilli (3)
[h]Within 1 year after discharge from index hospitalization
[i]Diagnosed with positive clinical culture and compatible clinical presentation
[j]Including *Serratia marcescens* (1) and unidentified nonfermentative gram-negative bacilli (1)
[k]Including *Klebsiella oxytoca* (2), *Serratia marcescens* (1), and unidentified non-fermentative gram-negative bacilli (2)

354) days for the 60 MDRGNB-CP patients, and 108 (range, 10–352) days for the 69 MDRGNB-CN patients. *E. coli* remained the most predominant causative microorganism of subsequent MDR-GNB infections in both MDRGNB-CP and MDRGNB-CN groups (Table 1). Among the 129 patients with subsequent MDRGNB infections, 5 had two concomitant MDRGNB infection foci (respiratory and urinary tracts [4], respiratory tract and intra-abdominal [1]). The lower respiratory tract was the most prevalent primary focus of subsequent MDRGNB infection (66.7% [86/129]), followed by urinary tract (24.8% [32/129]), intra-abdominal area (7.8% [10/129]), other infection foci (2.3% [3/129]), and primary bacteremia (2.3% [3/129]). Among the 60 subsequent MDRGNB infection episodes from the 125 MDRGNB-CP patients, 41 (68.3%) were caused by the same MDR bacterial species, 43 (71.7%) had the infection site concordant

to prior MDRGNB culture site, and 33 (55.0%) had the causative MDR bacterial species and culture site concordant to prior MDRGNB culture during index hospitalization. MDRGNB-CP patients had significantly higher cumulative probability of developing subsequent MDRGNB infection than MDRGNB-CN patients (log-rank test, $P < 0.001$) (Fig. 1a). Multivariate Cox regression analysis showed the positive MDRGNB culture during index hospitalization was an independent predictor for subsequent MDRGNB infection (hazard ratio [HR], 5.35; 95% confidence interval [CI], 3.72–7.71), after controlling other potential confounders, such as age (HR, 1.02; 95% CI, 1.01–1.03), malignancy (HR, 1.66; 95% CI, 1.12–2.47), congestive heart failure (HR, 1.70; 95% CI, 1.08–2.68), chronic obstructive pulmonary disease (HR, 1.60; 95% CI, 1.03–2.48), and antibiotics exposure during index hospitalization (HR, 2.20; 95% CI, 1.25–3.90) (Table 3).

Table 2 Clinical Characteristics of Study Patients by the Detection of Multidrug-resistant Gram-negative Bacteria (MDRGNB) in Either Surveillance of Clinical Culture during Index Hospitalization

Characteristics	MDRGNB culture positive group (n = 125)		MDRGNB culture negative group (n = 692)		p-value
Age, mean ± SD (year)	71.5 ± 14.8		64.1 ± 17.7		< 0.001
Male sex	76	(60.8)	399	(57.7)	0.51
LTCF or nursing-home residence	20	(16.0)	18	(2.6)	< 0.001
Long-term hemodialysis	7	(5.6)	17	(2.5)	0.06
Previous MDRGNB isolation[a]	44	(35.2)	27	(3.9)	< 0.001
Co-morbid medical conditions					
Diabetes mellitus	31	(24.8)	188	(27.2)	0.58
Malignancy	28	(22.4)	173	(25.0)	0.53
End-stage renal disease	7	(5.6)	24	(3.5)	0.25
Liver cirrhosis	7	(5.6)	72	(10.4)	0.09
Congestive heart failure	19	(15.2)	59	(8.5)	0.019
COPD	22	(17.6)	60	(8.7)	0.002
Cerebrovascular accident	37	(29.6)	88	(12.7)	< 0.001
Bed-ridden status	61	(48.8)	108	(15.6)	< 0.001
Presence of pressure sore	17	(13.6)	28	(4.1)	< 0.001
Central vascular catheter[b]	13	(10.4)	44	(6.4)	0.10
Long-term urinary catheter	18	(14.4)	37	(5.4)	< 0.001
Charlson comorbidity index, mean ± SD	3.8 ± 2.6		2.8 ± 2.7		< 0.001
High CCI (≥5)	47	(37.6)	174	(25.1)	0.004.
Index hospitalization treatment					
Antibiotics exposure[c]	115	(92.0)	471	(68.1)	< 0.001
3rd or 4th generation cephalosporin	52	(41.6)	156	(22.5)	< 0.001
Ampicillin-sulbactam	42	(33.6)	180	(26.0)	0.08
Piperacillin-tazobactam	41	(32.8)	77	(11.3)	< 0.001
Carbapenem	21	(16.8)	18	(2.6)	< 0.001
Fluoroquinolone	22	(17.6)	51	(7.4)	< 0.001
Aminoglycoside	4	(3.2)	6	(0.9)	0.05
ICU admission	14	(11.2)	21	(3.0)	< 0.001
Receiving of tracheal intubation	14	(11.2)	15	(2.2)	< 0.001
Length of hospital stay, median ± IRQ	19.0 ± 22.0		9.0 ± 12.0		< 0.001

Abbreviations: SD standard deviation, *MDRGNB* multidrug-resistant gram-negative bacteria, *COPD* chronic obstructive pulmonary disease, *CCI* Charlson comorbidity index, *ICU* intensive care unit, *IRQ* interquartile range
[a]Within 1 year prior to the index hospitalization
[b]Including Port-A catheter, Hickman catheter, permcath catheter, double-lumen catheter, and peripherally inserted central catheter
[c]Including oral and intravenous antibiotic exposure for > 48 h during index hospitalization

Analysis for species-specific risk for subsequent infection after index hospitalization discharge showed that the hazard risk in patients with initial MDR *Proteus mirabilis* culture was higher (HR, 231.29; 95% CI, 32.10–1666.31) than those without any MDRGNB culture, followed by MDR *P. aeruginosa* (HR, 56.99; 95% CI, 21.53–150.88), MDR *E. coli* (HR, 36.83; 95% CI, 17.59–77.14), MDR *K. pneumoniae* (HR, 15.83; 95% CI, 5.17–48.48), and MDR *A. baumannii* (HR, 15.25; 95% CI, 7.58–30.69). With respect to isolation

site, previous MDRGNB culture from urinary tract had the highest risk for subsequent MDRGNB urinary tract infection after discharge (HR, 18.45; 95% CI, 8.25–41.27) (Table 4).

A total of 148 in hospital mortality events were observed during the 12-month follow-up period after discharge from index hospitalization; 53 (35.8%) of them were associated with subsequent MDRGNB infections. MDRGNB-CP patients had significantly lower cumulative probability of survival than

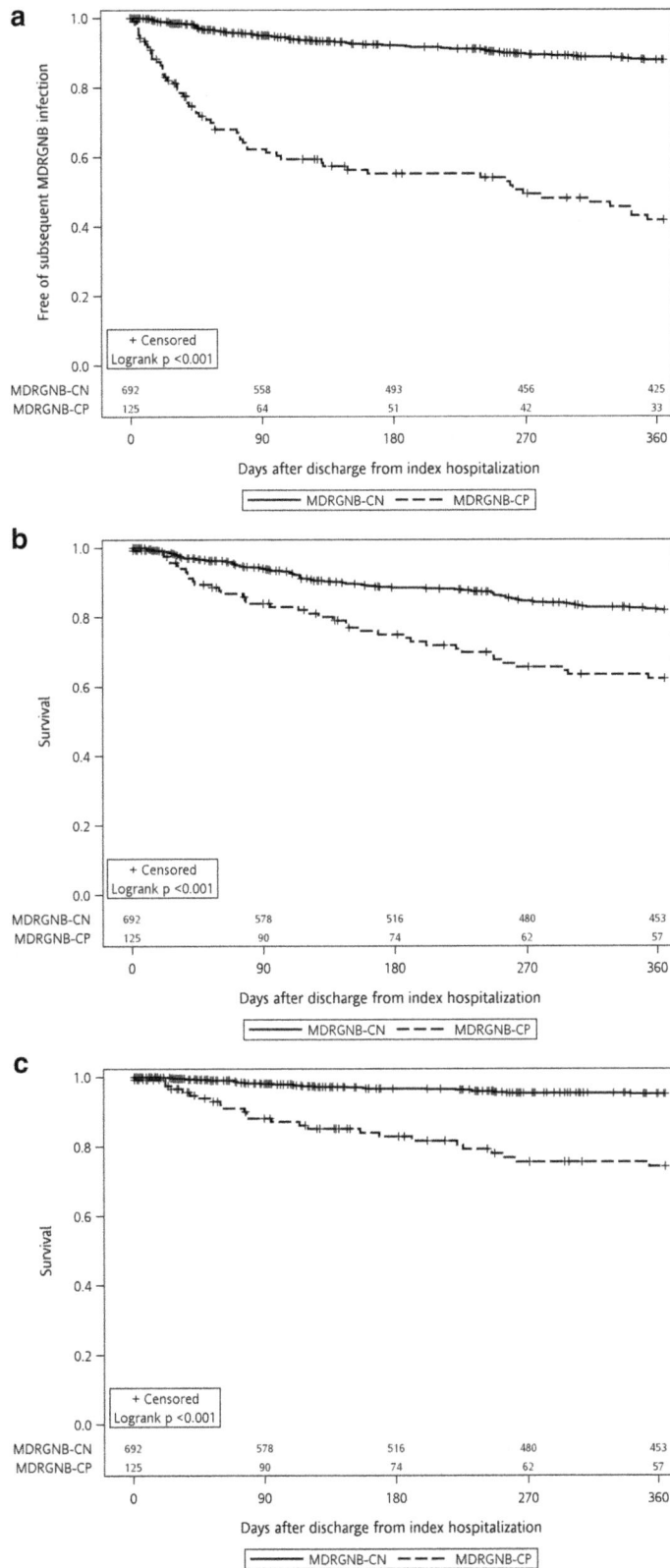

Fig. 1 (See legend on next page.)

> (See figure on previous page.)
> **Fig. 1** Kaplan–Meier curves at 1 year for **a** subsequent MDRGNB infection, **b** all-cause mortality, and **c** MDRGNB infection-associated mortality after discharge, stratified by index hospitalization MDRGNB culture result. Abbreviations: MDRGNB, multidrug-resistant gram-negative bacteria; MDRGNB-CN, multidrug-resistant gram-negative bacteria culture negative; MDRGNB-CP, multidrug-resistant gram-negative bacteria culture positive

MDRGNB-CN patients, irrespective of all-cause or subsequent MDRGNB infection-associated mortality (both log-rank tests, $P < 0.001$) (Fig. 1b and c). By Cox regression analysis, MDRGNB-CP during index hospitalization was an independent predictor for all-cause mortality (HR, 2.42; 95% CI, 1.67–3.50) and subsequent MDRGNB infection-associated mortality (HR, 4.88; 95% CI, 2.79–8.52), after controlling other potential confounders, such as age, malignancy, high Charlson comorbidity index, and long-term indwelling urinary catheter (Table 5).

We further divided our MDRGNB-CP patients into 2 subgroups: MDRGNB surveillance culture positive only patients and MDRGNB clinical culture positive patients (all patients with positive MDRGNB clinical culture, including those with both positive MDRGNB clinical and surveillance culture). After controlling for potential confounders, the risk for subsequent MDRGNB infection were both significantly higher in the MDRGNB surveillance culture positive only patients (HR, 4.63; 95% CI, 2.36–9.10) and MDRGNB clinical culture positive patients (HR, 5.56; 95% CI, 3.77–8.20), compared to that of MDRGNB-CN patients. The higher risk for all-cause mortality and subsequent MDRGNB infection-associated mortality after index hospitalization, compared to those of MDRGNB-CN patients, remained significant for the MDRGNB surveillance culture only patients (all-cause mortality, HR, 2.29; 95% CI, 1.19–4.41; subsequent MDRGNB infection-associated mortality, HR, 3.44; 95% CI, 1.20–9.90) and for the MDRGNB clinical culture positive patients (all-cause mortality, HR, 2.46; 95% CI,

Table 3 Univariate and Multivariate Cox Regression Analysis for the Risk for Subsequent Multidrug-resistant Gram-negative Bacteria (MDRGNB) Infection after Hospital Discharge

	Univariate analysis			Multivariate analysis		
	HR	(95% CI)	p-value	HR	(95% CI)	p-value
Age (per year increase)	1.03	(1.02–1.05)	< 0.001	1.02	(1.01–1.03)	0.007
Male sex	0.97	(0.68–1.37)	0.84	–	–	–
LTCF residence	2.59	(1.43–4.70)	0.002	–	–	–
Long-term hemodialysis	1.30	(0.53–3.19)	0.56	–	–	–
Diabetes mellitus	1.13	(0.77–1.64)	0.53	–	–	–
Malignancy	1.41	(0.95–2.09)	0.09	1.66	(1.12–2.47)	0.012
End-stage renal disease	0.96	(0.39–2.34)	0.93	–	–	–
Liver cirrhosis	0.65	(0.32–1.33)	0.24	–	–	–
Congestive heart failure	2.79	(1.83–4.27)	< 0.001	1.70	(1.08–2.68)	0.021
COPD	2.73	(1.80–4.15)	< 0.001	1.60	(1.03–2.48)	0.038
Cerebrovascular accident	1.75	(1.17–2.64)	0.007	–	–	–
Presence of pressure sore	2.32	(1.31–4.12)	0.004	–	–	–
Central vascular catheter[a,b]	1.83	(1.01–3.32)	0.046	–	–	–
Long-term urinary catheter[b]	1.72	(1.00–3.00)	0.05	–	–	–
Antibiotics exposure[c]	3.54	(2.03–6.17)	< 0.001	2.20	(1.25–3.90)	0.007
Intensive care unit admission[c]	1.26	(0.59–2.70)	0.55	–	–	–
Receiving tracheal intubation[c]	2.39	(1.25–4.56)	0.008	–	–	–
MDRGNB culture positive[c,d]	7.19	(5.08–10.19)	< 0.001	5.35	(3.72–7.71)	< 0.001

Abbreviations: *LTCF* long-term care facility, *COPD* chronic obstructive pulmonary disease
[a]Includes Port-A catheter, Hickman catheter, permcath catheter, double-lumen catheter, and peripherally inserted central catheter
[b]At the time of index hospitalization discharge
[c]During index hospitalization
[d]Including positive MDR-GNB culture from either surveillance or clinical culture of any anatomical site

Table 4 Species-Specific Risk for Subsequent Infection with Causative Multidrug-resistant Gram-negative Bacteria (MDRGNB) or Infection Site Identical to Prior MDRGNB Culture during Index Hospitalization

	Subsequent MDR-GNB infection of concordant species or isolation site		
	Hazard Ratio	(95% C.I.)[a]	P value
Initial MDRGNB species			
Proteus mirabilis	231.29	(32.10–1666.31)	< 0.001
Pseudomonas aeruginosa	56.99	(21.53–150.88)	< 0.001
Escherichia coli	36.83	(17.59–77.14)	< 0.001
Klebsiella pneumoniae	15.83	(5.17–48.48)	< 0.001
Acinetobacter species	15.25	(7.58–30.69)	< 0.001
Enterobacter species	5.83	(0.73–46.62)	0.10
Initial MDRGNB isolation site			
Urine	18.45	(8.25–41.27)	< 0.001
Respiratory tract	10.52	(6.81–16.26)	< 0.001
Blood	8.92	(1.14–69.83)	0.037

[a]Calculated as hazard risk between patients with positive culture for the indicated MDRGNB species or isolation site and those without any MDRGNB culture during index hospitalization

Table 5 Univariate and multivariate cox regression analysis for the risk for mortality after discharge from index hospitalization

	All-cause mortality						MDRGNB infection-associated mortality					
	Univariate analysis			Multivariate analysis			Univariate analysis			Multivariate analysis		
	HR	(95% CI)	p-value	HR	(95% CI)	p-value	HR	(95% CI)	p-value	HR	(95% CI)	p-value
Age (per year increase)	1.02	(1.01–1.03)	0.001	1.02	(1.01–1.03)	0.006	1.04	(1.02–1.06)	< 0.001	1.03	(1.01–1.05)	0.008
Male sex	1.34	(0.96–1.88)	0.09	–	–	–	1.24	(0.71–2.16)	0.45	–	–	–
LTCF residence	1.33	(0.65–2.71)	0.43	–	–	–	2.37	(0.94–5.95)	0.07	–	–	–
Long-term hemodialysis	1.10	(0.45–2.68)	0.84	–	–	–	1.86	(0.58–5.96)	0.30	–	–	–
Diabetes mellitus	0.89	(0.62–1.29)	0.89	–	–	–	0.93	(0.51–1.72)	0.82	–	–	–
Malignancy	6.28	(4.52–8.73)	< 0.001	5.30	(3.73–7.53)	< 0.001	2.32	(1.32–4.07)	0.004	2.34	(1.28–4.26)	0.006
End-stage renal disease	0.82	(0.34–2.00)	0.82	–	–	–	1.40	(0.44–4.48)	0.57	–	–	–
Liver cirrhosis	1.65	(1.04–2.61)	0.034	–	–	–	0.81	(0.29–2.23)	0.68	–	–	–
Congestive heart failure	1.25	(0.74–2.10)	0.41	–	–	–	2.38	(1.20–4.73)	0.014	–	–	–
COPD	1.40	(0.88–2.25)	0.16	–	–	–	2.62	(1.38–4.99)	0.003	–	–	–
Cerebrovascular accident	0.90	(0.57–1.43)	0.65	–	–	–	1.76	(0.94–3.28)	0.08	–	–	–
High CCI (≥5)	3.33	(2.41–4.60)	< 0.001	1.80	(1.27–2.55)	< 0.001	3.56	(2.08–6.12)	< 0.001	1.96	(1.10–3.49)	0.022
Presence of pressure sore	1.98	(1.13–3.41)	0.016	–	–	–	1.93	(0.77–4.85)	0.16	–	–	–
Central vascular catheter[a,b]	4.07	(2.66–6.22)	< 0.001	–	–	–	2.80	(1.26–6.21)	0.012	–	–	–
Long-term urinary catheter[b]	0.35	(0.13–0.94)	0.037	0.29	(0.11–0.80)	0.017	0.49	(0.12–2.02)	0.33	–	–	–
Antibiotics exposure[c]	1.70	(1.14–2.56)	0.010	–	–	–	3.96	(1.58–9.95)	0.003	–	–	–
MDRGNB culture positive[c,d]	2.40	(1.66–3.46)	< 0.001	2.42	(1.67–3.50)	< 0.001	5.91	(3.44–10.14)	< 0.001	4.88	(2.79–8.52)	< 0.001

Abbreviations: *MDRGNB* multidrug-resistant gram-negative bacteria, *LTCF* long-term care facility, *COPD* chronic obstructive pulmonary disease, *CCI* Charlson comorbidity index
[a]Including port-A catheter, Hickman catheter, permcath catheter, double-lumen catheter, and peripherally inserted central catheter
[b]At the time of index hospitalization discharge
[c]During index hospitalization
[d]Including positive MDRGNB culture from either surveillance or clinical culture of any anatomical site

1.62–3.74; subsequent MDRGNB infection-associated mortality, 5.33; 95% CI, 2.96–9.60).

Discussion

This study assessed the effects of prior MDRGNB colonization on subsequent infection risk and long-term outcome after hospital discharge and yielded three major findings. First, even in an environment that is expected to be free of or with low antibiotic selection pressure, the effect of previous MDRGNB colonization on the risk for subsequent MDRGNB infection remains significant and prolonged. Second, species-specific and isolation site-specific risks for the occurrence of subsequent MDRGNB infection were observed. The risk for subsequent infection was especially high for *P. mirabilis* and *P. aeruginosa* or genitourinary tract as colonization microorganisms or anatomical site, respectively. Third, prior MDRGNB colonization history independently predicted long-term survival of patients after hospitalization and directly contributed for more than one-third of late mortality. These findings are novel and important for first-line physicians to prepare for appropriate empirical antibiotics and timely infection control intervention in the treatment of previously hospitalized patients with community-onset infection.

Colonization and infection of antimicrobial-resistant bacteria are common in hospitalized patients and introduce significant risks for short-term morbidity and mortality. The effects of prolonged colonization and subsequent infections after hospital discharge should be comprehensively evaluated; however, only methicillin-resistant *Staphylococcus aureus* (MRSA) and vancomycin-resistant *Enterococcus* were previously reported [23–26]. A retrospective study by Huang et al. found that 17.4% (31/178) of patients with newly identified MRSA colonization or infection developed subsequent MRSA infections that were first manifested after discharge from the index hospitalization during an 18-month follow-up period [24]. In the current study, we demonstrated that 48% (60/125) of MDRGNB colonized or infected patients developed subsequent MDRGNB infections in a 12-month follow-up period, with more than half of these subsequent infections caused by the same MDR bacterial species and culture site. The risk for subsequent MDRGNB infection was especially high within 3 months after hospital discharge. Furthermore, our study found that patients harboring MDRGNB was an independent predictor for subsequent mortality after discharge from index hospitalization. Because previous studies never evaluate post-discharge events for patients with positive MDRGNB culture during hospitalization, the effect of MDRGNB on community disease burden and patient

outcome were therefore underestimated. This is the first study that demonstrated the prolonged effect of prior acquisition of antimicrobial-resistant bacteria on subsequent infections and mortality after initial hospitalization, with not only gram-positive bacteria but also GNB. As the prevalence of MDRGNB is continuously increasing in community and hospital environments [1, 2, 27, 28], our study findings highlight the urgent need for effective approaches to prevent the spread of MDRGNB in hospitals and to mitigate the MDRGNB colonization burden after hospitalization.

E. coli and *A. baumannii* were the most prevalent MDR species identified from patients during index hospitalization and at subsequent infections in this study. However, species-specific hazard risks for developing subsequent infection were higher for *P. mirabilis* and *P. aeruginosa* than those for *E. coli* and *A. baumannii*. This finding is important and deserves further exploration. A previous study by O'Fallone et al., which serial rectal surveillance cultures were obtained every 3–4 weeks from 33 elderly residents of a long-term care facility, found that multidrug-resistant *P. mirabilis* had significantly lower clearance rate (6.7%) and longer colonization duration than other non-*Proteus* MDR species [16]. However, they did not evaluate the effects from persistent colonization of *P. mirabilis* on the risk for subsequent infection. Our study results, by demonstrating the differential risk for subsequent infection after acquisition of different MDRGNB species, suggest the positive correlation between colonization persistence and risk for subsequent infection after hospital discharge. Further studies that explore the contributing factors for persistent MDRGNB colonization should be conducted to design effective decolonization strategies from infection control and prevention perspectives [29–31].

Though patients identified as harboring MDRGNB had significantly higher risk for developing subsequent MDRGNB infections, more than half of all subsequent MDRGNB infections occurred in patients who were not positive for MDRGNB in either initial surveillance cultures on admission or clinical cultures during hospitalization. These patients might have new MDRGNB colonization but were not detected by decision-driven clinical cultures during index hospitalization. This indicates the limitation of using clinical cultures alone in identifying patients with MDRGNB colonization. Other clinical characteristics, including old age, comorbid illnesses, and prior antibiotics exposure, also help clinicians in early suspicion of patients at risk for subsequent MDRGNB infections [10, 12, 13]. Clinicians should incorporate these data to guide their decision on using appropriate empirical antimicrobial therapy for patients with prior healthcare-associated exposure risk.

This study has several limitations. First, this was a single-center study. Thus, generalization from our findings requires further confirmation. Second, outcome data after index hospitalization were retrospectively collected and are therefore subject to information bias. Third, because not all study patients had completed a 12-month follow-up at our hospital, subsequent MDRGNB infection and mortality event that occurred elsewhere would not have been detected. Fourth, because the gastrointestinal tract is an important anatomical site harboring antimicrobial-resistant *Enterobacteriaceae* and *P. aeruginosa* [16, 32, 33], the lack of perianal swab cultures in active microbiological surveillance may have caused the underestimation of the MDR-GNB colonization rate and may have introduced an information bias and misclassification of study groups. Finally, we did not perform genotypic analysis for the 41 subsequent MDRGNB infection episodes that were caused by the same MDR bacterial species identified during index hospitalization. Therefore, the genotypic concordance between index hospitalization and subsequent infection isolates could not be confirmed.

Conclusions

The prolonged effects of prior MDRGNB colonization or infection significantly increase the risk for subsequent MDRGNB infection and mortality after hospitalization. *P. mirabilis* and *P. aeruginosa* as causative microorganisms or urinary tract as colonization site is a serious concern. Accurate assessment of the risk for MDRGNB-associated sequelae requires prolonged follow-up after discharge. Furthermore, studies aiming at the prevention of MDRGNB acquisition and eradication of colonization to reduce the prolonged effect of MDRGNB colonization are imperative.

Appendix

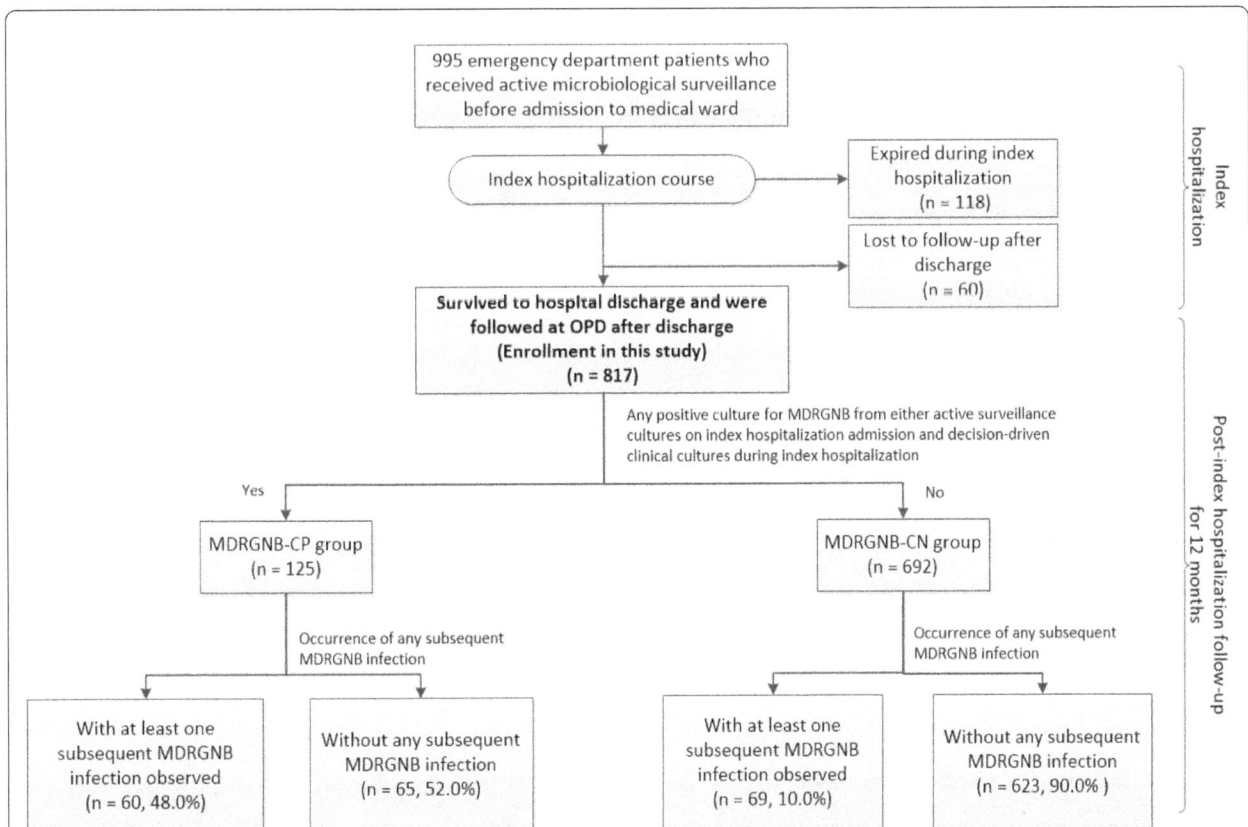

Fig. 2 Patient enrollment and classification flowchart. Abbreviations: OPD, outpatient department; MDRGNB, multidrug-resistant gram-negative bacteria; MDRGNB-CP, multidrug-resistant gram-negative bacteria culture positive; MDRGNB-CN, multidrug-resistant gram-negative bacteria culture negative

Abbreviations

HR: Hazard ratio; ICU: Intensive care unit; LOS: Length of hospital stay; MDRGNB: Multidrug-resistant gram-negative bacteria; MDRGNB-CN: Multidrug-resistant gram-negative bacteria culture negative; MDRGNB-CP: Multidrug-resistant gram-negative bacteria culture positive; NFGNB: Non-fermentative gram-negative bacilli; OPD: Outpatient Department

Funding

This study was supported partly by grants from the Department of Health, Taiwan (DOH98-DC-1005).

Authors' contributions

W-P T, Y-C C, S-Y C conceived and designed the studies. W-P T, Y-C C, S-Y C and S-Y C contributed to acquisition and analysis of the data. The manuscript was prepared by W-P T and S-Y C. Y-C C and S-C C supervised the conduction of the trial and data collection. S-Y C takes responsibility for the paper as a whole. All authors read and approved the final manuscript.

Competing interests

The authors declare that they have no competing interests.

Author details

[1]Department of Emergency Medicine, National Taiwan University Hospital, College of Medicine, National Taiwan University, No. 7, Zhongshan S. Rd., Zhongzheng Dist., Taipei 100, Taiwan. [2]Department of Internal Medicine, National Taiwan University Hospital, College of Medicine, National Taiwan University, No. 7, Zhongshan S. Rd., Zhongzheng Dist., Taipei 100, Taiwan. [3]Center for Infection Control, National Taiwan University Hospital, College of Medicine, National Taiwan University, No. 7, Zhongshan S. Rd., Zhongzheng Dist., Taipei 100, Taiwan.

References

1. Pop-Vicas AE, D'Agata EM. The rising influx of multidrug-resistant gram-negative bacilli into a tertiary care hospital. Clin Infect Dis. 2005;40:1792–8.
2. Bertrand X, Dowzicky MJ. Antimicrobial susceptibility among gram-negative isolates collected from intensive care units in North America, Europe, the Asia-Pacific rim, Latin America, the Middle East, and Africa between 2004 and 2009 as part of the Tigecycline evaluation and surveillance trial. Clin Ther. 2012;34:124–37.
3. Cosgrove SE. The relationship between antimicrobial resistance and patient outcomes: mortality, length of hospital stay, and health care costs. Clin Infect Dis. 2006;42(Suppl 2):S82–9.
4. Giske CG, Monnet DL, Cars O, Carmeli Y, ReAct-Action on Antibiotic Resistance. Clinical and economic impact of common multidrug-resistant gram-negative bacilli. Antimicrob Agents Chemother. 2008;52:813–21.
5. Gudiol C, Tubau F, Calatayud L, et al. Bacteraemia due to multidrug-resistant gram-negative bacilli in cancer patients: risk factors, antibiotic therapy and outcomes. J Antimicrob Chemother. 2011;66:657–63.
6. Lye DC, Earnest A, Ling ML, et al. The impact of multidrug resistance in healthcare-associated and nosocomial gram-negative bacteraemia on mortality and length of stay: cohort study. Clin Microbiol Infect. 2012;18:502–8.
7. Vardakas KZ, Rafailidis PI, Konstantelias AA, Falagas ME. Predictors of mortality in patients with infections due to multi-drug resistant gram negative bacteria: the study, the patient, the bug or the drug? J Inf Secur. 2013;66:401–14.
8. Reddy P, Malczynski M, Obias A, et al. Screening for extended-spectrum beta-lactamase producing Enterobacteriaceae among high-risk patients and rates of subsequent bacteremia. Clin Infect Dis. 2007;45:846–52.
9. Papadomichelakis E, Kontopidou F, Antoniadou A, et al. Screening for resistant gram-negative microorganisms to guide empirical therapy of subsequent infection. Intensive Care Med. 2008;34:2169–75.
10. Borer A, Saidel-Odes L, Eskira S, et al. Risk factors for developing clinical infection with carbapenem-resistant Klebsiella pneumoniae in hospital patients initially only colonized with carbapenem-resistant K pneumoniae. Am J Infect Control. 2012;40:421–5.
11. Hess AS, Kleinberg M, Sorkin JD, et al. Prior colonization is associated increased with increased risk of antibiotic-resistant gram-negative bacteremia in cancer patients. Diagn Microbiol Infect Dis. 2014;79:73–6.
12. Akturk H, Sutcu M, Somer A, et al. Carbapenem-resistant Klebsiella pneumoniae colonization in pediatric and neonatal intensive care units: risk factors for progression to infection. Braz J Infect Dis. 2016;20:134–40.
13. Gómez-Zorrilla S, Camoez M, Tubau F, et al. Prospective observational study of prior rectal colonization status as a predictor for subsequent development of Pseudomonas aeruginosa clinical infections. Antimicrob Agents Chemother. 2015;59:5213–9.
14. Harris AD, Jackson SS, Robinson G, et al. Pseudomonas aeruginosa colonization in the intensive care unit: prevalence, risk factors, and clinical outcomes. Infect Control Hosp Epidemiol. 2016;37:544–8.
15. Detsis M, Karanika S, Mylonakis E. ICU acquisition rate, risk factors, and clinical significance of digestive tract colonization with extended-spectrum beta-lactamase-producing Enterobacteriaceae: a systematic review and meta-analysis. Crit Care Med. 2017;45:705–14.
16. O'Fallon E, Gautam S, D'Agata EM. Colonization with multidrug-resistant gram-negative bacteria: prolonged duration and frequent cocolonization. Clin Infect Dis. 2009;48:1375–81.
17. Tseng WP, Chen YC, Yang BJ, et al. Predicting multidrug-resistant gram-negative bacterial colonization and associated infection on hospital admission. Infect Control Hosp Epidemiol. 2017;38:1216–25.
18. Siegel JD, Rhinehart E, Jackson M, Chiarello L. Management of multidrug-resistant organisms in health care settings, 2006. Am J Infect Control. 2007;35(Suppl 2):165–93.
19. Charlson ME, Pompei P, Ales KL, MacKenzie CR. A new method of classifying prognostic comorbidity in longitudinal studies: development and validation. J Chronic Dis. 1987;40:373–83.
20. Schneeweiss S, Wang PS, Avorn J, Glynn RJ. Improved comorbidity adjustment for predicting mortality in Medicare populations. Health Serv Res. 2003;38:1103–20.
21. Garner JS, Jarvis WR, Emori TG, Horan TC, Hughes JM. CDC definitions for nosocomial infections, 1988. Am J Infect Control. 1988;16:128–40.
22. Emori TG, Culver DH, Horan TC, et al. National Nosocomial Infections Surveillance System (NNIS): description of surveillance methods. Am J Infect Control. 1991;19:19–35.
23. Datta R, Huang SS. Risk of infection and death due to methicillin-resistant Staphylococcus aureus in long-term carriers. Clin Infect Dis. 2008;47:176–81.
24. Huang SS, Platt R. Risk of methicillin-resistant Staphylococcus aureus infection after previous infection or colonization. Clin Infect Dis. 2003;36:281–5.
25. Byers KE, Anglim AM, Anneski CJ, Farr BM. Duration of colonization with vancomycin-resistant Enterococcus. Infect Control Hosp Epidemiol. 2002;23:207–11.
26. Shenoy ES, Paras ML, Noubary F, Walensky RP, Hooper DC. Natural history of colonization with methicillin-resistant Staphylococcus aureus (MRSA) and vancomycin-resistant Enterococcus (VRE): a systematic review. BMC Infect Dis. 2014;14:177.
27. Ben-Ami R, Rodríguez-Baño J, Arslan H, et al. A multinational survey of risk factors for infection with extended-spectrum beta-lactamase-producing Enterobacteriaceae in nonhospitalized patients. Clin Infect Dis. 2009;49:682–90.
28. Chung DR, Song JH, Kim SH, et al. High prevalence of multidrug-resistant nonfermenters in hospital-acquired pneumonia in Asia. Am J Respir Crit Care Med. 2011;184:1409–17.
29. Septimus EJ, Schweizer ML. Decolonization in prevention of health care-associated infections. Clin Microbiol Rev. 2016;29:201–22.
30. Davido B, Batista R, Michelon H, et al. Is faecal microbiota transplantation an option to eradicate highly drug-resistant enteric bacteria carriage? J Hosp Infect. 2017;95:433–7.

31. Teerawattanapong N, Kengkla K, Dilokthornsakul P, Saokaew S, Apisarnthanarak A, Chaiyakunapruk N. Prevention and control of multidrug-resistant gram-negative bacteria in adult intensive care units: a systematic review and network meta-analysis. Clin Infect Dis. 2017;64(suppl_2):S51–60.
32. Villar HE, Baserni MN, Jugo MB. Faecal carriage of ESBL-producing *Enterobacteriaceae* and carbapenem-resistant gram-negative bacilli in community settings. J Infect Dev Ctries. 2013;7:630–4.
33. Wilson AP, Livermore DM, Otter JA, et al. Prevention and control of multi-drug-resistant gram-negative bacteria: recommendations from a joint working party. J Hosp Infect. 2016;92(Suppl 1):S1–44.

15

Myroides odoratimimus urinary tract infection in an immunocompromised patient: an emerging multidrug-resistant micro-organism

Giovanni Lorenzin[1,3], Giorgio Piccinelli[1], Lucrezia Carlassara[2], Francesco Scolari[2], Francesca Caccuri[1], Arnaldo Caruso[1] and Maria Antonia De Francesco[1*]

Abstract

Background: *Myroides* spp. are common environmental organisms and they can be isolated predominantly in water, soil, food and in sewage treatment plants. In the last two decades, an increasing number of infections such as urinary tract infections and skin and soft tissue infections, caused by these microorganisms has been reported. Selection of appropriate antibiotic therapy to treat the infections caused by *Myroides spp.* is difficult due to the production of a biofilm and the organism's intrinsic resistance to many antibiotic classes.

Case presentation: We report the case of a 69-year-old immunocompromised patient who presented with repeated episodes of macroscopic haematuria, from Northern Italy.
A midstream urine sample cultured a Gram negative rod in significant amounts (> 10^5 colony-forming units (cfu)/mL), which was identified as *Myroides odoratimimus*. The patient was successfully treated with trimethoprim/ sulfamethoxazole after antibiotic susceptibility testing confirmed its activity.

Conclusion: This case underlines the emergence of multidrug resistant *Myroides* spp. which are ubiquitous in the environment and it demands that clinicians should be more mindful about the role played by atypical pathogens, which may harbour or express multidrug resistant characteristics, in immunocompromised patients or where there is a failure of empiric antimicrobial therapy.

Background

The Myroides spp., which were previously classified as *Flavobacterium* spp., are Gram negative, non-fermentative and non-motile bacteria. They do not traditionally belong to the normal human flora. *Myroides* genus includes two species: *Myroides odoratus* and *Myroides odoratimimus* [1]. They are considered low-grade opportunistic pathogens and are rarely isolated from clinical samples but, occasionally, they are life-threatening [2]. Due to the presence of flexirubin, they are yellow pigmented on culture and they are obligated aerobic rod bacteria with a characteristic fruity odour (strawberry-like) [2, 3].

Despite the low pathogenicity potential, managing *Myroides odoratimimus* is difficult because most strains are multi-drug resistant [4, 5]. In addition, *Myroides* has different virulence factors [5], has the capacity of co-aggregation and self-aggregation to form biofilm [6]. and possess a polysaccharide capsule, which makes the bacterial surface extremely hydrophobic.

Case report

We present the case of a 69-year-old man with type II diabetes mellitus with ocular end-organ dysfunction, on oral hypoglycaemic agents, and with hypertension. He was also affected by an end stage renal failure requiring haemodialysis three times a week. Furthermore, he had other co-morbidities: ischaemic cardiomyopathy treated with oral anticoagulant therapy, mild chronic myelomonocytic leukemia (CMML), dyslipidemia and obesity.

* Correspondence: maria.defrancesco@unibs.it
[1]Institute of Microbiology, Department of Molecular and Translational Medicine, University of Brescia-Spedali Civili, P. le Spedali Civili 1, 25123 Brescia, Italy
Full list of author information is available at the end of the article

In June 2016, a permanent urinary Foley's catheter was positioned due to urinary retention.

In August 2017, the patient was seen to the emergency room (ER) of the Montichiari Hospital, Brescia, Italy. On admission, the patient was afebrile and upon physical examination, his vital signs (arterial pressure, heart rate and respiratory rate) were within normal limits. The patient gave a 3-day history of ongoing macroscopic haematuria and reported no lower urinary tract symptoms or other symptoms suggesting an inflammatory response or bleeding tendency. The patient had no history of abdominal or pelvic surgery. The international normalized ratio (INR) was 2.5 and hematologic parameters were within the normal range except red blood cell count, which was decreased (3×10^{6} /μL), related to kidney failure. Glycated haemoglobin (HbA1c) was 52 mmol/mol. Finally, he was discharged with a hemorrhagic cystitis diagnosis and he was empirically treated with ciprofloxacin at a renally-adjusted dose (250 mg 2/die for 1 week) with the complete resolution of the macroscopic heamaturia.

In September 2017, the patient was seen again to the ER for another episode of macro-hematuria. On admission, he had a temperature of 36.5 °C, the blood pressure and the heart rate were within the normal limits, and there weren't relevant findings on physical examination; blood cultures were performed but they were negative. Glycated haemoglobin (HbA1c) was 39 mmol/mol.

The patient had already started at home ciprofloxacin (250 mg 2/die) independently, so the clinician suggested that he continued this therapy for 1 week.

In the same month, the patient underwent a full urological investigation of haematuria, to exclude cancer or other abnormalities, a transrectal ultrasound, which identified a benign prostate adenoma, a cystoscopy which was negative for neoplasia, and a urinary cytology screening, which was negative for malignant cells. Despite the antibiotic therapy, the patient had symptoms related to urinary tract infection: bladder tenderness, hematuria and pelvic discomfort.

Therefore, a urine sample for culture was obtained by removing the indwelling catheter and obtaining a midstream specimen analysed by the laboratory of Microbiology and Virology of the Spedali Civili Hospital, Brescia, Italy; then, a new Foley's catheter has been replaced. Urinalysis showed the presence of nitrites, leukocyte esterase and 6–7 leukocytes per high power field by microscopy.

Patient was discharged with clear instructions given to him for a proper care of the urinary catheter and for a correct hand hygiene to prevent infections, and the prescription of an empirical antibiotic therapy. It comprised levofloxacin at 250 mg for 10 days, switched then to amikacin 500 mg intravenously for the following three dialysis sessions (for a total of one week) for cover against multi-drug resistant *Pseudomonas aeruginosa*, as guided by local epidemiology.

The urine culture grew a $> 10^{5}$ colony-forming units (cfu)/ml of a gram-negative rod. The bacterium was isolated from Columbia CNA agar (BioMérieux, Florence, Italy) after 24 h of incubation in aerobic conditions. The colonies appeared round, mucoid, yellow pigmented and with a fruity smell. The initial identification as *Myroides spp.* was performed using a matrix-assisted laser desorption ionization-time of flight mass spectrometry (MALDI-TOF MS) according to the manufacturer's instructions. The definitive identification was obtained with 16SrRNA gene sequencing. The obtained sequence was compared with the sequences in the GenBank database (http://ncbi.nlm.gov/blast) and it exhibited a 100% identity homology with *Myroides odoratimimus* strain BK21.

The antimicrobial susceptibility testing (AST) was first performed by using the standard disc diffusion on Mueller-Hinton agar. Then, the minimum inhibitory concentrations (MICs) were determined by automated microdilution broth test (BD-Phoenix NMIC-502, Becton Dickinson, Milan, Italy). The minimum inhibitory concentrations (MICs) were confirmed by Etest (BioMérieux). Since the breakpoints for *Myroides* spp. were unavailable, the interpretation of the results was performed according to the EUCAST guidelines for non-species related PK-PD breakpoints. The isolated strain was resistant to all beta-lactams, with and without inhibitors (Piperacillin/Tazobactam, MIC = 64; Ticarcillin/Clavulanate, MIC = 128; Ceftazidime/Avibactam, MIC = 32; Imipenem, MIC = 8; Meropenem, MIC = 4) and it was also resistant to fluoroquinolones, aminoglycosides, fosfomycin, nitrofurantoin and polymyxin. This conferred to the isolated strain a multi-drug resistance pattern. This strain was susceptible only to trimethoprim /sulfamethoxazole with a MIC of 1/19. A test was performed to assess beta-lactamase and carbapenemase production (ROSCO diagnostics, Biolife, Milan, Italy) according to the manufacturer's instructions. The results showed the absence of synergy between the meropenem disk and the dipicolinic acid, the phenylboronic acid, the EDTA and the cloxacillin.

In October 2017, due to the inadequacy of empiric therapy, the patient suffered from another hemorrhagic cystitis episode. Another urine culture confirmed the presence of a multi-drug resistant *Myroides odoratimimus* strain. According to the antibiotic susceptibility results, the patient was treated with trimethoprim/sulfamethoxazole at a renally-adjusted dose (160/800 mg daily for 2 weeks) which led to the resolution of macroscopic haematuria. In addition, in the same month, in order to reduce the possibility of recurrent UTIs, the urinary catheter was definitively removed.

Then, we tested its ability to grow in the form of biofilm. A Crystal Violet assay (CV) was performed to evaluate the production of biofilm at different concentrations of glucose and it was measured by spectrophotometry

(NanoDrop™ Spectrophotometer, Thermo Fisher). The results indicated that this strain could be classified as a "strong biofilm-producer" [7], which is able to produce a high amount of biofilm when it is compared to the reference strains (*Pseudomonas aeruginosa* PAO1, strain ATCC 15692). The increase of glucose concentration facilitates the production of biofilm by *Myroides odoratimimus*, contributing to an increase in vivo of its virulence. Therefore, a strong biofilm-producing bacteria, like *Myroides odoratimimus*, is well protected against antibiotics. A phylogenetic analysis was performed using the Quick Bioinformatics Phylogeny of Prokaryotes web-server and the data were then re-analysed using the Molecular Evolutionary Genetics Analysis software (MEGA 7.0.26) [8]. Geographical phylogeny was then extrapolated from the Gene-Bank database with a self-written programme. The results showed that our strain clustered with a strain isolated in Jena, Germany (Fig. 1a). The geographic analysis showed that this pathogen is poorly represented in Western Europe (Fig. 1b).

Discussion

Nowadays, the range of community and hospital acquired infections caused by atypical pathogens is continuously being updated. This increase in the number of newly described microorganisms is due to the use of both molecular identification, such as 16S rRNA sequencing and to the introduction in clinical microbiology laboratories of matrix-assisted laser desorption ionization–time of flight (MALDI-TOF) mass spectrometry.

The emergence of these microorganisms is associated with and impacted on by infection control and antimicrobial stewardship.

The antimicrobial resistance (AMR) has reached alarming levels in different parts of the world. As a result, many available treatment options are becoming ineffective. The major concern in AMR is the dissemination of bacteria with resistance to several antibiotics, also known as "superbugs".

The inappropriate, and often uncontrolled, use of antibiotics has led to a global AMR epidemic, as it is defined today.

Current antibiotic use in great amounts in humans and animals and subsequent release of antibiotic residues in the environment give rise to a selection pressure that leads to the increase in antibiotic resistant bacteria. In fact, once ingested, most antibiotics are eliminated not metabolized. They can move through sewage systems or directly into water and soil, and mix with environmental bacteria adding pressure for selection of antibiotic resistant organisms. Human exposure to environmental bacteria can occur through drinking water, eating food or by direct contact with the environment.

Myroides spp. can be classified as a multi-drug resistant environmental organism and can harbour different resistance mechanisms simultaneously, as demonstrated in this paper and in other studies [9]. Intrinsic resistance to β-lactamases is due to the presence of two metallo-β-lactamases, MUS-1 and TUS-1, which share a 73% of amino acid identity [4]. Furthermore, a resistance island was found on the chromosome of the bacterium [10]. This region has different types of resistance genes, including tetX (conferring tetracycline resistance), cat (chloramphenicol resistance) and bla-OXA-347 and bla-OXA-209 (conferring β-lactam resistance).

Moreover, it has been recently found that *Myroides odoratimimus* not only have common virulence factors, like *bauE* gene to acquire iron competing with the host and adherence factors (*DnaK, Hsp60*), but also can survive intracellularly (*katA, clpP, EF-Tu, and sodB*), even in human stomach (*ureA, ureB, ureG*), can disseminate easily and is able to destroy human tissues [5].

In addition, our strain is a strong biofilm producer. Biofilms are the sessile bacterial communities which adhere to both biotic and abiotic surfaces, such as medical devices. The bacteria are entrapped within a self-produced extracellular polymeric matrix [11]. Biofilm formation is an important virulence factor for many pathogens; in fact, it has become obvious that sessile bacterial cells in the biofilms express properties which are different from the properties of planktonic cells, for example, the ability to escape host defense, but also the higher resistance to antibacterial agents [12, 13]. The production of a strong biofilm is a serious problem because it increases pathogenicity in device-related infections and it is often associated with therapeutic failure, as well as persistence of infections [14]. The development of biofilm by *Myroides spp* can be of significant health hazard often leading to recurrent infections, as demonstrated in this paper and in other studies [6].

Our isolate was resistant to all the tested antibiotics except trimethoprim/sulfamethoxazole. The empirical therapy with fluoroquinolones and aminoglycoside was unsuccessful. The resistance observed might be due to an uncontrolled and excessive use of these drugs, in particular fluoroquinolones, which are used, when empirical clinical measures are required after taking urine samples for analysis and culture, as the first-choice drugs in treatment of patients with complicated UTI, according to the European guidelines [15].

In our patient, different risk factors played an important role in causing a multi-drug resistant *Myroides* urinary infection, such as the presence of prolonged urinary catheterisation and an immunocompromised condition. Repeated hospital admissions of the patient might represent an independent risk factor for colonization and infection with multi-resistant microorganisms such as

a

GU549435.1 M. odoratimimus strain Jiangsu China 2012
EU373415.1 M. odoratimimus strain Gyeongsangnamdo Korea 2007
68   KF017290.1 M. odoratimimus strain Sfax Tunisia 2013
KR349266.1 M. odoratimimus strain Fujian China 2015
9 69   EU331413.1 M. odoratimimus strain Zhejiang China 2007
89   GU570427.1 M. odoratimimus strain Chongqing China 2010
KJ401113.1 M. odoratimimus strain Xinjiang China 2014
98   KT163391.1 M. odoratimimus strain Kerala India 2015
98   EU660317.1 M. odoratimimus strain Tamil Nadu India 2013
73   KJ789156.1 M. odoratimimus strain Haikou Hainan China 2014
KT597573.1 M. odoratimimus strain Hubei China 2015
GQ383900.1 M. odoratimimus Nanjing Jiangsu China 2009
KT260524.1 M. odoratimimus strain Maharashtra India 2015
69   JQ396386.1 M. odoratimimus strain Fujian China 2012
JN700113.1 M. odoratimimus strain Yunnan China 2011
99   JQ229805.1 M. odoratimimus strain Yunnan China 2011
67 99   KC764979.1 M. odoratimimus strain Shandong China 2013
JF775418.1 M. odoratimimus strain Jiangsu China 2011
KF758445.1 M. odoratimimus strain Shandong China 2013
NR042354.1 M. odoratimimus strain Bonn Germany 2014
KC172018.1 M. odoratimimus strain Shandong China 2012
99   KR088355.1 M. odoratimimus strain Jena Thuringia Germany 2015
● Myroides odoratimimus Brescia 25123 2017

b

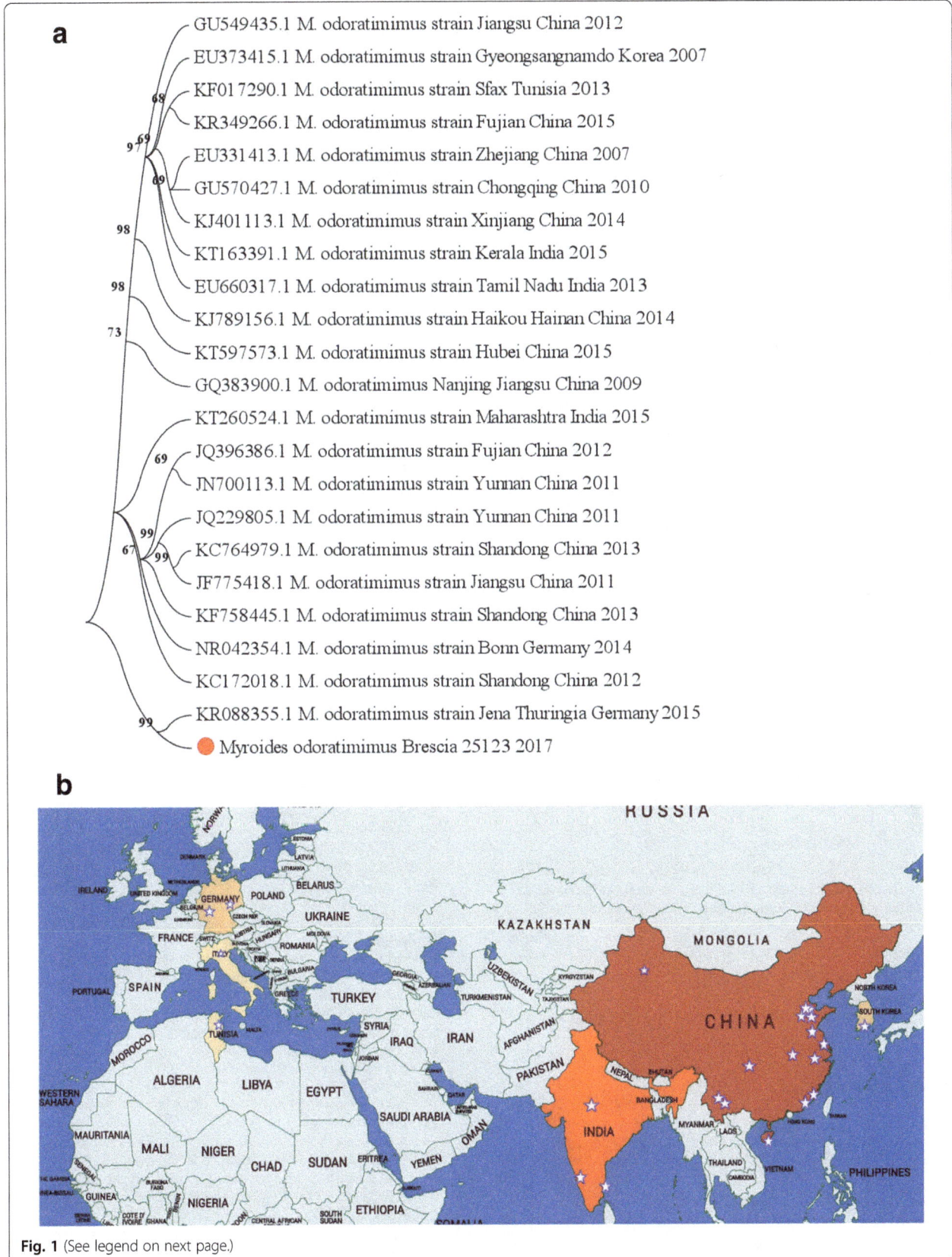

Fig. 1 (See legend on next page.)

(See figure on previous page.)
Fig. 1 Geographical analysis (**a**) and phylogenetic analysis (**b**) based on *Myroides odoratimumus* 16SrRNA gene sequences. The strain from the immunocompromised patient in Italy is indicated with the red point. Reference strains from GenBank with their accession number are shown. The tree was constructed by the neighbor-joining method based on Kimura's two-parameter model distance matrices with the MEGA program (version 7.0.26). Branch values are shown in the figure

Myroides spp. Outbreaks of UTIs due to *Myroides odoratimimus* and hospital acquired are already reported [16–18].

In this case, the source of the infection has not been determined, but our hypothesis is that the patient may have acquired the infection from an environmental source, maybe related to poor hand hygiene during the catheter care.

In literature there are several cases which associate *Myroides* spp. with different types of infections such as soft tissue infections [6, 19], UTI [16–18], sepsis [2, 20], bacteremia [21, 22], cellulitis [23, 24], pericardial effusion [25], pediatric severe burn injury [26], fulminant erysipelas [27] and urosepsis [28]. Many of these case reports were from India, Turkey, Syria Tunisia, Belgium, Italy and Greece. The phylogenetic analysis showed a small cluster of our strain with a European isolate.

Conclusions

Clinicians should be aware of atypical pathogens, in particular, in immunocompromised population, and urine culture should be considered at an earlier stage in these kind of patients due to the presence of less virulent organisms that may be harbouring important resistance mechanisms.

A well-designed antimicrobial stewardship associated with an efficient infection control are essential to limit the spread of these new emerging pathogens.

Abbreviations

CA-UTI: Catheter associated urinary tract infection; CNA: Columbia nalidixic acid; MIC: Minimal inhibitory concentration; PK-PD: Pharmacokinetic-pharmacodynamic

Acknowledgments
The Authors thank Dr. Buratti for reviewing the paper for English language.

Author's contributions
G.L performed the antibiotic susceptibility assays and the biofilm production assay; G.P. performed the sequence analysis; L.C. and F.S. collected and interpreted all the clinical data; F.C. and A.C. contributed to data analysis; M.A. D. F. analysed data and wrote the paper. All authors read and approved the final manuscript.

Competing interests
The authors declare that they have no competing interests.

Author details
[1]Institute of Microbiology, Department of Molecular and Translational Medicine, University of Brescia-Spedali Civili, P. le Spedali Civili 1, 25123 Brescia, Italy. [2]Department of Nephrology, University of Brescia, Hospital of Montichiari, Brescia, Italy. [3]Institute of Microbiology and Virology, Department of Biomedical, Surgical and Dental Sciences, University of Milan, Milan, Italy.

References
1. Vancanneyt M, Segers P, Torck U, Hoste B, Bernardet JF, Vandamme P, Kersters K. Reclassification of Flavobacterium odoratum (Stutzer 1929) strains to a new genus, Myroides, as Myroides odoratus comb. Nov. and Myroides odoratimimus sp. nov. Int J Syst Bacteriol. 1996;46:926–32.
2. Benedetti P, Rassu M, Pavan G, Sefton A, Pellizzer G. Septic shock, pneumonia, and soft tissue infection due to Myroides odoratimimus: report of a case and review of Myroides infections. Infection. 2011;39:161–5.
3. Holmes B, Snell JJ, Lapage SP. Revised description, from clinical isolates, of Flavobacterium, odoratum Stutzer and Kwaschnina 1929, and designation of the neotype strain. Int J Syst Bacteriol. 1977;27:330–6.
4. Mammeri H, Bellais S, Nordmann P. Chromosome-encoded beta-lactamases TUS-1 and MUS-1 from *Myroides odoratus* and *Myroides odoratimimus* (formerly Flavobacterium odoratum), new members of the lineage of molecular subclass B1 metalloenzymes. Antimicrob Agents Chemother. 2002;46(11):3561–7.
5. Hu S, Cao L, Wu Y, Zhou Y, Jiang T, Wang L, Wang Q, Ming D, Chen S, Wang M. Comparative genomic analysis of *Myroides odoratimimus* isolates. Microbiologyopen. 2018; https://doi.org/10.1002/mbo3.634.
6. Pompilio A, Galardi G, Gherardi G, Verginelli F, Geminiani C, Pilloni AP, Catalanotti P, Di Bonaventura G. Infection of recurrent calcaneal ulcer caused by a biofilm-producer Myroides odoratimimus strain. Folia Microbiol. 2018;63:203–7.
7. Stepanović S, Vuković D, Hola V, Di Bonaventura DS, Cirković I, Ruzicka F. Quantification of biofilm in microtiter plates: overview of testing conditions and practical recommendations for assessment of biofilm production by staphylococci. APMIS. 2007;115:891–9.
8. Tamura K, Peterson D, Peterson N, Stecher G, Nei M, Kuma S. MEGA 5: molecular evolutionary genetic analysis using maximum likelihood, evolutionary distance, and maximum parsimony methods. Mol Biol Evol. 2011;28:2371–9.
9. Gunzer F, Rudolph WW, Bunk B, Schober I, Peters S, Muller T, Oberheitmann B, Schröttner T. Whole-genome sequencing of a large collection of Myroides odoratimimus and Myroides odoratus isolated and antimicrobial susceptibility studies. Emerg Microbes Infect. 2018;7:61.
10. De Song M, Chen Q, Chen X. Analysis of resistance genes in pan-resistant Myroides odoratimimus clinical strain PR 63039 using whole genome sequencing. Microb Path. 2017;112:164–70.
11. Niveditha S, Pramodhini S, Umadevi S, Kumar S, Stephen S. The isolation and biofilm formation of uropathogens in the patients with catheter associated urinary tract infections (CAUTI). J Clin Diagn Res. 2012;6:1478–82.
12. O'Toole G, Kaplan HB, Kolter R. Biofilm formation as microbial development. Annu Rev Microbiol. 2000;54:49–79.
13. Singh S, Singh SK, Chowdhury I, Singh R. Understanding the mechanism of bacterial biofilms resistance to antimicrobial agents. Open Microbiol J. 2017; 11:53–62.

14. Donlan RM. Biofilm formation: a clinically relevant microbiological process. Clin Infect Dis. 2001;33:1387–92.
15. Bartoletti R, Cai T, Wagenlehner FM, Naber K, Bjerklund-Johansen TE. Treatment of urinary tract infections and antibiotic stewardship. Eur Urol Suppl. 2016;15:81–7.
16. Ktari S, Mnif B, Koubaa M, Mahioubi F, Ben Jemmaa M, Mhiri MN, Hammami A. Nosocomial outbreak of Myroides odoratimimus urinary tract infection in a Tunisian hospital. J Hosp Infect. 2012;80:77–51.
17. Yağci A, Cerikçioğlu N, Kaufmann ME, Malnick H, Söyletir G, Babacan F, Pitt TL. Molecular typing of Myroides odoratimimus (Flavobacterium odoratum) urinary tract infections in a Turkish hospital. Eur J Clin Microbiol Infect Dis. 2000;19:731–2.
18. Licker M, Sorescu T, Rus M, Cirlea N, Horhat F, Jurescu C, Botoca M, Cumpanas A, Timar R, Muntean D. Extensively drug-resistant Myroides odoratimimus-a case series of urinary tract infections in immunocompromised patients. Infect Drug Resist. 2018;11:743–9.
19. Maraki S, Sarchianaki E, Barabagadakis S. Myroides odoratimimus soft tissue infection in an immunocompetent child following a pig bite: case report and literature review. Braz J Infect Dis. 2012;16:390–2.
20. Jover-Sáenz A, Pérez-Villar F, Barcenilla-Gaite F. Severe sepsis caused by infected prosthesis joint due to Myroides odoratimimus. Medicina Clinica (English edition). 2016;147:276–7.
21. Endicott-Yazdani TR, Dhiman N, Benavides R, Spak CV. Myroides odoratimimus bacteremia in a diabetic patient. Proc (Bayl Univ Med Cent). 2015;28:342–3.
22. Belloir L, Billy PA, Hentgen C, Fille A, Barrans A. Myroides odoratimimus bacteremia. Med Mal Infect. 2016;46:396–7.
23. Bachmeyer C, Entressengle H, Khosrotehrani K, Goldman G, Delisle F, Arlet G, Grateaum G. Cellulitis due to Myroides odoratimimus in a patient with alcoholic cirrhosis. Clin Experim Dermatol. 2007;33:97–8.
24. Motwani B, Krezolek D, Symeonides S, Khayr W. Myroides odoratum cellulitis and bacteremia: a case report. Infect Dis Clin Pract. 2004;12:343–4. https://doi.org/10.1097/01.idc.0000144904.51074.79.
25. Prateek S, Gupta P, Mittal G, Singh AK. Fatal case of pericardial effusion due to Myroides odoratus: a rare case report. J Clin Diagn Res. 2015;9:DD01–2. https://doi.org/10.7860/JCDR/2015/15120.6740.
26. Soydan S, Ignak S, Demirei OU, Karadag G, Ocak Z. Myroides species in a Paediatric burn patient. J Clin Diagn Res. 2017;11:DD03–4.
27. Willems P, Muller J, Verhaegen J, Saegeman V, Desmet S. How to treat a fulminant erysipelas and sepsis caused by Myroides odoratimimus: case report and literature review. Acta Clin Belg. 2017;72:331–5.
28. Ranjan M, Karade S, Rahi P, Singh SP, Sen S. Urosepsis due to Multi Drug Resistant Myroides odoratimimus: A Case Report. Int J Curr Microbiol App Sci. 2017;6:1930–5.

16

Healthcare-associated infections in intensive care units in Taiwan, South Korea, and Japan: recent trends based on national surveillance reports

Cho-Han Chiang[1†], Sung-Ching Pan[2†], Tyan-Shin Yang[1], Keisuke Matsuda[3], Hong Bin Kim[4,5], Young Hwa Choi[6], Satoshi Hori[7], Jann-Tay Wang[1,2,8], Wang-Huei Sheng[1,2,8], Yee-Chun Chen[1,2,8,9*], Feng-Yee Chang[10] and Shan-Chwen Chang[1,2]

Abstract

Background: Sustainable systematic interventions are important for infection prevention and control (IPC). Data from surveillance of healthcare-associated infections (HAI) provides feedback for implementation of IPC programs. To address the paucity of such data in Asia, we searched for national HAI surveillance and IPC programs in this region.

Methods: Data were analysed from open access national surveillance reports of three Asian countries: Taiwan, South Korea and Japan from 2008 to 2015. National IPC programs were identified.

Results: There were differences among the countries in surveillance protocols, hospital coverage rates, and national IPC policies and programs. Nevertheless, there was a 53.0% reduction in overall HAI over the 8-year period. This consisted of a decrease from 9.34 to 5.03 infections per 1000 patient-days in Taiwan, from 7.56 to 2.76 in Korea, and from 4.41 to 2.74 in Japan (Poisson regression, all $p < 0.05$). Across the three countries, *Escherichia coli* and *Candida albicans* were the major pathogens for urinary tract infection. *Staphylococcus aureus*, *Acinetobacter baumannii* and *Enterococcus faecium* were common bloodstream pathogens. For pneumonia, *S. aureus*, *A. baumannii*, *Pseudomonas aeruginosa*, and *Klebsiella pneumoniae* were the predominant pathogens, with considerable country differences. There was a 64.6% decrease in the number of isolates of methicillin-resistant *S. aureus*, 38.4% decrease in carbapenem-resistant *P. aeruginosa* and 49.2% decrease in carbapenem-resistant *A. baumannii* (CRAB) in Taiwan (all $p < 0.05$), and similarly in Korea with the exception of CRAB (30.5 and 50.4% reduction, respectively, both $p < 0.05$).

Conclusion: We found a significant decrease in HAI across the three countries in association with sequential multifaceted interventions such as hand hygiene, care bundles, and antimicrobial stewardships. Further regional collaboration could be forged to develop joint strategies to prevent HAI.

Keywords: Healthcare-associated infections, National surveillance, Antimicrobial resistance, National policy, Infection prevention and control program

---

* Correspondence: yeechunchen@gmail.com
†Cho-Han Chiang and Sung-Ching Pan contributed equally to this work.
[1]College of Medicine, National Taiwan University, Taipei, Taiwan
[2]Department of Internal Medicine, National Taiwan University Hospital, Taipei, Taiwan
Full list of author information is available at the end of the article

Background

The European Healthcare-associated Infections Surveillance Network (HAI-net) is one of the most coordinated and comprehensive surveillance systems that monitors healthcare-associated infections (HAI). By centralizing data on antimicrobial use, HAI incidence, and HAI point prevalence, HAI-net builds a regional landscape that allows inter-country comparison and provides feedback for implementation of regional infection prevention and control (IPC) guidelines [1].

With its high burden of HAI, Asia stands to benefit by learning from such a surveillance network. A recent meta-analysis reported a pooled HAI incidence density of 20 cases per 1000 intensive care unit-days in Southeast Asia [2]; studies in India and China found pooled ventilator-associated pneumonia of 9.4 and 20.8 cases per 1000 ventilator-days, respectively [3, 4]. Establishing surveillance in Asian countries, either as national or regional collaborations, might help relevant stakeholders to identify systemic gaps and establish improvements in IPC.

The current understanding of HAI surveillance in Asia remains limited despite the relatively large numbers of IPC conducted in Asia [2, 5]. Likewise, national scale data documenting the regional HAI epidemiology in Asia is scarce [2]. To better understand the current state of HAI surveillance and IPC programs in Asia, we searched for data on existing national HAI surveillance programs. Three Asian countries: Taiwan [6, 7], South Korea [8–10], and Japan [11] were found to conduct nationwide HAI surveillance systems. The present study is based on data derived from open access reports from the surveillance systems of these countries. They include temporal trends of HAI in intensive care units (ICUs), the major causative pathogens and antimicrobial resistance (AMR). Nationally implemented IPC policies were also reviewed to gain insights on important interventions instituted in these three countries.

Methods
Study design and source of data
We performed a Google and PubMed search to determine the existing national HAI surveillance systems in Asian countries using the following terms "national nosocomial infection surveillance" or "national healthcare-associated infection surveillance" in combination with specific country names. The inclusion criteria were: English language, open access data or PubMed publications, annual data containing either point prevalence or yearly surveillance for 5 or more years. Data from the national HAI surveillance systems were retrospectively retrieved and analysed.

National surveillance systems of Taiwan, South Korea, and Japan
Three national HAI surveillance systems met the study criteria. These were the Taiwan Nosocomial Infection Surveillance (TNIS), Korean National Healthcare-associated Infection Surveillance (KONIS), and Japan Nosocomial Infection Surveillance (JANIS). Each system prospectively collects data on the incidence, causative pathogens, and antimicrobial resistance of HAI in ICUs. HAI data are stratified by infection site: urinary tract infection (UTI), bloodstream infection (BSI), hospital-acquired pneumonia (HAP); by device-use: catheter-associated urinary tract infection (CAUTI), central line-associated bloodstream infection (CLABSI), and ventilator-associated pneumonia (VAP); and by type of hospital (in Taiwan and South Korea). These HAI cases and categories are in accord with the definitions of the US National Healthcare Safety Network (NHSN) system with minor modifications to account for differences in clinical or laboratory practice and national policies.

Data collection
Demographic data for each country were retrieved from the World Bank and their respective national authorities. Hospital and ICU composition of each surveillance system were recorded from their official web portals. Annual data of overall HAI, device-associated HAI, causative pathogens, and rates of AMR of important bacteria were also retrieved from the three surveillance systems. We selected the study period as 2008 to 2015 because data for this period were accessible across all three systems. National-scale IPC policies and programs were obtained by online search or in consultation with experts from the three countries.

Data analysis
Incidence densities of overall HAI were determined as pooled means of UTI, BSI, and HAP rates, and calculated as overall HAI episodes per 1000 patient-days. Analysis of device-associated HAI included CAUTI, CLABSI, and VAP. For Taiwan and Korea, incidence densities of device-associated HAI were calculated as device-associated infection episodes per 1000 device-days. For Japan, device-associated HAI were analysed by device-associated infection episodes per 1000 patient-days which made Japanese data incompatible with data from other countries. Causative pathogens were classified at the species level. AMR proportions of selected pathogens were calculated as number of antimicrobial-resistant isolates divided by the total number of isolates of the same species.

Statistical analysis
A Poisson regression model was used to assess the temporal trends of HAI incidence. Linear regression was used to analyse the trends in AMR isolates, using the STATA statistical program (version 14.0 Texas, USA). A P value < 0.05 was considered statistically significant.

Results

Characteristics of Taiwan, South Korea and Japan's National Surveillance Systems

The characteristics of the national HAI surveillance systems of Taiwan, South Korea, and Japan are summarised in Table 1 [6, 8, 11]. The type, size and proportion of hospitals enrolled in the national surveillance varied among the countries. Taiwan included medical centres and regional hospitals classified according to hospital accreditation. Most of them had hospital beds of 300 beds or more. Korea and Japan included hospitals with more than 300 and 200 beds, respectively. The hospital coverage and participation rates were 21.2 and 100.0% in Taiwan, 18.0 and 38.6% in Korea, and 1.9 and 6.8% in Japan, respectively. A total of 472, 169 and 163 ICUs were enrolled in Taiwan, Korea and Japan, respectively. The number of participating hospitals and ICUs in all three countries during the study period has expanded (Additional file 1: Table S1) [6, 8, 11]. Categorization of HAI was different in JANIS, which presented only UTI, CLABSI and VAP. Infection incidence was also calculated differently as episodes per 1000 patient-days.

National infection control policies or programs and HAI trends across Taiwan, South Korea, and Japan

Numerous independent changes, aimed at improving surveillance and compliance, were made for national IPC policies, programs, or practices in each country (Fig. 1). Additional file 2: Table S2 summarised the details of national IPC programs in the past two decades by country. For example, during the study period hand hygiene, care bundles, hospital environment hygiene program and antimicrobial stewardship were the main interventions implemented in Taiwan. The hand hygiene program adapted the WHO multimodal strategies with particular emphasis on alcohol-based hand rub at the point of care. The care bundles program aimed to prevent CAUTI, CLABSI, and VAP. On the other hand, Korea and Japan enforced IPC practices by legislating and mandating IPC in hospitals. Incentives in terms of reimbursement 1.8–2.7 US dollars and 10 US dollars per admission were given to hospitals who met IPC standards in Korea and Japan, respectively. All three countries mandated assignment of infection control personnel. They also implemented formal and structured antimicrobial stewardship programs, which include surveillance of AMR pathogens and regulations of antimicrobial use.

Overall HAI rates

All three countries experienced a significant reduction of approximately 50% in HAI rates by the end of the study period. The incidence density in Taiwan decreased by 46.2% from 9.3 to 5.0 infections per 1000 patient-days; in Korea HAI declined by 63.1% from 7.6 to 2.8, and in Japan by 38.6% from 4.4 to 2.7 (Poisson regression, all $p < 0.05$) (Fig. 1).

There was a significant reduction in device-associated HAI at all sites of infection in Taiwan and Korea ($p < 0.05$) (Fig. 2). Japan had low rates of CAUTI and CLABSI (presented as infections per 1000 patient-days) that persisted over the 8-year period. The most remarkable change was noted for CAUTI in Korea, with an 81.3% decrease from 4.8 to 0.9 infections per 1000 device-days ($P < 0.05$). All three countries experienced a similar trend in VAP during the study period with a 57.7% reduction from 2.6 to 1.1 infections per 1000 device-days in Taiwan.

Causative pathogens

The distributions of the top five (or four for Japan) causative pathogens according to country and site of infection in 2015 are shown in Table 2. For Taiwan and Korea, UTI, BSI and HAP data were presented; for Japan, UTI, CLABSI and VAP data were presented. A more comprehensive list of pathogens is shown in Additional file 3: Table S3, Additional file 4: Table S4, and Additional file 5: Table S5.

Escherichia coli and *Candida albicans* were included in the top five organisms causing UTI in all three countries. *E. coli* and *C. albicans* constituted 19.8 and 16.9%, 17.6 and 12.6, 37.6 and 7.9% of UTI for Taiwan, Korea, and Japan, respectively (Table 2). Along with *Candida albicans*, non-*albicans Candida* species and yeast-like organisms constituted 31.4% of the urinary tract pathogens in Taiwan. In Korea, 23.4% of the UTI were due to *Candida* species (Additional file 3: Table S3).

Staphylococcus aureus was a major pathogen of BSI. The rates were 14.2% in Korea, 13.0% in Japan, and 6.5% in Taiwan (Table 2). Along with *S. aureus*, *Staphylococcus epidermidis* and coagulase-negative staphylococci constituted 38.8% of the CLABSI isolates in Japan. There were major differences among the countries in the distribution of other predominant pathogens. *Acinetobacter baumannii* and *E. faecium* were the predominant BSI pathogens in Taiwan and Korea. Major *Candida* species constituted 12.1% of the BSI isolates in Taiwan and 12.9% in Korea (Additional file 4: Table S4).

S. aureus, *P. aeruginosa* and *K. pneumoniae* were the predominant pathogens for HAP across all three countries (Table 2). Interestingly, *A. baumannii* was predominant in Taiwan and Korea but not in Japan, similar to the observation for BSI. For Taiwan and Korea, these four pathogens comprised 65.7 and 81.2% of the HAP isolates, respectively.

Antimicrobial resistance

Higher AMR rates were noted in Korea than in Taiwan (Fig. 3). The data for Japan were incomplete for several study years and are not shown in the figures. There was

Table 1 Demographics and national surveillance systems of Taiwan, South Korea and Japan

Parameter	Taiwan	South Korea	Japan
Country background			
Population[a]	23,433,753[b]	50,746,659[c]	127,276,000[d]
Income bracket[e]	High income	High income	High income
GDP, US dollars	571,736 million[f]	1,530,750.92 million[g]	4,872,136.95 million[g]
Share of GDP on national health expenditure	6.3%[f]	7.6%[h]	10.7%[h]
Number of hospitals[a]	486[i]	534[j]	7426[k]
Surveillance system	Taiwan Nosocomial Infection Surveillance (TNIS)	Korean National Healthcare-associated Infection Surveillance System (KONIS)	Japan Nosocomial Infection Surveillance (JANIS)
Year established	2001	2006	2000
Authority	Centers for Disease Control, Ministry of Health and Welfare, Taiwan	Korea Centers for Disease Control and Prevention	Ministry of Health, Labor and Welfare, Japan
ICU Surveillance[a]			
Number of hospitals enrolled	103	96	143
Number of ICUs enrolled	472	169	163
Types of hospitals enrolled (total number in the country)	Medical Centers and Regional hospitals [l] ($n = 103$)	Bed size > 900, 700–899, 300–699 ($n = 249$)[n]	Bed size > 200 ($n = 2100$)
Hospital coverage rate	21.2% (103/486)	18.0% (96/534)	1.9% (143/7426)
Hospital participation rate[m]	100.0% (103/103)	38.6% (96/249)	6.8% (143/2100)
Mandated standard ratio of infection control personnel	1 dedicated full-time certificated IC nurse per 300 beds (basic) or per 250 beds (optimal) 1 FTE qualified IC doctor per 500 beds (basic) or per 300 beds (optimal)[o] For hospitals > 500 beds: 1 FTE IC medical technician (basic) or 1 dedicated full-time certificated IC medical technician (optimal); 1 FTE IC medical technician for hospitals with 300–499 beds (optimal)	1 dedicated full-time IC nurse per 200 beds (basic) or per 150 beds (optimal)[n] 1 qualified IC doctor per 300 beds	1 dedicated full-time certificated IC nurse (at > 0.8 FTE)[p] 1 part-time IC doctor (at > 0.5 FTE) 1 part-time IC medical technician and 1 part-time pharmacist (at > 0.5 FTE) Additional manpower for antimicrobial stewardship[p]
Healthcare-associated infection data provided			
Site-specific HAIs	UTI, BSI, HAP: episode per 1000 patient-day	UTI, BSI, HAP: episode per 1000 patient-day	UTI: episode per 1000 patient-day
Device-associated HAIs	CAUTI, CLABSI, VAP: episode per 1000 device-day	CAUTI, CLABSI, VAP: episode per 1000 device-day	CLABSI, VAP: episode per 1000 patient-day
Causative pathogens	Top 10 of the most common pathogens	99% of all the causative pathogens	Top 5 of the most common pathogens[q]
Antimicrobial-resistant pathogens	MRSA, VRE, CRAB, CRPA, CRE, CREC, CRKP	MRSA, VRE, IRAB, IRPA, CefR-KP, CipR-KP, CefR-EC, CipR-EC	MRSA

Abbreviations: BSI bloodstream infections, *CAUTI* catheter-associated urinary tract infection, *CefR-EC* cefotaxime-resistant *Escherichia coli*, *CefR-KP* cefotaxime-resistant *Klebsiella pneumoniae*, *CipR-EC* ciprofloxacin-resistant *E. coli*, *CipR-KP* ciprofloxacin-resistant *K. pneumoniae*, *CLABSI* central line-associated bloodstream infections, *CRAB* carbapanem (imipenem or meropenem)-resistant *Acinetobacter baumannii*, *CRE* carbapanem (imipenem, meropenem, or ertapenem)-resistant Enterobacteriaceae, *CREC* carbapanem (imipenem, meropenem, or ertapenem)-resistant *E. coli*, *CRKP* carbapanem (imipenem, meropenem, or ertapenem)-resistant *K. pneumoniae*, *CRPA* carbapanem (imipenem or meropenem)-resistant *Pseudomonas aeruginosa*, *FTE* full-time equivalent, *GDP* gross domestic product, *HAI* Healthcare-associated infections, *HAP* hospital-acquired pneumonia, *IC* infection control, *IRAB* imipenem-resistant *A. baumannii*, *IRPA* imipenem-resistant *P. aerugonisa*, *MRSA* methicillin-resistant *Staphylococcus aureus*, *MSSA* methicillin-susceptible *S. aureus*, *UTI* urinary tract infections, *VAP* ventilator-associated pneumonia, *VRE* vancomycin-resistant enterococci (*Enterococcus faecalis* or *E. faecium*)
[a]2014 data
[b]Data retrieved from http://www1.stat.gov.tw/ct.asp?xItem=15408&CtNode=4692&mp=3. Assessed 14 April 2018.
[c]Data retrieved from https://data.worldbank.org/country/korea-rep. Assessed 14 April 2018
[d]Data retrieved from https://data.worldbank.org/country/japan?view=chart. Assessed 14 April 2018
[e]Data retrieved from World Bank Country and Lending Groups at https://datahelpdesk.worldbank.org/knowledgebase/articles/906519-world-bank-country-and-lending-groups. Accessed 10 September 2018. For the current 2019 fiscal year, high-income economies are those with a gross national income per capita, calculated using the World Bank Atlas method of $12,056 or more

[f]2016 data. Raw data NT dollars 17,152,093 million, converted to US dollars by ratio 30:1. Retrieved from https://www.mohw.gov.tw/lp-3781-2.html. Accessed 10 September 2018

[g]2017 data based on World Bank national accounts data, and Organization for Economic Co-operation and Development (OECD) National Accounts data. Retrieved from https://data.worldbank.org/indicator/NY.GDP.MKTP.CD. Accessed 10 September 2018

[h]2017 data based on Organization for Economic Co-operation and Development (OECD) estimated data for Japan and provisional data for Korea. Retrieved from https://stats.oecd.org/Index.aspx?DataSetCode=SHA. Accessed 10 September 2018

[i]Data retrieved from https://www.mohw.gov.tw/dl-40542-045687b7-aa43-458c-ab70-e8ff24c5b1b3.html. Accessed 10 September 2018

[j]Data retrieved from http://kosis.kr/eng/statisticsList/statisticsList_01List.jsp?vwcd=MT_ETITLE&parentId=D#SubCont. Accessed 10 September 2018

[k]Data retrieved from http://www.mhlw.go.jp/english/database/db-hh/2-2.html. Accessed 10 September 2018

[l]The data for Taiwan included medical centers and regional hospitals, which were classified according to hospital accreditation and covered only acute care hospitals

[m]The hospital coverage rate was calculated as the number of participating hospitals divided by the total number of hospitals in the same year in each country. The hospital participation rate was calculated as the number of participating hospitals divided by the total number of hospitals to be enrolled in each surveillance system

[n]In terms of surveillance, the requirement for participation in KONIS was 1 full-time infection control nurse over 200-bed size hospital. Regarding the mandatory personnel requirement, this regulation has been launched as a financial incentive program since 2016, as described in Additional file 2: Table S2

[o]Data available at https://www.cdc.gov.tw/professional/info.aspx?treeid=beac9c103df952c4&nowtreeid=bd387fa55fef03f0&tid=FED32554F2B55D11. Accessed September 10, 2018

[p]Infection prevention and control incentive through reimbursement policies was revised in 2010, 2012 and 2018, as described in Additional file 2: Table S2. Since 2012, each hospital is reimbursed 1000 JPY (about 10 USD) per patient per admission if it fulfills the Ministry of Health, Labor and Welfare requirements which mandated one dedicated full-time certificated ICN (at > 0.8 FTE), one part-time ICD (at > 0.5 FTE), one part-time IC pharmacist and one part-time medical technician/microbiologist (at > 0.5 FTE). Since 2018, reimbursement policies per admission included three parts. It provides 3900 JPY (about 39 USD) per admission for infection prevention and control incentive at a major hospital, or 1000 JPY for a small hospital. Additional 1000 JPY was reimbursed if this hospital participates a local IPC network incentive. Another 1000 JPY was reimbursed for AS incentive. For hospitals with AS incentive, it mandates the following manpower in addition to 2012 requirements: one part-time doctor mainly for AS (at > 0.5 FTE), one full-time ICP either a certificated ICN or IC pharmacist or medical technician

[q]MRSA and MSSA are listed as separate pathogens

a significant decrease in the number of isolates of methicillin-resistant *S. aureus* (MRSA) from 2008 to 2015. This included a 64.6% reduction in Taiwan and 30.5% in Korea ($p < 0.05$) (Fig. 3a). The proportion of MRSA among all *S. aureus* isolates in 2015 remained high in Korea (83.1%), while it decreased in Taiwan by 12.3% from 79.9% in 2008 to 70.1% over the 8-year period. There was also a significant decrease in the number of isolates of carbapenem-resistant *P. aeruginosa* (CRPA) during the study period with a reduction of 50.4% in Korea and 38.4% in Taiwan ($p < 0.05$) (Fig. 3b).

Carbapenem-resistant *A. baumannii* (CRAB) was more commonly isolated in Taiwan than in South Korea. The number of CRAB isolates initially increased in Taiwan and then decreased significantly with a total reduction of 49.2% from 2010 to 2015 ($p < 0.05$). In contrast, the number of CRAB isolates in Korea increased by 91.8% by the end of the study period (Fig. 3c). The proportion of CRAB among *A. baumannii* isolates was higher in Korea than in Taiwan, and increased from 2008 to 2015 in both countries.

Discussion

In the current study, we described the surveillance and IPC programs of Taiwan, South Korea and Japan. A variation in surveillance protocol, such as HAI case definition and surveillance items was found among the three countries although these protocols were similar to those employed by the HAI-net and NHSN. There were also common IPC strategies shared by the three countries, but each with special emphasis on different aspects of IPC. We also compared the rates of HAI and the most common causative pathogens as reported by the three surveillance systems. There was a 53% decline in overall HAI in the surveyed ICUs of all three countries over the

8-year period. The overall incidence densities of HAI in Taiwan, Korea, and Japan in 2015 were 5.0, 2.8, and 2.7 per 1000 patient-days, respectively. These rates are comparable to HAI-net (2.6 per 1000 patient-days), and substantially lower than those of developing countries, as shown in Table 3 [2, 12–15].

We believe that essential elements that contributed to the sustained decrease in the incidence of HAI in Taiwan, Korea and Japan were the national surveillance programs combined with improvement in IPC practices [16]. In Korea, there was a significant decline in device-associated HAI in association with the implementation of the KONIS program [17]. National IPC programs such as hand hygiene, care bundles, antimicrobial stewardships, and environmental hygiene have been shown to effectively reduce HAI and infections caused by AMR pathogens [7, 18–20]. In Taiwan, hand hygiene program over a 4-year period were found to reduce HAI in ICU by 17.2% and BSI by 12.7% [20], and care bundles to further reduce CAUTI and CLABSI by 22.7 and 12.2%, respectively [21, 22]. In Korea, a multicentre study found that VAP rate decreased from 4.08 to 1.16 cases per 1000 ventilator-days following 3 months of bundle intervention [23]. Evidence-based IPC practices have been shown to be cost-saving and effective in preventing HAI [20, 24]. Adoption of these practices to reduce HAI burden might be helpful for many Asian countries, which are facing problems such as rising healthcare costs and inefficient healthcare insurance systems [25].

Appointment of infection control professionals or infection control committees is a common strategy across the three countries (Fig. 1, Additional file 2: Table S2). In Japan, one serious fundamental obstacle before 2010 was the lack of personnel dedicated to IPC. In 2010, Japan revised medical reimbursement system and provided 10

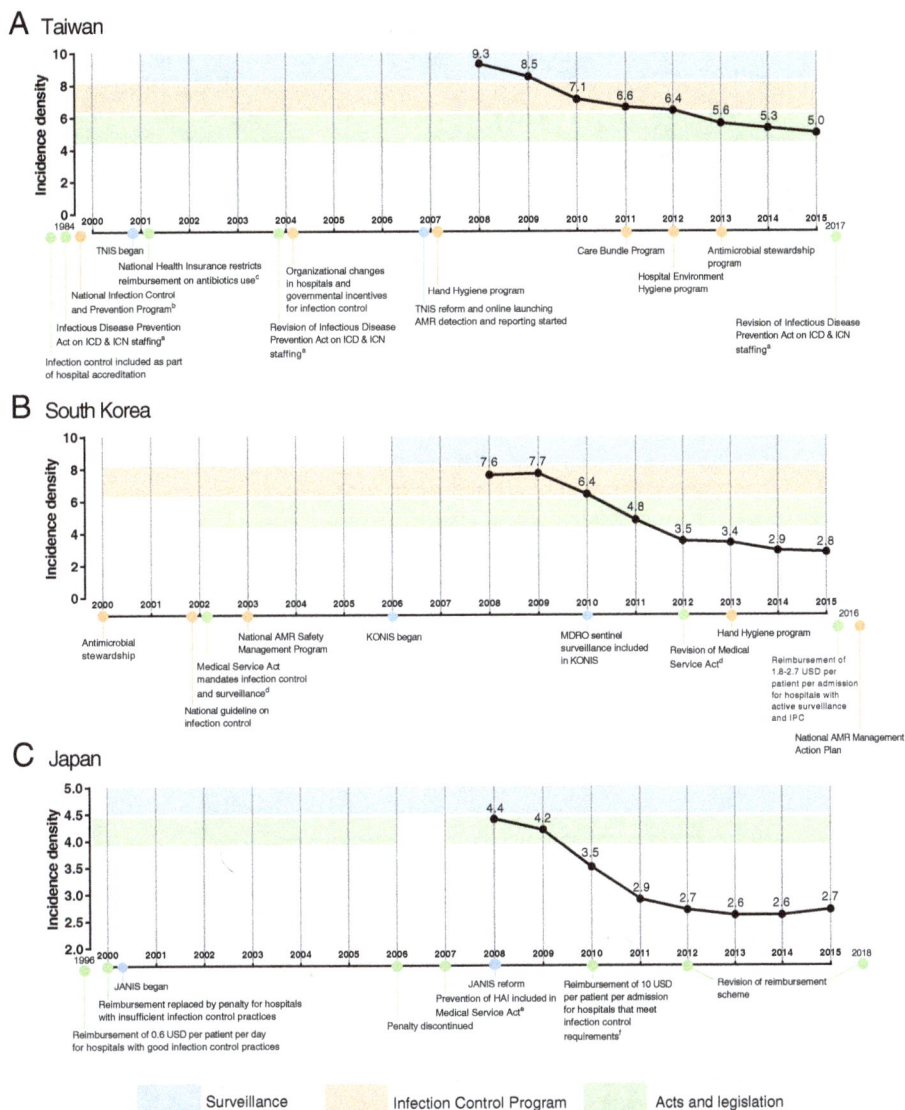

Fig. 1 Incidence densities of healthcare-associated infections in intensive care units across Taiwan, South Korea, and Japan from 2008 to 2015. Abbreviations: AMR: antimicrobial-resistance; HAI: healthcare-associated infections; ICN: infection control nurse; ICP: infection control personnel; IPC: infection prevention and control; JANIS: Japan Nosocomial Infection Surveillance; ICD: infection control doctor; KONIS: Korean National Healthcare-associated Infection Surveillance; MDRO: multi-drug resistant organisms; TNIS: Taiwan Nosocomial Infection Surveillance. [a] In 1984, every teaching hospital in Taiwan was required to have one ICN per 300 hospital beds. In 2004, hospitals with more than 500 beds are required to have at least one ICD, and hospitals with more than 300 beds are required to have at least one ICN per 250 beds. In 2017, hospitals with more than 500 beds are encouraged to have one ICD for every 300 beds and one ICN for every 250 beds (Table 1). [b] Included training healthcare staff, establishing infection control committees, and formulating hospital policies. [c] Restricts use of antimicrobials in ambulatory patients with upper respiratory infections but without evidence of bacterial infection. [d] Act 29 specifies that IPC are the duties of hospitals with more than 300 beds. Act 47 mandates IPC as part of hospital accreditation. In 2012, hospitals with more than 200 beds are required to appoint an infection control committee and at least one full-time experienced staff (Table 1). [e] Japanese medical law obligated all health care institutions to implement operational safety measures against HAI, which includes IPC guidelines, IPC training, and disease reporting. [f] Hospitals should have an infection control team that consists of ICN, ICD, infection control pharmacist and infection control microbiology technologist. Hospitals should also have an IPC policy and antimicrobial stewardship program (Table 1). **a** Taiwan; **b** South Korea; **c** Japan

USD per patient per admission if a hospital payed the annual cost for the designated work hours for infection control personnel which included certified nurse, doctor, pharmacist and medical technician/microbiologist. IPC incentives through reimbursement policies were revised in 2012 and 2018, as described in Additional file 2: Table S2. Such a scheme encourages hospitals dedicated certificated personnel to participate in IPC (Table 1). Other than manpower, personnel training and resource infrastructure are essential for surveillance and prevention of HAI [26, 27].

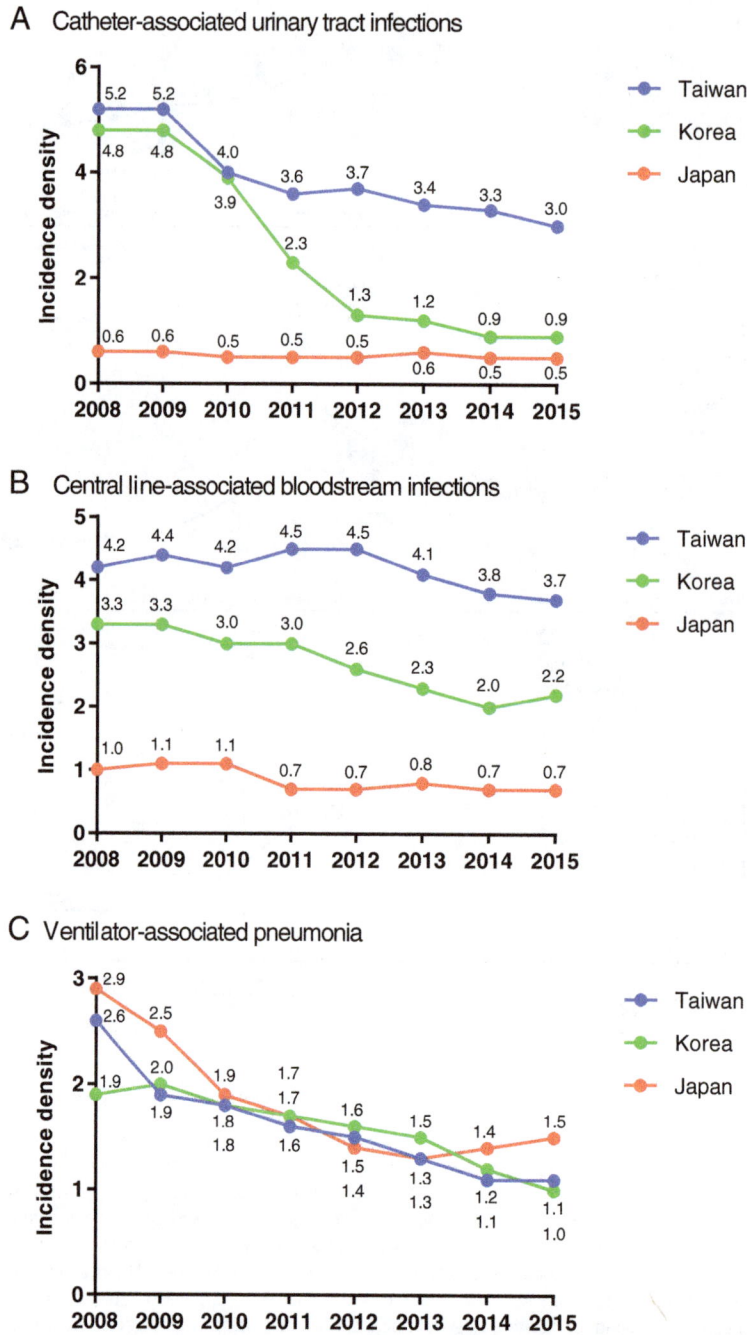

Fig. 2 Annual trends of device-associated infections in intensive care units from 2008 to 2015. Data are presented as episodes per 1000 device-days (Taiwan, Korea) or episodes per 1000 patient-days (Japan; data comprised urinary tract infections, central line-associated bloodstream infections and ventilator-associated pneumonia). **a** Catheter-associated urinary tract infections; **b** Central line-associated bloodstream infections; **c** Ventilator-associated pneumonia

During the study period, financial incentives to support IPC programs were employed by Korea and Japan. Japan switched its reimbursement system to a penalty system in 2000, and then changed it back to the current reward system in 2010. This suggests that a supportive environment that encourages IPC practices might be better than one that punishes for wrongdoing, and should be fostered by national authorities for effective prevention of HAI [27]. Correspondingly, such a difference in reimbursement may have well influenced the outcomes of HAI in Taiwan, Korea and Japan.

Changes in case definition might have contributed to the observed HAI trends. For example, the newer definition for UTI established in 2009 would probably have

Table 2 Common causative pathogens of healthcare-associated infections in intensive care units enrolled in the national surveillance systems of Taiwan, South Korea, and Japan in 2015

Rank	Organism	Proportion	Organism	Proportion	Organism	Proportion
Urinary Tract Infections[a]	Taiwan (N = 3990)		South Korea (N = 760)		Japan (N = 202)	
1	Escherichia coli	19.8%	Escherichia coli	17.6%	Escherichia coli	37.6%
2	Candida albicans	16.9%	Candida albicans	12.6%	Pseudomonas aeruginosa	16.3%
3	Enterococcus faecium	8.5%	Enterococcus faecalis	9.5%	Candida albicans	7.9%
4	Pseudomonas aeruginosa	7.4%	Enterococcus faecium	9.3%	Klebsiella pneumoniae	6.9%
5	Klebsiella pneumoniae	7.3%	Klebsiella pneumoniae	8.6%	Enterococcus faecalis	6.4%
Bloodstream Infections	Taiwan (N = 4138)		South Korea (N = 1288)		Japan[b] (N = 268)	
1	Acinetobacter baumannii	10.4%	Enterococcus faecium	14.7%	Staphylococcus epidermidis	15.7%
2	Klebsiella pneumoniae	9.6%	Staphylococcus aureus	14.2%	Staphylococcus aureus	13.0%
3	Enterococcus faecium	7.2%	Acinetobacter baumannii	12.6%	Coagulase negative staphylococci	10.1%
4	Staphylococcus aureus	6.5%	Coagulase negative staphylococci	12.0%	Serratia marcescens	5.6%
5	Candida albicans	6.2%	Enterococcus faecalis	7.3%		
Pneumonia	Taiwan (N = 1397)		South Korea (N = 554)		Japan[c] (N = 650)	
1	Pseudomonas aeruginosa	22.5%	Acinetobacter baumannii	34.5%	Staphylococcus aureus	21.8%
2	Acinetobacter baumannii	18.0%	Staphylococcus aureus	28.5%	Pseudomonas aeruginosa	18.6%
3	Klebsiella pneumoniae	16.2%	Klebsiella pneumoniae	9.4%	Klebsiella pneumoniae	7.8%
4	Staphylococcus aureus	9.0%	Pseudomonas aeruginosa	8.8%	Stenotrophomonas maltophilia	6.8%
5	Enterobacter species	6.2%	Enterobacter aerogenes	3.2%		

[a]The National Healthcare Safety Network definition of catheter-associated urinary tract infections was updated in 2015, and excluded Candida, yeasts or molds as potential pathogens. Nevertheless, TNIS, KONIS and JANIS kept these pathogens and data are provided
[b]Japan's data on bloodstream infection represents central line-associated bloodstream infections
[c]Japan's data on pneumonia represents ventilator-associated pneumonia

excluded cases that might have been classified as HAI under the older definition [28]. Nevertheless, based on the consistent decline of HAI incidence across all infection categories, it is unlikely that modifications in case definition can explain the remarkable decrease in HAI trends.

Substantial variation exists for causative pathogens of HAI across the three countries. This variability could be due to a number of factors, including baseline characteristics of participating hospitals and ICUs, variation in diagnostic standards and case definitions, geography and climate, and IPC practices. For example, Japan's BSI was dominated by staphylococci (39.9%) possibly because its reports were limited to device-associated modules in BSI. An interesting variation that is likely not attributable to systemic differences was noted for A. baumannii, which was isolated commonly from Taiwan and Korea but rarely from Japan. Results from HAI-net seem to support this notion, with higher proportions of HAI caused by Acinetobacter spp. in some countries [13].

Our study showed a general decrease in isolates of important AMR species: MRSA, CRPA and CRAB even though the number of participating ICUs has expanded from 2008 to 2015. This downward trend is likely due to hand hygiene to prevent cross-transmission of AMR

pathogens, care bundles to prevent device- or procedure-associated infections, and antimicrobial stewardship programs to mitigate the selection pressure implemented in these countries [7, 18–20, 29]. A recent meta-analysis reported that antimicrobial stewardship programs in Asia reduced overall antimicrobial consumption by 9.74% and incidence density of important AMR pathogens such as MRSA by 0.9 to 1.4 isolates per 1000 patient-days [19]. Expenditure associated with antimicrobial prescription and hospitalization were also found to decrease by a range of 9.7 to 58.1%. These findings highlight the efficacy and importance of antimicrobial stewardship programs in combating the rise of AMR pathogens.

While surveillance of HAI may provide important feedback for IPC efforts, the high costs in establishing and maintaining the system may preclude many countries from undertaking such an ordeal. Introducing information technology in surveillance systems may help reduce labor intensive and increase the efficiency of surveillance [30–33]. In Asia, National Taiwan University Hospital has established a web-based real-time surveillance system based on algorithms for AMR pathogens, UTI and BSI. The surveillance system is sophisticated in its ability to integrate and analyse several data sources [32, 33]. Their studies and a recent

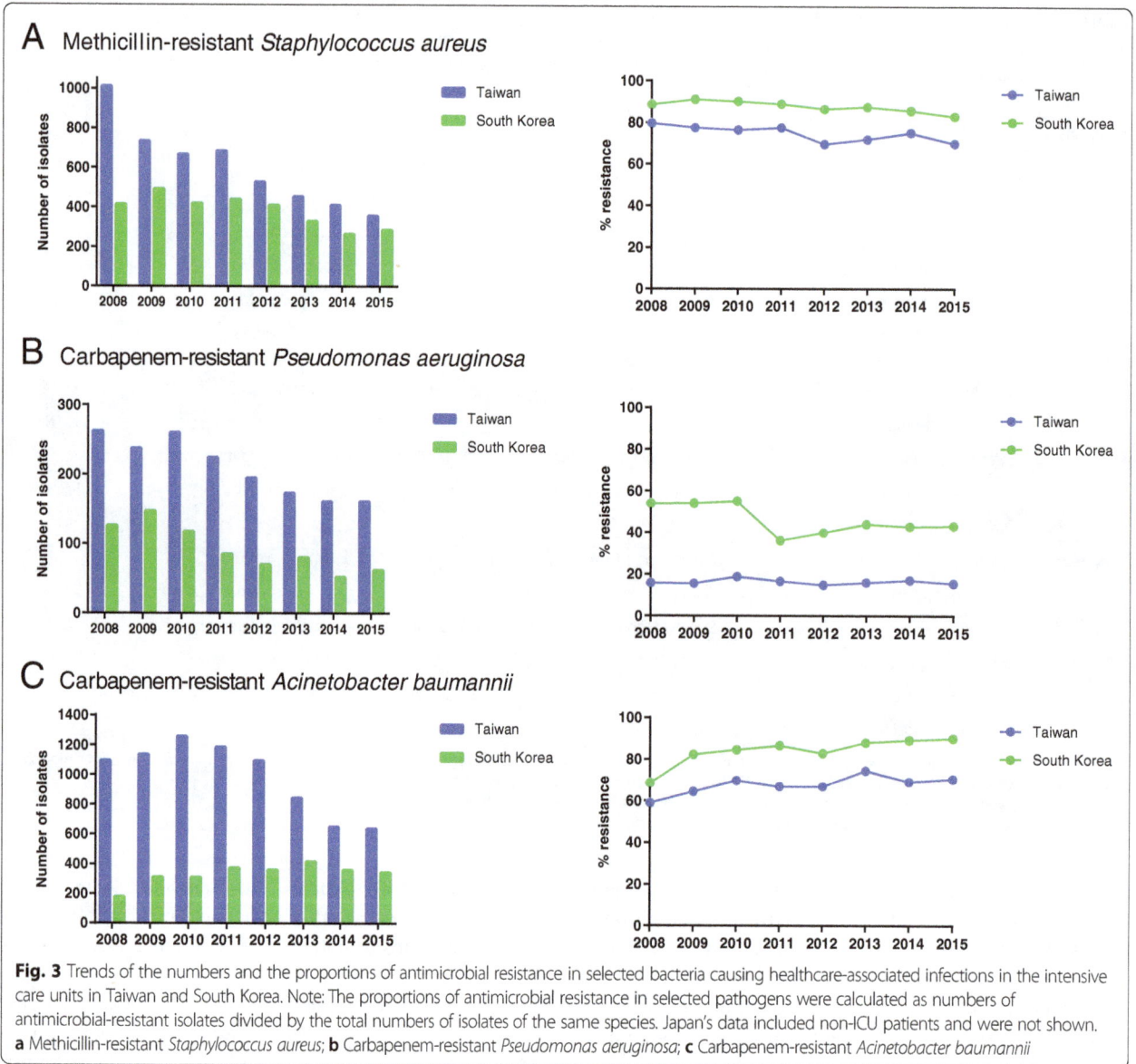

Fig. 3 Trends of the numbers and the proportions of antimicrobial resistance in selected bacteria causing healthcare-associated infections in the intensive care units in Taiwan and South Korea. Note: The proportions of antimicrobial resistance in selected pathogens were calculated as numbers of antimicrobial-resistant isolates divided by the total numbers of isolates of the same species. Japan's data included non-ICU patients and were not shown. **a** Methicillin-resistant *Staphylococcus aureus*; **b** Carbapenem-resistant *Pseudomonas aeruginosa*; **c** Carbapenem-resistant *Acinetobacter baumannii*

systematic review of the literature demonstrated that adopting electronic surveillance software yields considerable time savings pertaining to case findings, data collection, case ascertainment and classification while maintaining high levels of sensitivity and specificity [31–33]. Thus, information technology may represent an opportunity for countries seeking to establish HAI surveillance and overcome the gaps of human resources.

Our study provides a framework for other countries to establish or improve surveillance and IPC programs. Further studies on cost-effectiveness of these strategies will be helpful to relevant stakeholders as they allocate and prioritize budget for infection control. Our work also serves as the foundation for possible regional collaborations in East Asia or in greater Asia. Standardization of protocols will allow inter-country comparison and benchmarking.

For Europe, the similarities and differences in HAI trends between our study and the HAI-net re-affirmed the need for continual surveillance and IPC efforts.

The strengths of this study were our ability to obtain an overview of the surveillance and IPC programs of Taiwan, Korea, and Japan that were seldom described in past reports. We were also able to obtain comprehensive HAI data from their surveillance systems and compare these data with Western developed countries and developing countries worldwide. The limitations were the need to use open access datasets. This restricted our ability to assess and compare HAI epidemiology comprehensively across the three countries. JANIS only releases data on UTI, CLABSI, and VAP in its surveillance reports. Information on the other infection modules: CAUTI, BSI, and HAP were unavailable. We were unable to comprehensively

Table 3 Comparison of healthcare-associated infections in intensive care units across different geographic regions

Countries/Regions (surveillance system)	Data source or type of study	Year	Overall[a]	Site-specific HAI (per 1000 patient-days)			Device-associated HAI (per 1000 device-days)		
				UTI [b]	BSI	HAP	CAUTI[b]	CLABSI	VAP
Taiwan (TNIS)	National surveillance	2015	5.0 (8514/1692998)	2.1	2.1	0.8	3.0	3.7	1.1
South Korea (KONIS)	National surveillance	2015	2.8[c] (2608/945605)	0.8	1.3	0.7	0.9	2.2	1.0
Japan (JANIS)	National surveillance	2015	2.7[d] (952/347386)	0.5	–	–	–	0.7[e]	1.5[e]
USA (NHSN) [12]	National surveillance	2012	1.6[f] (37872/23344616)	–	–	–	2.1	1.1	1.4
Europe (HAI-net) [13]	National surveillance	2015	2.6 (15821/6177114)	1.1	2.0	4.0	3.6	3.6	10.0
Southeast Asia [2]	Meta-analysis[g]	2000–2012	20.0[h] (16.9450/26681)	–	–	–	8.9	4.7	14.7
Developing countries worldwide [14]	Meta-analysis[g]	1995–2008	47.9[h] (28.54250/148893)	–	–	–	9.8	11.3	22.9
Developing countries worldwide (INICC)[i] [15]	Multi-center study	2010–2015	–				5.1	4.1	13.1

Abbreviations: BSI bloodstream infections, *CAUTI* catheter-associated urinary tract infections, *CLABSI* central line-associated bloodstream infections, *HAI* healthcare-associated infections, *HAI-net* Healthcare-associated Infections Surveillance Network (Europe), *HAP* hospital-acquired pneumonia, *ICU* intensive care units, *INICC* International Nosocomial Infection Control Consortium (developing countries worldwide), *NHSN* National Healthcare Safety network (USA), *UTI* urinary tract infections, *VAP* ventilator-associated pneumonia
[a]Data are pooled mean of site-specific HAI such as UTI, BSI, and HAP or otherwise specified, and computed from raw data provided in the reports. Thus, all these data should be interpreted appropriately
[b]The NHSN CAUTI definition was updated in 2015 and excluded *Candida*, yeasts or molds as potential CAUTI pathogens. Nevertheless, TNIS, KONIS and JANIS kept these pathogens and data are provided
[c]Data were collected during July 2015–June 2016
[d]Data are pooled means of UTI, CLABSI and VAP
[e]Data were calculated by episodes/1000 patient-day
[f]Data are pooled means of CAUTI, CLABSI and VAP
[g]Infection frequencies reported in high-quality studies were greater than those from low-quality studies
[h]Weights were given to different studies to compute the final data. Unweighted raw data were derived from the original article and denoted in parenthesis
[i]Data were prospectively collected from 861,284 patients in 703 ICUs from 50 countries

describe the complete pathogen rankings and AMR profiles for each country, because these data were unavailable on some surveillance systems. There are differences in protocols employed by each surveillance system, such as JANIS, which calculated device-associated infections differently. Standardization of protocols should allow for inter-country comparison. Furthermore, we need to include antibiotic use in future studies because of their critical impact on development of resistance. Finally, there were differences in the types of the hospitals enrolled in the three systems, wide variation of hospital participation rates (6.8% in Japan and 100% in Taiwan), and thus, discrepancies in hospital coverage rates (1.9% in Japan and 21.2% in Taiwan). Therefore, data presented here cannot be generalized to the entire 3 countries.

Conclusions

We found that national surveillance data obtained from Taiwan, South Korea, and Japan from 2008 to 2015 was associated with a 53.0% reduction in HAI in surveyed ICUs. There were differences among the countries in surveillance protocols, hospital coverage rates, national IPC programs, distribution of invading microorganisms and antibiotic resistance. The overall decrease in HAI appears to be due to improved surveillance coupled with a series of interventions in each country. We propose

that a regional HAI network be established in East Asia similar to Europe's HAI-net. Such a coordinated effort should enable greater regional collaborations and development of joint strategies as we learn from one another.

Additional files

Additional file 1: Table S1. The number of participating hospitals and intensive care units of national healthcare-associated infection surveillance system in each country from 2008 to 2015. (DOCX 33 kb)

Additional file 2: Table S2. National infection prevention and control policies and programs initiated, implemented or extended in Taiwan, South Korea, and Japan. (DOCX 59 kb)

Additional file 3: Table S3. Common causative pathogens of healthcare-associated urinary tract infections in intensive care units enrolled in national surveillance systems in Taiwan, South Korea, and Japan in 2015. (DOCX 36 kb)

Additional file 4: Table S4. Common causative pathogens of healthcare-associated bloodstream infections in intensive care units enrolled in national surveillance systems in Taiwan, South Korea, and Japan in 2015. (DOCX 36 kb)

Additional file 5: Table S5. Common causative pathogens of healthcare-associated pneumonia in intensive care units enrolled in national surveillance systems in Taiwan, South Korea, and Japan in 2015. (DOCX 36 kb)

Abbreviations
AMR: Antimicrobial resistance; AS: Antimicrobial stewardship; BSI: Bloodstream infection; CAUTI: Catheter-associated urinary tract infection; CLABSI: Central line-associated bloodstream infection; CRPA: Carbapenem-resistant *Pseudomonas aeruginosa*CRABCarbapenem-resistant *Acinetobacter baumannii*; FTE: Full-time equivalent; HAI: Healthcare-associated infections; HAI-net: European Healthcare-associated Infections Surveillance Network; HAP: Hospital-acquired pneumonia; IC: Infection control; ICD: Infection control doctor; ICN: Infection control nurse; ICP: Infection control personnel; ICU: Intensive care units; INICC: International Nosocomial Infection Control Consortium; IPC: Infection prevention and control; JANIS: Japan Nosocomial Infection Surveillance; KONIS: Korean National Healthcare-associated Infection Surveillance; MRSA: Methicillin-resistant *Staphylococcus aureus*; NHSN: National Healthcare Safety Network; TNIS: Taiwan Nosocomial Infection Surveillance; UTI: Urinary tract infection; VAP: Ventilator-associated pneumonia

Acknowledgements
We thank Calvin M. Kunin for his critical review of the manuscript.

Funding
No funding support.

Authors' contributions
Part of data were presented by CH Chiang at the International Conference on Prevention and Infection Control, 20–23 June 2017, Geneva, Switzerland. YC Chen coordinated and designed the study, and proofread the manuscript. CH Chiang, TS Yang and K Matsuda collected and analysed the data. SC Pan supervised statistical analysis. CH Chiang, SC Pan and YC Chen prepared the manuscript. FY Chang and SC Chang were involved in national infection control and prevention programs during the study period. HB Kim, YH Choi and other authors provided relevant information to consolidate the contents of the manuscript.

Competing interests
The authors declare that they have no competing interests.

Author details
[1]College of Medicine, National Taiwan University, Taipei, Taiwan. [2]Department of Internal Medicine, National Taiwan University Hospital, Taipei, Taiwan. [3]Faculty of Medicine, Osaka University, Osaka, Japan. [4]Department of Internal Medicine, Seoul National University College of Medicine, Seoul, Republic of Korea. [5]Division of Infectious Diseases, Seoul National University Bundang Hospital, Seongnam, Republic of Korea. [6]Department of Infectious Diseases, Ajou University School of Medicine, Suwon, Republic of Korea. [7]Department of Infection Control Science, Juntendo University Faculty of Medicine, Tokyo, Japan. [8]Center for Infection Control, National Taiwan University Hospital, Taipei, Taiwan. [9]National Institute of Infectious Diseases and Vaccinology, National Health Research Institutes, Miaoli County, Taiwan. [10]Division of Infectious Diseases and Tropical Medicine, Department of Internal Medicine, Tri-Service General Hospital, National Defense Medical Center, Taipei, Taiwan.

References
1. European Centre for Disease Prevention and Control. Healthcare-associated Infections Surveillance Network. Available at: https://ecdc.europa.eu/en/about-us/partnerships-and-networks/disease-and-laboratory-networks/hai-net. Assessed 14 Apr 2018.
2. Ling ML, Apisarnthanarak A, Madriaga G. The burden of healthcare-associated infections in Southeast Asia: a systematic literature review and meta-analysis. Clin Infect Dis. 2015;60(11):1690–9.
3. Mehta Y, Jaggi N, Rosenthal VD, Kavathekar M, Sakle A, Munshi N, et al. Device-associated infection rates in 20 cities of India, data summary for 2004–2013: findings of the international nosocomial infection control consortium. Infect Control Hosp Epidemiol. 2016;37(2):172–81.
4. Tao L, Hu B, Rosenthal VD, Gao X, He L. Device-associated infection rates in 398 intensive care units in Shanghai, China: international nosocomial infection control consortium (INICC) findings. Int J Infect Dis. 2011;15(11):e774–80.
5. World Health Organization. Report on the burden of endemic health care-associated infection worldwide: clean care is safer care. Available at: http://apps.who.int/iris/bitstream/handle/10665/80135/9789241501507_eng.pdf;jsessionid=D87704F8824B725B0E90EBA22DE3BAAE?sequence=1. Accessed 14 Apr 2018.
6. Centers for Disease Control, R.O.C (Taiwan). Nosocomial Infections Surveillance System. Available at: http://www.cdc.gov.tw/english/info.aspx?treeid=00ed75d6c887bb27&nowtreeid=f0131176aa46d5db&tid=1A8C498AF5F8AF5D. Accessed 14 Apr 2018.
7. Tseng SH, Lee CM, Lin TY, Chang SC, Chuang YC, Yen MY, et al. Combating antimicrobial resistance: antimicrobial stewardship program in Taiwan. J Microbiol Immunol Infect. 2012;45(2):79–89.
8. Korean Society for Healthcare-associated Infection Control and Prevention. Korean Nosocomial Infections Surveillance System. Available at: http://www.koshic.org/main/main.html. Accessed 14 Apr 2018.
9. Choi JY, Kwak YG, Yoo H, Lee SO, Kim HB, Han SH, et al. Trends in the incidence rate of device-associated infections in intensive care units after the establishment of the Korean nosocomial infections surveillance system. J Hosp Infect. 2015;91(1):28–34.
10. Choi JY, Kwak YG, Yoo H, Lee SO, Kim HB, Han SH, et al. Trends in the distribution and antimicrobial susceptibility of causative pathogens of device-associated infection in Korean intensive care units from 2006 to 2013: results from the Korean nosocomial infections surveillance system (KONIS). J Hosp Infect. 2016;92(4):363–71.
11. Ministry of Health, Labour and Welfare, Japan. Japan Nosocomial Infections Surveillance. Available at: https://janis.mhlw.go.jp/report/icu.html. Accessed 14 Apr 2018.
12. Centers for Disease Control and Prevention, USA. National Healthcare Safety Network Reports. Available at: https://www.cdc.gov/nhsn/datastat/index.html. Accessed 14 Apr 2018.
13. European Centre for Disease Prevention and Control. Healthcare-associated infections acquired in intensive care units - Annual Epidemiological Report for 2015. Available at: https://ecdc.europa.eu/en/publications-data/healthcare-associated-infections-acquired-intensive-care-units-annual. Accessed 14 Apr 2018.
14. Allegranzi B, Bagheri Nejad S, Combescure C, Graafmans W, Attar H, Donaldson L, et al. Burden of endemic health-care-associated infection in developing countries: systematic review and meta-analysis. Lancet. 2011;377(9761):228–41.
15. Rosenthal VD, Al-Abdely HM, El-Kholy AA, AlKhawaja SAA, Leblebicioglu H, Mehta Y, et al. International nosocomial infection control consortium report, data summary of 50 countries for 2010-2015: device-associated module. Am J Infect Control. 2016;44(12):1495–504.
16. Haley RW, Culver DH, White JW, Morgan WM, Emori TG, Munn VP, et al. The efficacy of infection surveillance and control programs in preventing nosocomial infections in US hospitals. Am J Epidemiol. 1985;121(2):182–205.
17. Kim EJ, Kwak YG, Park SH, Kim SR, Shin MJ, Yoo HM, et al. Trends of device utilization ratios in intensive care units over 10-year period in South Korea: Device utilization ratio as a new aspect of surveillance. J Hosp Infect. 2017. doi: https://doi.org/10.1016/j.jhin.2017.10.007. [Epub ahead of print]. pii: S0195-6701(17)30547-9.
18. Price L, MacDonald J, Melone L, Howe T, Flowers P, Currie K, et al. Effectiveness of national and subnational infection prevention and control interventions in high-income and upper-middle-income countries: a systematic review. Lancet Infect Dis. 2018;18(5):e159–71.
19. Honda H, Ohmagari N, Tokuda Y, Mattar C, Warren DK. Antimicrobial stewardship in inpatient settings in the Asia Pacific Region: a systematic review and meta-analysis. Clin Infect Dis. 2017;64(suppl_2):S119–26.
20. Chen YC, Sheng WH, Wang JT, Chang SC, Lin HC, Tien KL, et al. Effectiveness and limitations of hand hygiene promotion on decreasing healthcare–associated infections. PLoS One. 2011;6(11):e27163.

21. Lai CC, Lee CM, Chiang HT, Hung CT, Chen YC, Su LH, et al. Implementation of a national bundle care program to reduce catheter-associated urinary tract infection in high-risk units of hospitals in Taiwan. J Microbiol Immunol Infect. 2017;50(4):464–70.

22. Lai CC, Cia CT, Chiang HT, Kung YC, Shi ZY, Chuang YC, et al. Implementation of a national bundle care program to reduce central line-associated bloodstream infections in intensive care units in Taiwan. J Microbiol Immunol Infect. 2017. doi: https://doi.org/10.1016/j.jmii.2017.10.001. [Epub ahead of print]. pii: S1684–1182(17)30231–1.

23. Eom JS, Lee MS, Chun HK, Choi HJ, Jung SY, Kim YS, et al. The impact of a ventilator bundle on preventing ventilator-associated pneumonia: a multicenter study. Am J Infect Control. 2014;42(1):34–7.

24. Umscheid CA, Mitchell MD, Doshi JA, Agarwal R, Williams K, Brennan PJ. Estimating the proportion of healthcare-associated infections that are reasonably preventable and the related mortality and costs. Infect Control Hosp Epidemiol 2011;32(2):101–1.

25. Organisation for Economic Co-operation and Development. Health at a Glance 2017 OECD Indicators. Available at: https://doi.org/10.1787/health_glance-2017-en. Accessed 14 Apr 2018.

26. Kwak YG, Lee SO, Kim HY, Kim YK, Park ES, Jin HY, et al. Risk factors for device-associated infection related to organisational characteristics of intensive care units: findings from the Korean nosocomial infections surveillance system. J Hosp Infect. 2010;75(3):195–9.

27. Sakamoto F, Sakihama T, Saint S, Greene MT, Ratz D, Tokuda Y. Health care-associated infection prevention in Japan: the role of safety culture. Am J Infect Control. 2014;42(8):888–93.

28. Healthcare Infection Control Practices Advisory Committee. Guideline for prevention of catheter-associated urinary tract infections 2009. Available at: https://www.cdc.gov/infectioncontrol/pdf/guidelines/cauti-guidelines.pdf. Accessed 14 Apr 2018.

29. Krein SL, Greene MT, Apisarnthanarak A, Sakamoto F, Tokuda Y, Sakihama T, et al. Infection Prevention Practices in Japan, Thailand, and the United States: Results From National Surveys. Clin Infect Dis. 2017;64(suppl_2):S105–11.

30. Van Mourik MSM, Perencevich EN, Gastmeier P, Bonten MJM. Designing surveillance of healthcare-associated infections in the era of automation and reporting mandates. Clin Infect Dis. 2018;66(6):970–6.

31. Russo PL, Shaban RZ, Macbeth D, Carter A, Mitchell BG. Impact of electronic healthcare-associated infection surveillance software on infection prevention resources: a systematic review of the literature. J Hosp Infect. 2018;99(1):1–7. https://doi.org/10.1016/j.jhin.2017.09.002 Epub 2017 Sep 8.

32. Tseng YJ, Wu JH, Ping XO, Lin HC, Chen YY, Shang RJ, et al. A web-based multidrug-resistant organism surveillance and outbreak detection system with rule-based classification and clustering. J Med Internet Res. 2012;14(5):e131.

33. Tseng YJ, Wu JH, Lin HC, Chen MY, Ping XO, Sun CC, et al. A web-based, hospital-wide health care-associated bloodstream infection surveillance and classification system: development and evaluation. JMIR Med Inform. 2015; 3(3):e31.

17

Urinary tract infection caused by a small colony variant form of capnophilic *Escherichia coli* leading to misidentification and non-reactions in antimicrobial susceptibility tests

Yu Jin Park[1], Nguyen Le Phuong[1], Naina Adren Pinto[1], Mi Jeong Kwon[1], Roshan D'Souza[1,2], Jung-Hyun Byun[1*], Heungsup Sung[3] and Dongeun Yong[1]

Abstract

Background: Small colony and capnophilic variant cases have been separately reported, but there has been no reports of their simultaneous presence in one isolate. We report a case of *Escherichia coli* with coexpressed small colony and capnophilic phenotypes causing misidentification in automated biochemical kits and non-reactions in antimicrobial susceptibility test cards.

Case presentation: An 86-year-old woman developed urinary tract infection from a strain of *Escherichia coli* with SCV and capnophilic phenotypes in co-existence. This strain did not grow without the presence of CO_2, and therefore proper identification from automated system was not possible. 16 s rRNA sequencing and matrix-assisted laser desorption/ionization time-of-flight mass spectrometry was able to identify the bacteria.

Conclusion: As these strains do not grow on culture parameters defined by CLSI or on automated systems, proper identification using alternative methods are necessary.

Keywords: Small colony variant, Capnophilic, *Escherichia coli*, Misidentification

Background

Small colony variants (SCV) can be defined as a naturally occurring sub-population of bacteria characterized by their reduced colony size and distinct biochemical properties [1]. Capnophilic *E. coli*, which thrive in the presence of high concentrations of carbon dioxide, have rarely been reported [2, 3]. SCV and capnophilic variant cases have never been reported in co-existence. Herein, we report the first case of *E. coli* with coexpressed SCV and capnophilic phenotypes isolated from a urinary tract infection.

* Correspondence: jhbyun@yuhs.ac; JHBYUN@yuhs.ac
[1]Department of Laboratory Medicine and Research Institute of Bacterial Resistance, Severance Hospital, Yonsei University College of Medicine, 50-1 Yonsei-ro, Seodaemun-gu, Seoul 03722, Republic of Korea
Full list of author information is available at the end of the article

Case report

An 86-year-old woman visited our hospital with foamy urine and foul odor. Urinalysis showed many WBCs (163.7 WBCs/μL) and bacteria (11,343.7 bacteria/uL), and positivity for nitrite. Gram-negative coccobacilli were revealed upon microscopic examination. The sample was cultured on sheep blood agar plate (BAP) and MacConkey agar plates at 35 °C in a 5% CO_2 atmosphere for 24 h. After one day of incubation, > 100,000 CFU/ml of pinpoint Gram-negative colonies grew on the BAP with 10,000 CFU/ml of Gram-positive cocci. After isolation of pinpoint colonies and another 24-h incubation, the pinpoint Gram-negative colonies were irregularly divided into large colonies and pinpoint SCV colonies on BAP (Table 1).

While the VITEK 2 system (bioMerieux, Durham, USA) identified the pinpoint colony as *Burkholderia cepacia* group, the Bruker Biotyper (Bruker Daltonics, Leipzig,

Table 1 Bacterial identification and antimicrobial susceptibility testing results

		Small colonies ▲		Wild type, large colonies △	
Morphology					
Bacterial identification by	VITEK 2 GN ID card	*Burkholderia cepacia* group		*Escherichia coli*	
	Bruker Biotyper	*Escherichia coli*		*Escherichia coli*	
	VITEK MS	*Escherichia coli*		*Escherichia coli*	
VITEK 2 AST card		Terminated		Terminated	
MicroScan AST/ID panel		Terminated		Terminated	
Disk diffusion method*					
in ambient air		No growth		No growth	
in 5% CO_2					
Amikacin		23	S	19	S
Ampicillin		24	S	23	S
Ampicillin-sulbactam		26	S	28	S
Aztreonam		40	S	42	S
Cefazolin		30	S	45	S
Cefepime		37	S	33	S
Cefotaxime		37	S	45	S
Cefoxitin		34	S	30	S
Ceftazidime		35	S	39	S
Ertapenem		39	S	42	S
Gentamicin		24	S	19	S
Levofloxacin		**6**	**R**	**6**	**R**
Meropenem		37	S	43	S
Piperacillin-tazobactam		29	S	33	S
Tigecycline		28	S	32	S
16s rRNA sequencing		*Escherichia coli* with 100.0% identity		*Escherichia coli* with 99.7% identity	

*Disk diffusion method results are given as measured zone diameters [8] and interpretive category. *S* susceptible, *R* resistant

Germany) and VITEK MS (bioMerieux, Marcy-l'Étoile, France) matrix-assisted laser desorption/ionization time-of-flight mass spectrometry (MALDI-TOF MS) systems identified both colonies as *E. coli*. The 16 s rRNA sequencing concluded both isolates were *E. coli*. As automated systems in an ambient air were unable to grow capnophilic SCVs, antimicrobial susceptibility testing profile was determined through disk diffusion method [4]. With the exception of levofloxacin resistance, bacteria was susceptible to all other antimicrobials. From these findings, we concluded that this isolate was CO_2-dependent and had the ability to revert to its natural large form in the presence of CO_2.

Whole genome sequencing analysis by the MiSeq® system (Illumina, San Diego, USA) was performed to inspect assumed genes that contained previously-reported causative mutations for the *E. coli* SCV phenotype (*hemB*, *menC*, and *lipA* gene) [1, 5], but no genetic mutational variations

were observed between the two strains. The *yadF* gene was not present in either strain, which is consistent with previous reports about capnophilic *E. coli* strains [6].

Discussion

The first *E. coli* SCV was reported in 1931, but there have been only few reports from clinical specimens [7–9]. Interestingly, this SCV strain was also capnophilic. The bacterial growth for reported capnophilic *E. coli* strains formed either large colonies in the presence of CO_2 or no colonies in the absence of CO_2 [2, 3]. To the best of our knowledge, this is the first report of *E. coli* with coexpressed SCV and capnophilic phenotype. Fortunately, this strain was susceptible to all other antimicrobials with the exception of levofloxacin, and therefore did not cause any severe outcome clinically. However, if this strain was to acquire drug resistance in the future, it is diagnostically crucial not to misidentify or neglect such strain for proper therapeutic purposes.

Additional criteria including CO_2 conditions are needed because CLSI guidelines defining incubation conditions for *Enterobacteriaceae* involve 35 °C ambient air [4], which are unsuitable for growing capnophilic SCVs. We advise that all urine cultures should be incubated in an environment containing 5% CO_2 to avoid overlooking of such strains. Proper identification using alternative methods such as MALDI-TOF MS systems are necessary for these capnophilic strains.

Abbreviations
BAP: Blood agar plate; MALDI-TOF MS: Matrix-assisted laser desorption/ionization time-of-flight mass spectrometry; SCV: Small colony variants

Acknowledgements
Not applicable.

Funding
None received.

Authors' contributions
The study was planned and designed by YP, NP, NAP, MK, RD, JB, HS, and DY. MK collected the samples. YP, JB, HS, and DY conducted the experiments. The interpretation of the genetic results was done by NP, NAP, and RD. The manuscript was prepared by YP and JB. All authors contributed to and commented on the manuscript. All authors read and approved the final manuscript.

Competing interests
The authors declare that they have no competing interests.

Author details
[1]Department of Laboratory Medicine and Research Institute of Bacterial Resistance, Severance Hospital, Yonsei University College of Medicine, 50-1 Yonsei-ro, Seodaemun-gu, Seoul 03722, Republic of Korea. [2]J.Craig Venter Institute (JCVI), 9605 Medical Center Dr #150, Rockville, MD 20850, USA. [3]Department of Laboratory Medicine, Asan Medical Center, University of Ulsan College of Medicine, 88 Olympic-ro 43-gil, Songpa-gu, Seoul 05505, Republic of Korea.

References
1. Santos V, Hirshfield I. The physiological and molecular characterization of a small colony variant of Escherichia coli and its phenotypic rescue. PLoS One. 2016. https://doi.org/10.1371/journal.pone.0157578.
2. Lu W, Chang K, Deng S, Li M, Wang J, Xia J, et al. Isolation of a capnophilic Escherichia coli strain from an empyemic patient. Diagn Microbiol Infect Dis. 2012. https://doi.org/10.1016/j.diagmicrobio.2012.03.020.
3. Tena D, González-Praetorius A, Sáez-Nieto JA, Valdezate S, Bisquert J. Urinary tract infection caused by capnophilic Escherichia coli. Emerg Infect Dis. 2008. https://doi.org/10.3201/eid1407.071053.
4. Clinical and Laboratory Standards Institute. Performance standards for antimicrobial susceptibility testing. 28th edition ed. In: CLSI document M100: clinical and laboratory standards institute; 2018.
5. Tashiro Y, Eida H, Ishii S, Futamata H, Okabe S. Generation of small colony variants in biofilms by Escherichia coli harboring a conjugative F plasmid. Microbes Environ. 2017. https://doi.org/10.1264/jsme2.ME16121.
6. Sahuquillo-Arce JM, Chouman-Arcas R, Molina-Moreno JM, Hernandez-Cabezas A, Frasquet-Artes J, Lopez-Hontangas JL. Capnophilic Enterobacteriaceae. Diagn Microbiol Infect Dis. 2017. https://doi.org/10.1016/j.diagmicrobio.2017.01.010.
7. Roggenkamp A, Sing A, Hornef M, Brunner U, Autenrieth IB, Heesemann J. Chronic prosthetic hip infection caused by a small-colony variant of Escherichia coli. J Clin Microbiol. 1998;36(9):2530–4.
8. Sendi P, Frei R, Maurer TB, Trampuz A, Zimmerli W, Graber P. Escherichia coli variants in periprosthetic joint infection: diagnostic challenges with sessile bacteria and sonication. J Clin Microbiol. 2010. https://doi.org/10.1128/jcm.01562-09.
9. Tappe D, Claus H, Kern J, Marzinzig A, Frosch M, Abele-Horn M. First case of febrile bacteremia due to a wild type and small-colony variant of Escherichia coli. Eur J Clin Microbiol Infect Dis. 2006. https://doi.org/10.1007/s10096-005-0072-0.

18

Incidence of infections due to third generation cephalosporin-resistant *Enterobacteriaceae* - a prospective multicentre cohort study in six German university hospitals

Anna M. Rohde[1,2]* ⓘ, Janine Zweigner[1,2,3], Miriam Wiese-Posselt[1,2], Frank Schwab[1,2], Michael Behnke[1,2], Axel Kola[1,2], Birgit Obermann[1,4], Johannes K.-M. Knobloch[1,4,11], Susanne Feihl[1,5], Christiane Querbach[1,5], Friedemann Gebhardt[1,5], Alexander Mischnik[1,6], Vera Ihle[1,6], Wiebke Schröder[1,7], Sabina Armean[1,7], Silke Peter[1,8], Evelina Tacconelli[1,7], Axel Hamprecht[1,9], Harald Seifert[1,9], Maria J. G. T. Vehreschild[1,10], Winfried V. Kern[1,6], Petra Gastmeier[1,2] and on behalf of the DZIF-ATHOS study group[1]

Abstract

Background: Infections caused by third generation cephalosporin-resistant *Enterobacteriaceae* (3GCREB) are an increasing healthcare problem. We aim to describe the 3GCREB infection incidence and compare it to prevalence upon admission. In addition, we aim to describe infections caused by 3GCREB, which are also carbapenem resistant (CRE).

Methods: In 2014–2015, we performed prospective 3GCREB surveillance in clinically relevant patient specimens (screening specimens excluded). Infections counted as hospital-acquired (HAI) when the 3GCREB was detected after the third day following admission, otherwise as community-acquired infection (CAI).

Results: Of 578,420 hospitalized patients under surveillance, 3367 had a 3GCREB infection (0.58%). We observed a similar 3GCREB CAI and HAI incidence (0.28 and 0.31 per 100 patients, respectively). The most frequent pathogen was 3GCR *E. coli*, in CAI and HAI (0.15 and 0.12 per 100 patients). We observed a CRE CAI incidence of 0.006 and a HAI incidence of 0.008 per 100 patients (0.014 per 1000 patient days).

Conclusions: Comparing the known 3GCREB admission prevalence of the participating hospitals (9.5%) with the percentage of patients with a 3GCREB infection (0.58%), we conclude the prevalence of 3GCREB in university hospitals to be about 16 times higher than suggested when only patients with 3GCREB infections are considered. Moreover, we find the HAI and CAI incidence caused by CRE in Germany to be relatively low.

Keywords: Fluoroquinolone, Carbapenem, Gram-negative, ESBL, *Enterobacter* spp., *Klebsiella* spp., *E. coli*, CRE, Hospital-acquired infections, Community-acquired infections

* Correspondence: Anna.rohde@charite.de
[1]German Center for Infection Research (DZIF), Inhoffenstraße 7, 38124 Braunschweig, Germany
[2]Charité – Universitätsmedizin Berlin, Institute of Hygiene and Environmental Medicine, Hindenburgstraße 27, 12203 Berlin, Germany
Full list of author information is available at the end of the article

Background

Emerging multidrug-resistant Gram-negative bacteria are a global health concern, especially those harbouring extended-spectrum beta-lactamases (ESBL), which render *Enterobacteriaceae* resistant to third generation cephalosporins (3GC) and extended-spectrum penicillins [1]. Third generation cephalosporin resistant *Enterobacteriaceae* (3GCREB) infections are a special threat to patient safety, as resistance may cause a delay in effective antimicrobial therapy and thereby lead to worsening patient outcomes [2]. EU surveillance data shows that the 3GC resistance rate of *E. coli* in blood and cerebrospinal fluid samples has increased in many EU countries (EU mean 2012: 11.9%, 2015: 13.1%) [3]. The incidence density of 3GCREB in clinical specimens in German intensive care units (ICUs) rose from 2001 to 2015 (*E. coli*: 0.16 to 3.83/1000 patient days, *K. pneumoniae*: 0.25 to 1.41/1000 patient days) [4]. The percentage of hospital-acquired infections (HAI) caused by ESBL-producing *Enterobacteriaceae* in German ICUs and surgical departments increased as well (2007: 10.9% to 2012: 15.5%) [5].

The ATHOS (Antibiotic Therapy Optimization Study) project aimed at assessing the 3GCREB admission prevalence and 3GCREB incidence of community-acquired and hospital-acquired infections (CAI, HAI) in six German university hospitals in 2014 and 2015. The prevalence data was published previously [6]. Here, we describe the incidence of 3GCREB infections in the same hospitals and relate the data to the 3GCREB admission prevalence. Furthermore, we analyse the distribution of additional resistance phenotype patterns in those 3GCREB that caused infections.

Methods

Study design and data sources

The ATHOS project was a prospective observational cohort study that monitored hospitalized patients in general wards and ICUs for their first 3GCREB detection in clinical specimens (active surveillance). Each microbiology finding was followed by checking the health record or by contacting the wards and clinicians directly. The study was performed in six German university hospitals from January 1, 2014 to December 31, 2015. Patients hospitalized in the departments of dermatology, gynaecology/obstetrics, ophthalmology, otorhinolaryngology, paediatrics and psychiatry were excluded from surveillance.

Microbiological analysis

Gram-negative bacteria were identified down to species level using either MALDI-TOF MS or VITEK®2 (bioMérieux, Nürtingen, Germany). Antimicrobial susceptibility testing was performed using VITEK®2. *Enterobacteriaceae* were classified as susceptible or resistant based on minimal

inhibitory concentrations according to EUCAST breakpoints [7]. Non-susceptibility was regarded as resistance. Indicator antimicrobials for third generation cephalosporin resistance were cefotaxime and ceftazidime, indicators for carbapenem resistance were imipenem and meropenem.

Definitions

A 3GCREB case was defined as the first 3GCREB isolate detected in clinical specimens (e.g. urine, wound swab, blood culture, tracheobronchial secretion or other clinical specimens) in a patient during a single hospital stay. Readmission followed by another 3GCREB detection created a new case.. Cases were distinguished in colonisations and cases with infections. Infections were defined as the detection of 3GCREB in a clinical specimen with additional signs and symptoms of infection as determined by a clinician followed by adequate antimicrobial therapy. A single case could present several 3GCREB species, each with several infections (though counting only by infection type). Acquisition was defined as follows: detection on day 1–3 (admission day = day 1) counted as community-acquired (CA), later detections counted as hospital-acquired (HA) [8]. We stratified for the following infection types: urinary tract infection (UTI), lower respiratory tract infection (LRTI), surgical site infection (SSI) and bloodstream infection (BSI). Other infection types were pooled in the category "other infections". We analysed HAI caused by HA-3GCREB and CAI caused by CA-3GCREB. Cases with an ambiguous acquisition (CA-3GCREB with HAI and HA-3GCREB on top of existing CAI) were discarded.

Statistical analysis

Infection incidence was calculated as infections per 100 patients, incidence density as infections per 1000 patient days. Both were stratified by species, resistance phenotype and infection type. Then 95% confidence intervals were calculated. The species distribution over infection types was tested with X^2 test (R x C table). The comparison of resistance phenotypes among 3GCREB responsible for different infection types was tested with Fisher's exact test (2 × 2 table, carbapenem-resistant versus -susceptible). *P*-values < 0.05 were considered significant. Statistical analysis was performed with SAS 9.4 (SAS Institute, Cary, NC, USA) and OpenEpi (Open Source Epidemiologic Statistics for Public Health, V3.01 http://www.openepi.com).

Ethics and data protection

3GCREB surveillance was performed in accordance with the German Infection Protection Act [9]. The ethics committee at Charité, University Medicine Berlin, Germany, approved this study (EA/018/14). Data from the six hospitals was entered into an online accessible database approved by the data protection commissioner.

Results

The ATHOS project was conducted at six German university hospitals comprising a total of 283 wards and 4957 beds in the surveillance area. The majority were general wards with surgical specialty ($n = 104$) followed by medical specialty ($n = 83$), intensive care units (ICU, $n = 49$), haematology/oncology ($n = 35$) and intermediate care wards ($n = 12$).

In the period 2014–2015, 578,420 patient admissions with 3,385,112 patient days were under surveillance. After excluding invalid data and cases of colonization ($n = 2262$), 3367 clinical cases with one or more 3GCREB infections (0.58% of the patients) were analysed (Fig. 1a). The median age was 69 (IQR 58–77 years) and 55% of the cases were male. Of the cases, 92% had one infection, 7% had two infections and 1% had three or four infections.

To compare different infection types, cases were broken down into single infections and those with ambiguous acquisition were discarded, yielding 3370 single infections. The majority of infections were hospital-acquired (3GCREB HAI, Fig. 1b). We observed a difference in infection incidence among the university hospitals, e.g. the 3GCREB HAI incidence ranged from 0.17–0.42 per 100 patients. Therefore, the data of the individual hospitals was pooled for further analysis. The absolute numbers of infections stratified by species, resistance phenotype, and infection type are shown in Table 1, the infection incidences and incidence densities in Table 2. The 3GCREB CAI incidence was 0.28 per 100 patients, and that of HAI 0.31 per 100 patients. The majority of CAI were caused by 3GCREB which were also fluoroquinolone resistant (FQR, 0.17 per 100 patients), in HAI that incidence was lower (0.14 per 100

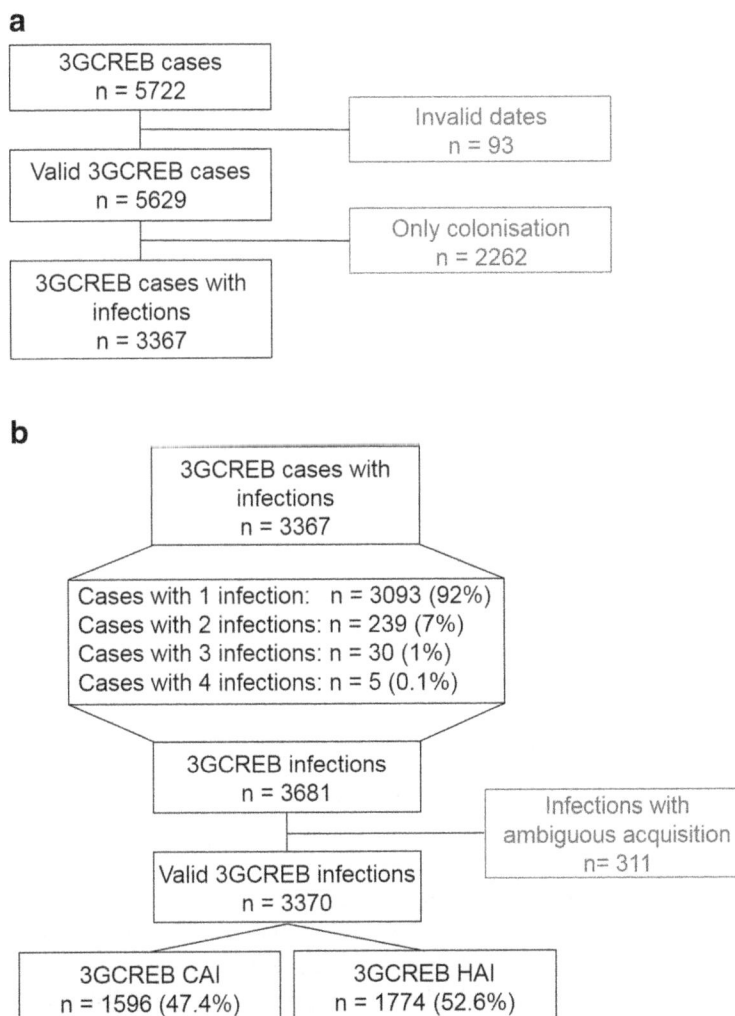

Fig. 1 Flow chart of third generation cephalosporin resistant *Enterobacteriaceae* (3GCREB) cases (**a**) and infections (**b**). **a**) Readmission followed by 3GCREB detection created a second case. **b**) Each case could represent several infections but only one per infection type

Table 1 Distribution of third generation cephalosporin resistant *Enterobacteriaceae* (3GCREB) infections in the ATHOS project, 2014–2015, Germany

Parameter	Category	3GCREB infections n (%)	3GCREB CAI n (%)	3GCREB HAI n (%)
3GCREB	total	3370 (100%)	1596 (100%)	1774 (100%)
Species	*E. coli*	1624 (48%)	910 (57%)	714 (40%)
	Enterobacter spp.	702 (21%)	221 (14%)	481 (27%)
	Klebsiella spp.	562 (17%)	264 (17%)	298 (17%)
	Citrobacter spp.	209 (6%)	76 (5%)	133 (7%)
	Other species [a]	273 (8%)	125 (8%)	148 (8%)
Resistance	all 3GCREB			
	only 3GCR	1488 (44%)	580 (36%)	908 (51%)
	+ FQR	1796 (53%)	979 (61%)	817 (46%)
	+ CR	86 (3%)	37 (2%)	49 (3%)
	E. coli	1624 (100%)	910 (100%)	714 (100%)
	only 3GCR	409 (25%)	209 (23%)	200 (28%)
	+ FQR	1203 (74%)	698 (77%)	505 (71%)
	+ CR	12 (1%)	3 (0%)	9 (1%)
	Enterobacter spp.	702 (100%)	221 (100%)	481 (100%)
	only 3GCR	553 (79%)	168 (76%)	385 (80%)
	+ FQR	122 (17%)	45 (20%)	77 (16%)
	+ CR	27 (4%)	8 (4%)	19 (4%)
	Klebsiella spp.	562 (100%)	264 (100%)	298 (100%)
	only 3GCR	157 (28%)	59 (22%)	98 (33%)
	+ FQR	362 (64%)	181 (69%)	181 (61%)
	+ CR	43 (8%)	24 (9%)	19 (6%)
Infections	SSI	401 (12%)	99 (6%)	302 (17%)
	UTI	1528 (45%)	872 (55%)	656 (37%)
	LRTI	571 (17%)	158 (10%)	413 (23%)
	BSI	459 (14%)	220 (14%)	239 (13%)
	Other infections [b]	411 (12%)	247 (15%)	164 (9%)
Year	2014	1784 (53%)	847 (53%)	937 (53%)
	2015	1586 (47%)	749 (47%)	837 (47%)
Ward type	General ward	2174 (65%)	1102 (69%)	1072 (60%)
	ICU/interm. Care	1196 (35%)	494 (31%)	702 (40%)
Specialty	Surgical	1407 (42%)	522 (33%)	885 (50%)
	Non-surgical	1963 (58%)	1074 (67%)	889 (50%)

3GCREB infections among 578,420 patient admissions and 3,385,112 patient days in six German university hospitals. [a] "Other *Enterobacteriaceae* species" include *Cedecea, Hafnia, Morganella, Pantoea, Proteus, Providencia, Raoultella,* and *Serratia* species. [b] "Other infections" includes all other infection types. 3GCREB = third generation cephalosporin-resistant *Enterobacteriaceae*, 3GCR third generation cephalosporin resistance, FQR fluoroquinolone resistance, CR carbapenem resistance, CA community-acquired, HA hospital-acquired, SSI surgical site infection, UTI urinary tract infection, LRTI lower respiratory tract infection, BSI bloodstream infection, ICU intensive care unit, interm. Care intermediate care. Column percentages were calculated for each parameter with respect to "3GCREB total"

patients). 3GCREB that were also carbapenem resistant caused 0.006 CAI and 0.008 HAI per 100 patients.

Among 3GCREB species, *E. coli* caused the highest incidence of CAI (0.15 per 100 patients) and HAI (0.12 per 100 patients). The most frequent infections were UTIs irrespective of the acquisition; the incidence of 3GCREB CA-UTI exceeded that of 3GCREB

HA-UTI (0.15 vs. 0.11 per 100 patients). For SSI and LRTI, the incidence of 3GCREB HAI exceeded that of CAI (Table 2).

Figure 2 shows the distribution of 3GCREB infections stratified by CAI/HAI and by species. Species distribution differed significantly in UTI, LRTI and BSI: HA-UTI, -LRTI and -BSI were caused more frequently

Table 2 Incidence (densities) of infections with third generation cephalosporin-resistant *Enterobacteriaceae* (3GCREB), ATHOS project, 2014–2015, Germany

Parameter	Category	3GCREB CAI incidence per 100,000 admissions (95% CI)	3GCREB CAI incidence per 100 admissions (95% CI)	3GCREB HAI incidence per 100 admissions (95% CI)	3GCREB HAI incidence density per 1000 patient days (95% CI)
3GCREB	total	276 (263–290)	0.28 (0.26–0.29)	0.31 (0.29–0.32)	0.52 (0.50–0.55)
Species	*E. coli*	157 (147–168)	0.16 (0.15–0.17)	0.12 (0.12–0.13)	0.21 (0.20–0.23)
	Enterobacter spp.	38 (33–44)	0.04 (0.03–0.04)	0.08 (0.08–0.09)	0.14 (0.13–0.16)
	Klebsiella spp.	45 (40–52)	0.05 (0.04–0.05)	0.05 (0.05–0.06)	0.09 (0.08–0.10)
	Citrobacter spp.	13 (10–16)	0.01 (0.01–0.02)	0.02 (0.02–0.03)	0.04 (0.03–0.05)
	Other species [a]	22 (18–26)	0.02 (0.02–0.03)	0.03 (0.02–0.03)	0.04 (0.04–0.05)
Resistance	all 3GCREB				
	only 3GCR	100 (92–109)	0.10 (0.09–0.11)	0.16 (0.15–0.17)	0.27 (0.25–0.29)
	+ FQR	169 (159–180)	0.17 (0.16–0.18)	0.14 (0.13–0.15)	0.24 (0.23–0.26)
	+ CR	6 (5–9)	0.006 (0.005–0.009)	0.008 (0.006–0.011)	0.014 (0.011–0.019)
	E. coli				
	only 3GCR	36 (31–41)	0.04 (0.03–0.04)	0.04 (0.03–0.04)	0.06 (0.05–0.07)
	+ FQR	121 (112–130)	0.12 (0.11–0.13)	0.09 (0.08–0.10)	0.15 (0.14–0.16)
	+ CR	1 (0–2)	0.001 (0.000–0.002)	0.002 (0.001–0.003)	0.003 (0.001–0.005)
	Enterobacter spp.				
	only 3GCR	29 (25–34)	0.03 (0.03–0.03)	0.07 (0.06–0.07)	0.11 (0.10–0.13)
	+ FQR	8 (6–10)	0.01 (0.01–0.01)	0.01 (0.01–0.02)	0.02 (0.02–0.03)
	+ CR	1 (1–3)	0.001 (0.001–0.003)	0.003 (0.002–0.005)	0.006 (0.003–0.009)
	Klebsiella spp.				
	only 3GCR	10 (8–13)	0.01 (0.01–0.01)	0.02 (0.01–0.02)	0.03 (0.02–0.04)
	+ FQR	31 (27–36)	0.03 (0.03–0.04)	0.03 (0.03–0.04)	0.05 (0.05–0.06)
	+ CR	4 (3–6)	0.004 (0.003–0.006)	0.003 (0.002–0.005)	0.006 (0.003–0.009)
Infections	SSI	17 (14–21)	0.02 (0.01–0.02)	0.05 (0.05–0.06)	0.09 (0.08–0.10)
	UTI	151 (141–161)	0.15 (0.14–0.16)	0.11 (0.11–0.12)	0.19 (0.18–0.21)
	LRTI	27 (23–32)	0.03 (0.02–0.03)	0.07 (0.07–0.08)	0.12 (0.11–0.13)
	BSI	38 (33–43)	0.04 (0.03–0.04)	0.04 (0.04–0.05)	0.07 (0.06–0.08)
	Other infections [b]	43 (38–48)	0.04 (0.04–0.05)	0.03 (0.02–0.03)	0.05 (0.04–0.06)

[a] "Other *Enterobacteriaceae* species" include *Cedecea, Hafnia, Morganella, Pantoea, Proteus, Providencia, Raoultella,* and *Serratia* species. [b] "Other infections" includes all other infection types. 3GCREB = third generation cephalosporin-resistant *Enterobacteriaceae*, *3GCR* third generation cephalosporin resistance, *FQR* fluoroquinolone resistance, *CR* carbapenem resistance, *3GCR + CR* carbapenem resistant *Enterobacteriaceae* (CRE), *CAI* community-acquired infection, *HAI* hospital-acquired infection, *SSI* surgical site infection, *UTI* urinary tract infection, *LRTI* lower respiratory tract infection, *BSI* bloodstream infection, *95% CI* 95% confidence interval

by *Enterobacter* spp.. HA-BSI were also caused to a higher percentage by *Klebsiella* spp. than CA-BSI. Figure 3 shows the distribution of resistance phenotypes by infection type. The resistance phenotypes of 3GCR *E. coli* isolates did not differ between CAI and HAI (Fig. 3a). In contrast, 3GCR *Klebsiella* spp. showed a higher proportion of carbapenem resistance in all CAI except UTI. Twenty percent of the 3GCR *Klebsiella* spp. that caused CA-BSI and 28% of those that caused CA-LRTI were carbapenem resistant. A high percentage of 3GCR *Klebsiella* spp. that caused surgical site infections were also carbapenem resistant, irrespective of the acquisition (15% in CA-SSI and 13% in HA-SSI) (Fig. 3b).

Discussion

The incidence of 3GCREB infections among patients admitted to German university hospitals in 2014/15 was < 1%. Additional fluoroquinolone resistance was frequent in particular in CAI, while additional carbapenem resistance was rare, both in CAI and HAI (0.006 and 0.008 per 100 patients; HAI incidence density 0.014 per 1000 patient days). An interesting finding was that among CA-LRTI caused by 3GCR *Klebsiella* spp., the percentage of additional carbapenem resistance (28%) was substantial and significantly higher than in 3GCR *Klebsiella* spp. causing HA-LRTI (6%, $p = 0.015$).

In an admission prevalence study performed in parallel, we screened a minimum of 500 patients per hospital for

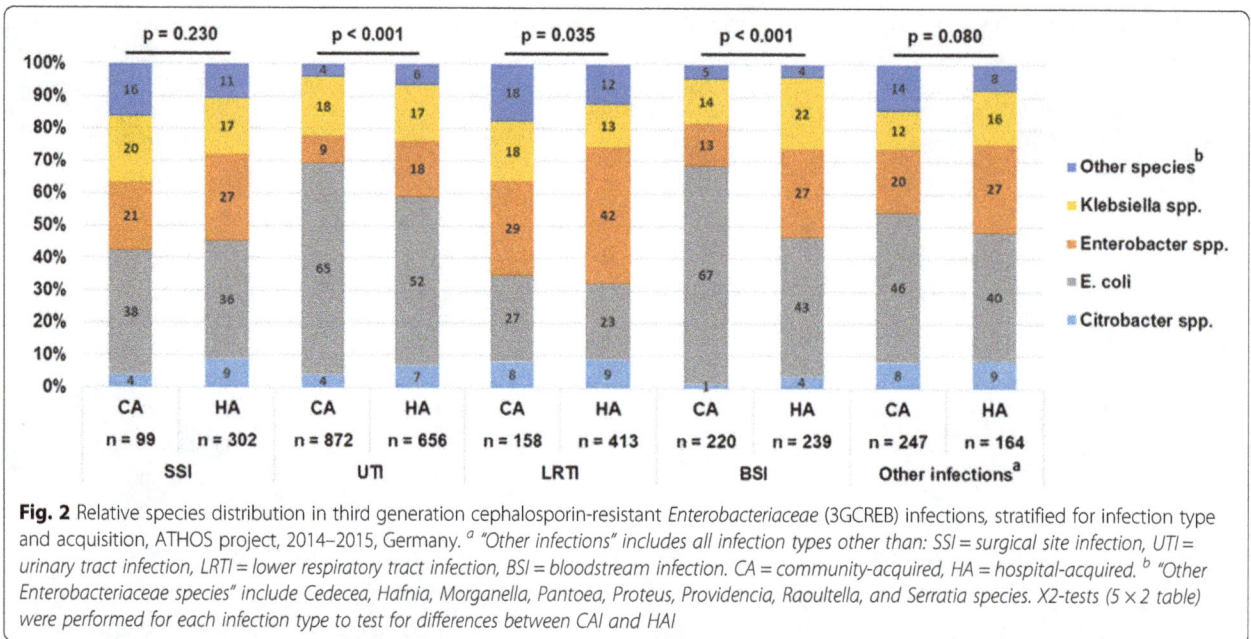

Fig. 2 Relative species distribution in third generation cephalosporin-resistant *Enterobacteriaceae* (3GCREB) infections, stratified for infection type and acquisition, ATHOS project, 2014–2015, Germany. [a] *"Other infections" includes all infection types other than: SSI = surgical site infection, UTI = urinary tract infection, LRTI = lower respiratory tract infection, BSI = bloodstream infection. CA = community-acquired, HA = hospital-acquired.* [b] *"Other Enterobacteriaceae species" include Cedecea, Hafnia, Morganella, Pantoea, Proteus, Providencia, Raoultella, and Serratia species. X2-tests (5 × 2 table) were performed for each infection type to test for differences between CAI and HAI*

rectal 3GCREB carriage on admission (day 1–3, admission day = day 1). This study showed a 3GCREB colonization prevalence of 9.5% [6]. Therefore, we conclude that the colonization rate of patients in university hospitals is about 16 times higher (=9.5%/0.58% patients with 3GCREB infection) than suggested when only patients with 3GCREB infections are considered. The reason for this high colonization prevalence and for a CAI incidence comparable to HAI is most likely the case mix in tertiary care university hospitals due to their position at the end of the treatment chain. On admission, many patients most likely have received previous antimicrobial treatment and have higher co-morbidity scores than patients in other hospital types.

The incidence of CAI causing 3GCREB that were also resistant to fluoroquinolones exceeded that of HAI (Table 2). One reason for this may be the high antibiotic use reported by patients admitted to the participating hospitals (34% of the 3GCREB-negative and 53% of the 3GCREB-positive patients) [6]. Another reason may be an enhanced use of fluoroquinolones in outpatient care [10]. This excess of fluoroquinolone use might be caused (among other reasons) by over prescription and non-adherence to antibiotic prescription guidelines in outpatient care [11–13]. A reduction of fluoroquinolone prescriptions would be desirable.

In 2013/14, the EU mean of carbapenemase-producing (CP) *E. coli* and *K. pneumoniae* was found to be 0.025 per 1000 patient days and 0.006 per 1000 patient days were reported for Germany (EuSCAPE study) [14]. We observed a CRE HAI incidence density for *Klebsiella* spp. of 0.006 (95% CI 0.000–0.008) and for *E. coli* of 0.003 per 1000 patient days (95% CI 0.001–0.005). The

EuSCAPE study showed that among CRE, 70% of the *K. pneumoniae* and 30% of the *E. coli* produced carbapenemases [14]. Combining these percentages of CPE among CRE with our CRE data yields an estimated CPE incidence density for *Klebsiella* spp. and *E. coli* of 0.005 per 1000 patient days (*Klebsiella* spp. 0.004 and *E. coli* 0.001 per 1000 patient days). Thus, our data is comparable to the EuSCAPE data for Germany [14].

In contrast to other *Enterobacteriaceae* species, 3GCR *Klebsiella* spp. showed a high percentage of carbapenem resistance among CA infections, especially in LRTI and BSI. In a UK study, the prevalence of carbapenem resistance in clinically relevant *K. pneumoniae* specimens was also due primarily to community-acquired isolates (70%) [15]. The EU mean of carbapenem resistance in invasive *K. pneumoniae* isolates increased from 2012 to 2015 to 8%. In two European countries, carbapenem resistance was observed in over 25% of *K. pneumoniae* (Italy 34% and Greece 62%). In isolates from Germany, carbapenem resistance was rare (0.1%) [3]. Surveillance in German ICUs showed that the carbapenem resistance rate of *K. pneumoniae* in clinically relevant specimens increased from 2001 to 2015 to 1.5% [4]. A large admission prevalence study found a low CRE admission prevalence in Germany (comparable to UK, both 0.1%) [6, 16]. In light of this data, we conclude that even with increasing trends Germany currently still is a low CRE prevalence region.

The ATHOS project was a prospective observational study. One major limitation is the lack of patient-based information on previous healthcare contacts. Therefore, a classification into the important "healthcare-associated"

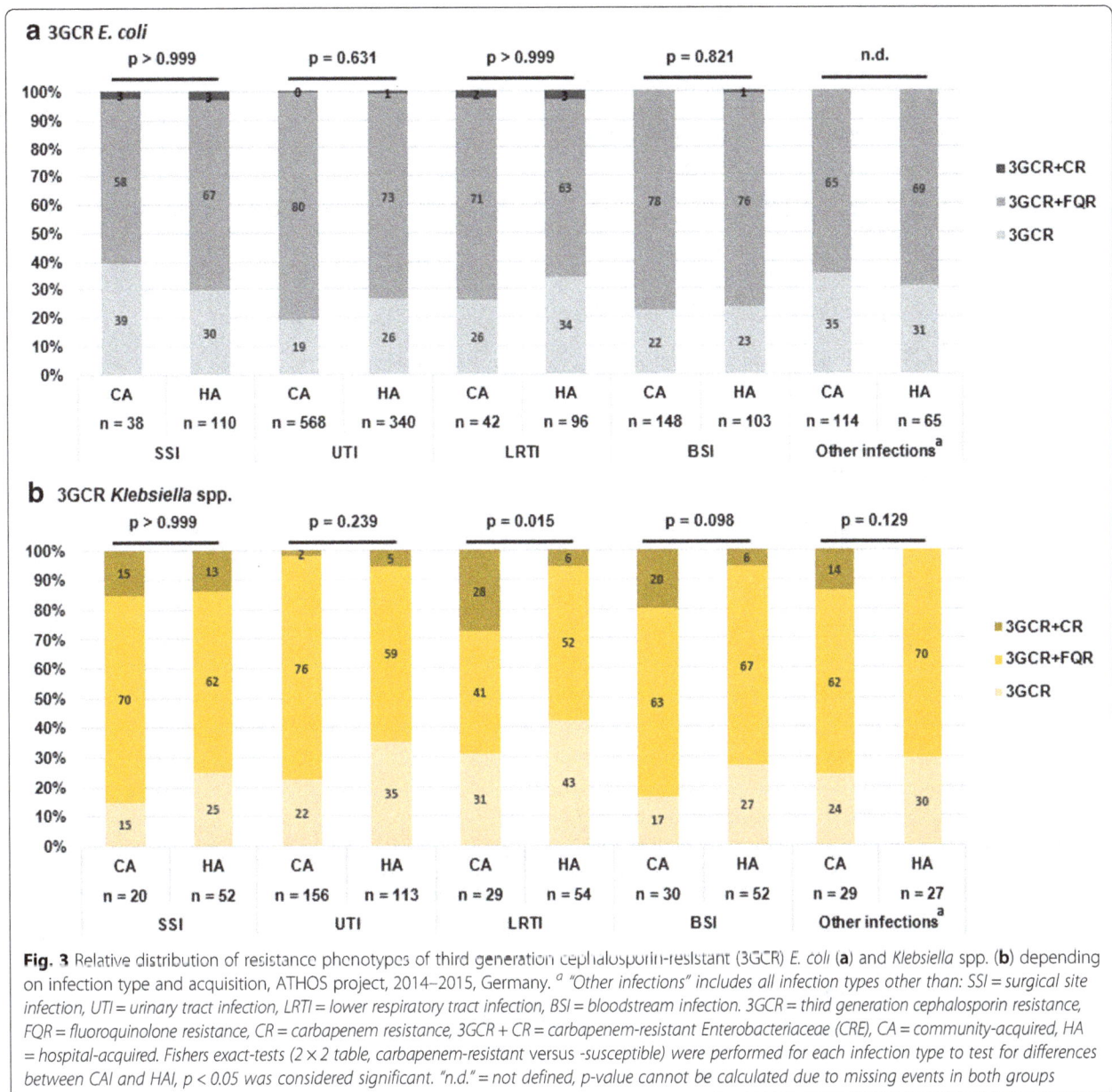

Fig. 3 Relative distribution of resistance phenotypes of third generation cephalosporin-resistant (3GCR) *E. coli* (**a**) and *Klebsiella* spp. (**b**) depending on infection type and acquisition, ATHOS project, 2014–2015, Germany. [a] "Other infections" includes all infection types other than: SSI = surgical site infection, UTI = urinary tract infection, LRTI = lower respiratory tract infection, BSI = bloodstream infection. 3GCR = third generation cephalosporin resistance, FQR = fluoroquinolone resistance, CR = carbapenem resistance, 3GCR + CR = carbapenem-resistant Enterobacteriaceae (CRE), CA = community-acquired, HA = hospital-acquired. Fishers exact-tests (2 × 2 table, carbapenem-resistant versus -susceptible) were performed for each infection type to test for differences between CAI and HAI, $p < 0.05$ was considered significant. "n.d." = not defined, p-value cannot be calculated due to missing events in both groups

category was not possible. Instead, the somewhat arbitrary day 3 limit for classification into CA and HA was applied, as it is commonly used for surveillance of HAI [8]. Nonetheless, we have some insight into the healthcare contacts of our patient mix from our patients in the admission prevalence study sample, 9% of whom had stayed in a rehabilitation centre, 5% in a long-term care facility and 26% in another hospital in the 6 months prior to admission [6]. Some CAI may, in fact, be healthcare-associated and thus the incidence of CAI may be overestimated in our analysis. This CA/HA classificiation was also used for SSI. We cannot exclude that some CA-SSI cases may be readmitted cases. An advantage of the study is the inclusion of general wards. We can describe the incidence of

3GCREB infections in German university hospitals comprehensively and are not limited to ICU data. However, due to the hospital-wide surveillance, we lack ward-specific denominator data and are not able to calculate department-specific incidences.

One strength of the study is the inclusion of most *Enterobacteriaceae* species, since other studies are often restricted to *E. coli* or *K. pneumoniae*. Such studies are likely to underestimate the real incidence of CRE. We found a major part of CRE-HAI caused by *Enterobacter* spp. (0.006 per 1000 patient days, 95% CI 0.000–0.008). Imipenem resistance of *E. cloacae* complex has increased over the last years in German ICUs [4]. In addition, long-term surveillance by the US Veterans Health

Administration of CRE in patients also showed a steady increase of carbapenem resistance in *E. cloacae* [17]. However, we have noticed that Vitek®2 frequently over-reported imipenem resistance. For future CRE studies, we suggest including *Enterobacter* spp. and using additional, more reliable diagnostic methods (e.g. disk diffusion test or agar gradient diffusion) to determine if the high frequency of Vitek®2 imipenem resistance represents the true epidemiology. Another drawback of using routine diagnostic methods is that we were unable to compare sequence types of 3GCREB causing CAI and HAI.

As a result of the 3GCREB admission prevalence study performed in parallel [6] and the surveillance data for infections, we can for the first time estimate the 3GCREB prevalence to be about 16-times higher than indicated by the 3GCREB infection incidence (0.58%). This will enable other university hospitals with a similar patient mix to estimate roughly the dimension of colonization prevalence present in their patients. Furthermore, we conclude that very few 3GCREB carriers are identified using clinically indicated diagnostic procedures. Therefore, we believe the majority of hospitals underestimate the extent of 3GCREB prevalence. This study gives a comprehensive description of the incidence of CRE found in German university hospitals.

Conclusion

Overall, our analysis showed that German university hospitals have a low 3GCREB infection incidence when compared to the admission prevalence. As we observed a comparable incidence of 3GCREB CAI and HAI, it is important that clinicians consider cephalosporin resistance in their empirical treatment decisions, irrespective of the acquisition type (CA vs. HA) of the infection.

Abbreviations
3GC (3GCR): 3rd generation cephalosporin (–resistant); 3GCREB: 3rd generation cephalosporin-resistant *Enterobacteriaceae*; ATHOS: Antibiotic therapy optimisation study; BSI: Bloodstream infection; CA (CAI): Community-acquired (infection); CP (CPE): Carbapenemase-producing (*Enterobacteriaceae*); CR (CRE): Carbapenemase-resistant (*Enterobacteriaceae*); *E. cloacae: Enterobacter cloacae; E. coli: Escherichia coli*; ESBL: extended spectrum β-lactamase; EU: European Union; EUCAST: European committee on antimicrobial susceptibility testing; HA (HAI): Hospital-acquired (infection); ICU: Intensive care unit; IQR: Interquartile range; *K. pneumonia: Klebsiella pneumonia*; LRTI: Lower respiratory tract infection; MALDI-TOF MS: Matrix-assisted laser desorption/ionization-time of flight mass spectrometry; spp.: species; SSI: Surgical site infection; UK: United Kingdom; US: United States; UTI: Urinary tract infection

Acknowledgements
We would like to acknowledge all other members of the ATHOS study group:
Michael Buhl, Tübingen; Dirk Busch, Munich; Simone Eisenbeis, Tübingen; Gesche Först, Freiburg; Federico Foschi, Tübingen; Meyke Gillis, Cologne; Dorothea Hansen, Cologne; Georg Häcker, Freiburg; Markus Heim, Munich; Martin Hug, Freiburg; Klaus Kaier, Freiburg; Fabian Küpper, Freiburg; Georg Langebartels, Cologne; Andrea Liekweg, Cologne; Hans-Peter Lipp, Tübingen; Nayana Märtin, Berlin; Mathias Nordmann, Berlin; Andrea Pelzer, Cologne;

Luis-Alberto Peña-Diaz, Berlin; Jan Rupp, Lübeck; Christin Schröder, Berlin; Katrin Spohn, Tübingen; Michaela Steib-Bauert, Freiburg; Jörg J. Vehreschild, Cologne; Ulrich vor dem Esche, Freiburg and Solvy Wolke, Berlin.

Funding
The German Centre for Infection Research (DZIF) funded the ATHOS project (TTU 08.801).

Authors' contributions
AMR local site coordinator, local data collection, supervision of data collection in partner sites, data analysis, drafting and revising manuscript. JZ study design, surveillance protocol, local site coordinator. MWP study design, surveillance protocol, local site coordinator. FS study design, data analysis. MB database setup, supervision of data collection in partner sites. AK microbiological analysis. BO local data collection. JKMK local principal investigator, microbiological analysis. SF microgiological analysis, local data collection. CQ local data collection. FG local site coordinator. AM microbiological analysis. VI local data collection. WS local site coordinator, local data collection. SA local data collection. SP microbiological analysis. ET local principal investigator. AH microbiological analysis. HS principal investigator of the study, study design, surveillance protocol. MJGTV local site coordination, local data collection. WVK principal investigator of the project, study design, surveillance protocol. PG principal investigator of the study, study design, surveillance protocol. All authors contributed to writing the manuscript through commenting and approved the final document.

Competing interests
No competing interests unless stated.
MJGTV is a consultant to: Alb Fils Kliniken, Astellas Pharma, MaaT Pharma, MSD/Merck; has served with the speakers' bureau of: Astellas Pharma, Basilea, Gilead Sciences, Merck/MSD, Organobalance and Pfizer; received research funding from: 3 M, Astellas Pharma, DaVolterra, Gilead Sciences, Merck/MSD, Morphochem, Organobalance, and Seres Therapeutics.
HS reports grants from Bundesministerium für Bildung und Forschung (BMBF), the German Center for Infection Research (DZIF), Cubist, and Novartis, and personal fees from Astellas-Basilea, Cubist, Durata, Genentech, Gilead, MSD, Roche Pharma, and Tetraphase.
JKMK received research and travel grants from Novartis, bioMérieux, Bayer Vital, and Alere and served as consultant or speaker for bioMérieux, Novartis,and Pfizer.
JZ received a speaker's honorarium from Pfizer.

Author details
[1]German Center for Infection Research (DZIF), Inhoffenstraße 7, 38124 Braunschweig, Germany. [2]Charité – Universitätsmedizin Berlin, Institute of Hygiene and Environmental Medicine, Hindenburgstraße 27, 12203 Berlin, Germany. [3]Department of Infection Control and Hygiene, University Hospital Cologne, Kerpener Straße 62, 50937 Köln, Germany. [4]Department of Infectious Diseases and Microbiology, Institute for Medical Microbiology, University Hospital Schleswig-Holstein, Ratzeburger Allee 160, 23562 Lübeck, Germany. [5]Institute for Medical Microbiology, Immunology and Hygiene, Klinikum Rechts der Isar, Technische Universität München, Munich, Germany. [6]Division of Infectious Diseases, Department of Medicine II, Medical Center and Faculty of Medicine, University of Freiburg, Hugstetter Strasse 55, 79106

Freiburg, Germany. [7]Division of Infectious Diseases, Department of Internal Medicine 1, University Hospital Tübingen, Otfried-Müller-Straße 12, 72076 Tübingen, Germany. [8]Institute for Medical Microbiology and Hygiene, University Hospital Tübingen, Elfriede-Aulhorn-Straße 6, 72076 Tübingen, Germany. [9]Institute for Medical Microbiology, Immunology and Hygiene, University Hospital Cologne, Goldenfelsstrasse 19-21, 50935 Köln, Germany. [10]Department I of Internal Medicine, University Hospital of Cologne, Herderstraße 52-54, 50931 Köln, Germany. [11]Institute for Medical Microbiology, Virology and Hygiene, University Medical Center Hamburg-Eppendorf, Martinistraße 52, 20246 Hamburg, Germany.

References

1. World Health Organization: Antimicrobial resistance: global report on surveillance. In. WHO Library Cataloguing-in-Publication Data: World Health Organisation 2014.
2. Rottier WC, Ammerlaan HS, Bonten MJ. Effects of confounders and intermediates on the association of bacteraemia caused by extended-spectrum beta-lactamase-producing Enterobacteriaceae and patient outcome: a meta-analysis. J Antimicrob Chemother. 2012;67(6):1311–20.
3. European Centre for Disease Prevention and Control: Antimicrobial resistance surveillance in Europe 2015. Annual Report of the European Antimicrobial Resistance Surveillance Network (EARS-Net). In. Stockholm: ECDC; 2017.
4. Remschmidt C, Schneider S, Meyer E, Schroeren-Boersch B, Gastmeier P, Schwab F. Surveillance of antibiotic use and resistance in intensive care units (SARI). Dtsch Arztebl Int. 2017;114(50):858–65.
5. Leistner R, Schroder C, Geffers C, Breier AC, Gastmeier P, Behnke M. Regional distribution of nosocomial infections due to ESBL-positive Enterobacteriaceae in Germany: data from the German National Reference Center for the surveillance of nosocomial infections (KISS). Clin Microbiol Infect. 2015;21(3):255 e251–5.
6. Hamprecht A, Rohde AM, Behnke M, Feihl S, Gastmeier P, Gebhardt F, Kern WV, Knobloch JK, Mischnik A, Obermann B, et al. Colonization with third-generation cephalosporin-resistant Enterobacteriaceae on hospital admission: prevalence and risk factors. J Antimicrob Chemother. 2016;71(10):2957–63. https://doi.org/10.1093/jac/dkw216.
7. Breakpoint tables for interpretation of MICs and zone diameters. Version 4.0. http://www.eucast.org.
8. Multidrug-Resistant Organism & Clostridium difficile Infection (MDRO/CDI) Module. https://www.cdc.gov/nhsn/pdfs/pscmanual/12pscmdro_cdadcurrent.pdf.
9. Federal Ministry of Justice and Consumer Protection: German Infection Protection Act, §23. In.; 2001.
10. Dingle KE, Didelot X, Quan TP, Eyre DW, Stoesser N, Golubchik T, Harding RM, Wilson DJ, Griffiths D, Vaughan A, et al. Effects of control interventions on Clostridium difficile infection in England: an observational study. Lancet Infect Dis. 2017;17(4):411–21.
11. Pouwels KB, Dolk FCK, Smith DRM, Robotham JV, Smieszek T. Actual versus 'ideal' antibiotic prescribing for common conditions in English primary care. J Antimicrob Chemother. 2018;73(suppl_2):19–26.
12. Smieszek T, Pouwels KB, Dolk FCK, Smith DRM, Hopkins S, Sharland M, Hay AD, Moore MV, Robotham JV. Potential for reducing inappropriate antibiotic prescribing in English primary care. J Antimicrob Chemother. 2018;73(suppl_2):ii36–43.
13. Zweigner J, Meyer E, Gastmeier P, Schwab F. Rate of antibiotic prescriptions in German outpatient care - are the guidelines followed or are they still exceeded? GMS Hyg Infect Control. 2018;13 Doc04.
14. Grundmann H, Glasner C, Albiger B, Aanensen DM, Tomlinson CT, Andrasevic AT, Canton R, Carmeli Y, Friedrich AW, Giske CG, et al. Occurrence of carbapenemase-producing Klebsiella pneumoniae and Escherichia coli in the European survey of carbapenemase-producing Enterobacteriaceae (EuSCAPE): a prospective, multinational study. Lancet Infect Dis. 2017;17(2):153–63.
15. Trepanier P, Mallard K, Meunier D, Pike R, Brown D, Ashby JP, Donaldson H, Awad-El-Kariem FM, Balakrishnan I, Cubbon M et al: Carbapenemase-producing Enterobacteriaceae in the UK: a national study (EuSCAPE-UK) on prevalence, incidence, laboratory detection methods and infection control measures. J Antimicrob Chemother. 2017;72(2):596–603.
16. Otter JA, Dyakova E, Bisnauthsing KN, Querol-Rubiera A, Patel A, Ahanonu C, Tosas Auguet O, Edgeworth JD, Goldenberg SD. Universal hospital admission screening for carbapenemase-producing organisms in a low-prevalence setting. J Antimicrob Chemother. 2016;71(12):3556–61.
17. Kaase M, Schimanski S, Schiller R, Beyreiss B, Thurmer A, Steinmann J, Kempf VA, Hess C, Sobottka I, Fenner I, et al. Multicentre investigation of carbapenemase-producing Escherichia coli and Klebsiella pneumoniae in German hospitals. Int J Med Microbiol. 2016.

19

Characteristics of the antibiotic regimen that affect antimicrobial resistance in urinary pathogens

Boudewijn Catry[1*†], Katrien Latour[1,2†], Robin Bruyndonckx[3,4], Camellia Diba[3], Candida Geerdens[3] and Samuel Coenen[4]

Abstract

Background: Treatment duration, treatment interval, formulation and type of antimicrobial (antibiotic) are modifiable factors that will influence antimicrobial selection pressure. Currently, the impact of the route of administration on the occurrence of resistance in humans is unclear.

Methods: In this retrospective multi-center cohort study, we assessed the impact of different variables on antimicrobial resistance (AMR) in pathogens isolated from the urinary tract in older adults. A generalized estimating equations (GEE) model was constructed using 7397 *Escherichia coli* (*E. coli*) isolates.

Results: Resistance in *E. coli* was higher when more antibiotics had been prescribed before isolation of the sample, especially in women (significant interaction $p = 0.0016$) and up to nine preceding prescriptions it was lower for higher proportions of preceding parenteral prescriptions (significant interactions $p = 0.0067$). The laboratory identity, dying, and the time between prescription and sampling were important confounders ($p < 0.001$).

Conclusions: Our model describing shows a dose-response relation between antibiotic use and AMR in *E. coli* isolated from urine samples of older adults, and, for the first time, that higher proportions of preceding parenteral prescriptions are significantly associated with lower probabilities of AMR, provided that the number of preceding prescriptions is not extremely high (≥10 during the 1.5 year observation period; 93% of 5650 included patients).

Trial registration: Retrospectively registered.

Keywords: Route of administration, Drug resistance, Uropathogens, Elderly

Background

The bacterium *Escherichia coli* (*E. coli*) is by far the most common uropathogen in older adults [1]. Investigations in residents from long-term care facilities also revealed that the primary indication for antimicrobial (antibiotic) use is a urinary tract infection (UTI) [2]. If a lower UTI spreads to the kidneys or, via a blood stream infection, to other organs, life threatening organ failure can occur [3].

An antimicrobial therapy consists of a specific product, synergies with other agents, its route of administration (formulation), a dose, a treatment interval, treatment duration, and they all can have an effect on the selection of antimicrobial resistance (AMR) [4, 5]. A vast amount of studies has been focusing on synergies, the ideal dose (pharmacokinetic/pharmacodynamic parameters [6]), treatment interval and the impact of duration on resistance [7], to maintain clinical efficacy while minimizing resistance. In contrast, limited research has been done on the importance of the route of administration on the occurrence of resistance. The purpose of the present research was to study the influence of different variables of the antimicrobial prescription on the occurrence of resistance in *E. coli* isolated from urine samples in Belgian older adults (≥65 years).

* Correspondence: Boudewijn.Catry@sciensano.be
†Boudewijn Catry and Katrien Latour contributed equally to this work.
[1]Healthcare-associated infections & Antimicrobial resistance (https://www.nsih.be), Sciensano, Ruy Juliette Wytsmanstraat 14, Brussels 1050, Belgium
Full list of author information is available at the end of the article

Methods
Data
Microbiological results for individual patient samples, retrieved from 15 voluntary participating clinical laboratories (2005) were linked with individual antimicrobial consumption and sociodemographic data (July 2004 – December 2005). The latter were retrieved from the Intermutualistic Agency (IMA), which bundles national reimbursement information from the seven Belgian health insurance funds. These data were collected within a large retrospective cohort study assessing the link between antimicrobial consumption and resistance in the individual patient [8]. In the current study, we focused on the resistance status (i.e. susceptible versus non-susceptible) of *E. coli* isolates found in the urine of retired adults (aged 65 or above) in relation to the consumption of antibacterials for systemic use (substances with Anatomic Therapeutic Chemical (ATC) code J01) [9]. Patients for whom antimicrobial consumption data were available but no urine sample was analyzed, or for whom a sample was analyzed but no antimicrobials were prescribed during the study period, were excluded for the here described analysis.

Antimicrobial susceptibility testing results for *E. coli* were obtained from Kirby Bauer disk diffusion tests with a wide variety of number and agents examined. The majority of labs applied Clinical Laboratory Standards Institute (CLSI) guidelines for inoculum standardization, incubation conditions and breakpoint interpretation criteria. An isolate's resistance status (Antimicrobial Resistance Iindex; ARI) was calculated as the number of non-susceptible test results divided by the total number of antimicrobials tested (expressed as the proportion of non-susceptible test results) [10]. Antimicrobial consumption was summarized as the total dose of prescribed antimicrobials (expressed as the number of defined daily doses; DDD), the number of unique preceding prescriptions (N_prescriptons) and the proportion of unique preceding prescriptions for a parenteral antimicrobial (%Injectable). Antimicrobial agents had to be purchased minimally 2 days before the sample was taken to ensure that patients started taking the purchased antibiotic at the moment of sampling. Prescriptions for the same antimicrobial (identical ATC level 4 code) within 7 days were considered as one unique prescription. Other covariates that were considered are gender (male or female), age category (65–84 or 85 and above), whether the patient died during the year of the study or was still alive at the end of 2005 (yes or no; death), and the log(time). For the log(time), the logarithmic value of the time was calculated, with time defined as the number of days between sampling and the last prescription. Previous antimicrobial consumption was not restricted to antimicrobials only prescribed for urinary tract infections.

Statistical analysis
Because multiple samples from the same patient were potentially taken, observations within the same patient are expected to be correlated. To account for the correlated nature of the data, a generalized estimating equations (GEE) model [11] was used. Because the explanatory covariates are time-dependent, we used an independent working correlation [12]. Note that although this working correlation might be incorrect, parameter estimates and empirical standard errors are deemed consistent due to the use of a sandwich estimator [13]. A GEE model with ARI as the outcome variable and a logit link function was constructed. To account for the fact that one lab analyzed multiple samples and determined the number of antibiotics tested, we included laboratory identification code (Lab ID) as a covariate in the GEE model. Because the remaining covariates considered to explain antimicrobial resistance were numerous (7 covariates and their two-way interactions), we conducted model building in two steps. In a first step, we removed all insignificant ($p > 0.15$) covariates in a backward fashion. In a second step, we included significant two-way interactions between remaining covariates in a forward fashion, using $\alpha = 0.05$. Due to collinearity between the dose and the number of preceding prescriptions (Pearson correlation = 0.73), we decided to continue with the latter.

Ethics statement
Data from laboratories and reimbursement organizations were encrypted by a trusted third party to ensure patient confidentiality. The procedure and the study protocol were approved by the Sectorial committee of the Belgian Federal Social Security as well as by the jointed ethical committee of the Scientific Institute of Public Health (WIV-ISP) and the Centres for Veterinary and Agrochemical Research (CODA-CERVA) (both institutes merged on April 2018 into Sciensano).

Results
The final data used in this study contained information on resistance status for 7397 isolates retrieved from 5650 patients (Table 1). The majority of patients were female (79%), were aged 65–84 years (76.8%) and survived 2005 (82.2%). The number of isolates per patient widely varied (Additional file 1: Table S1) and the ARI showed differences according to the gender, partly related to the different compounds tested (Additional file 2: Figure S1).

Descriptive statistics of prescribed antibiotics
Table 1 shows the antimicrobial prescriptions reported in the cohort. The mean (standard deviation) number of prescriptions and DDD per patient was 4.4 (4.1), and 44.4 (59.2), respectively (see for extra information Additional file 1: Table S2).

Table 1 Characteristics of the antimicrobial prescriptions in 5650 older adults prior to (minimum 2 days) an isolation of *Escherichia coli* (*n* = 7379) from a urine sample as retrieved from 15 voluntary participating Belgian clinical laboratories (January 2005 – December 2005)

Variable	Men (1551 isolates)		Women (5846 isolates)	
	Median	IQR	Median	IQR
Time	24	[10–79]	41	[13–125]
DDD	27.8	[10.3–64.1]	23	[9.5–53.0]
N_prescriptions	4	[2–6]	3	[2–6]
%Injectable	25	[0–57]	11	[0–50]
ARI *E. coli*	0.17	[0–0.35]	0.13	[0–0.31]

IQR: interquartile range *Time*: time in days between sampling and start of preceding antimicrobial (antibiotic) prescription. *DDD*: sum of defined daily dose (DDD) prior to sampling. *N_prescriptions*: number of prescriptions (If the same antimicrobial formulation (substance) was delivered within 7 days this was defined as one prescription). *%Injectable*: route of administration (modeled as the ratio of preceding injectable over preceding orally administered antimicrobial prescriptions, i.e. the proportion of preceding parenteral prescriptions). *ARI*: Antimicrobial Resistance Index calculated as proportion of non-susceptible antimicrobial resistance test results as defined by Kirby Bauer disk diffusion test

Statistical model building

Backward model building (using α = 0.15) resulted in the inclusion of covariates related to gender, log(time), the number of preceding prescriptions, route of administration (modeled as the proportion of non-oral antimicrobials prescribed), the lab in which the isolates were analyzed and whether or not the patient survived 2005. Subsequent forward model building (using α = 0.05) resulted in the inclusion of the interactions between the number of preceding prescriptions on the one hand and the proportion of non-oral antimicrobials prescribed or the patient's gender on the other hand. The odds ratios (95% Wald confidence intervals) of the final model are reported in Table 2.

The final model revealed that the odds of resistance (non-susceptibility, i.e. a higher ARI) decreased when the patient was still alive at the end of 2005 and when time between sampling and prescribing increased. The formulation (%Injectable; proportion of preceding parenteral prescriptions) effect depended on the number of preceding prescriptions and the patient's gender. When the number of preceding prescriptions is below 10, the odds of non-susceptibility is higher for men. When the number of preceding prescriptions is high (> 9), the odds of non-susceptibility is higher for women (Fig. 1). As seen in Fig. 2, if the number of preceding prescriptions is below 10, the predicted ARI is lower for a higher

proportion of preceding parenteral prescriptions. If the number of preceding prescriptions is high (> 9), the predicted ARI is lower for a lower proportion of preceding parenteral prescriptions. In other words, up to nine preceding prescriptions the higher the proportion of preceding parenteral prescription the lower the odds for AMR. When exposed to more than nine preceding prescriptions this effect is no longer present (calculated over the time frame of 1.5 year).

Discussion

This retrospective multicenter study showed a dose-response relationship between antimicrobial use and resistance in uropathogens in older adults. Our results demonstrate, for the first time in human clinical isolates, that the oral route of administration is associated with an increased likelihood of resistance compared to the parenteral route, provided the number of prescriptions (week courses) is below 10 (over one and a half year observation time). This is in full agreement with animal experimental studies in rodents for *E. coli* exposed to betalactams and tetracyclines [14], and earlier findings in a randomized control field trial in cattle [15]. The effect of route of administration moreover interacted with the number of preceding prescriptions. Up to 9 prescriptions, when other variables held constant, probability of resistance decreased by increase in proportion of preceding parenteral antibiotic

Table 2 Odds ratios (95% Wald confidence intervals) for covariates in the final model* that determine antimicrobial resistance (higher Antimicrobial Resistance Index, ARI) in *Escherichia coli* from retired patients that have been prescribed antimicrobials at least 2 days prior to sampling

Co-variate	Odds ratio [95%CI]	Co-variate	Odds ratio [95%CI]
Gender (male)	1.29 [1.14–1.45]	Log(time)	0.83 [0.81–0.85]
N_prescriptions	1.05 [1.04–1.06]	Survival (yes)	0.84 [0.78–0.92]
%Injectable	1.00 [0.99–1.00]	N_prescriptions * %Injectable	1.0004 [1.0001–1.0007]
		N_prescriptions * gender (male)	0.97 [0.956–0.99]

N_prescriptions: number of preceding antimicrobial prescriptions received 2 days or more before each sample; %Injectable: proportion of parenteral (non-oral) preceding antimicrobial prescriptions. *Laboratory identity (*n* = 15) was controlled for in the final model (*p* < 0.0001), but individual values were not included in the Table

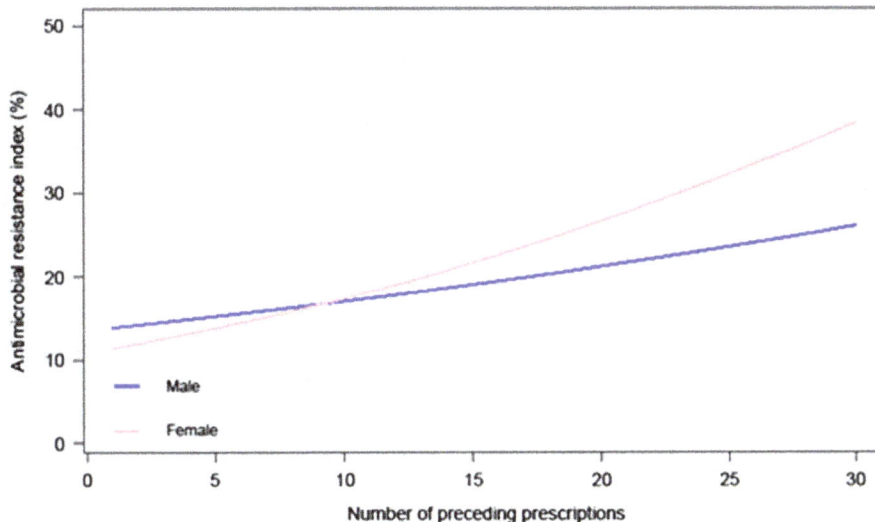

Fig. 1 Predicted antimicrobial resistance index (ARI) as reported for *Escherichia coli* isolated from the urinary tract of retired patients (Belgium, 2005) when varying the number of preceding prescriptions (1–30) for male and female patients. Estimates were obtained from a generalized estimating equations (GEE) model (fitted for a patient that was alive at the end of the study and was tested 33 (median) days after the most recent prescription in reference laboratory 15)

prescriptions. Since, seemingly, resistance gets organized after some threshold, possibly by reorganization of resistance at the molecular level, a different pattern was observed for samples with more than 9 prescriptions.

Comparison with the literature
Recently, a study comparing resistance in faecal *E. coli* from different groups of children (healthy, cancer, cystic fibrosis), suggested that aminopenicillin administered intravenously had only a modest effect on selection of intestinal resistance in cancer patients and possibly less impact than oral administration, which was the main route of administration of aminopenicillin to children with cystic fibrosis [16].

Apart from these studies, relatively little attention has been recently given to the route of administration and its particular influence on antimicrobial resistance. One exception is the stimulation to switch from intravenous to oral formulations (IV/PO switch) as soon as possible

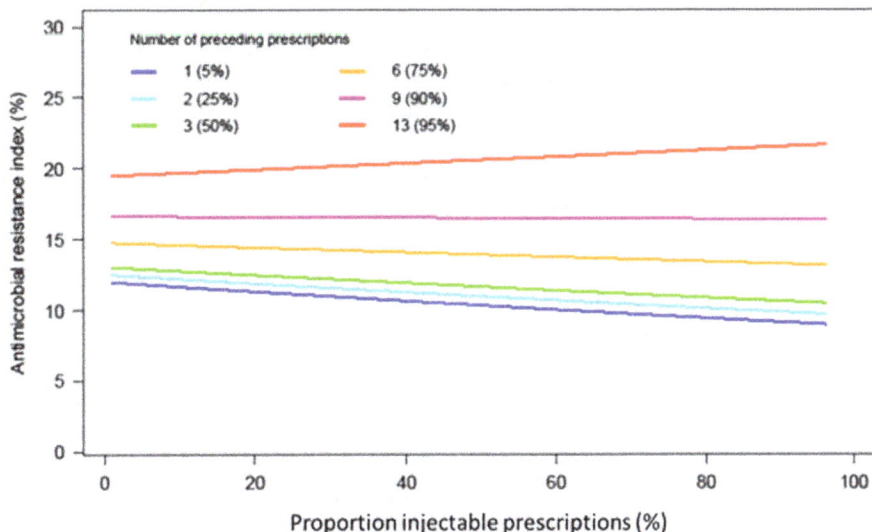

Fig. 2 Probability of resistance as estimated by the antimicrobial resistance index (ARI) as reported for *Escherichia coli* isolates from urinary tract infections in retired patients (Belgium 2005), when varying the proportion of injectable (% non-oral) prescriptions and the number of preceding prescriptions. Estimates were obtained using the final generalized estimating equations (GEE) model (fitted for a female patient that was alive at the end of the study and was tested 33 (median) days after her antibiotic prescription in lab 15)

in acute care hospitals to reduce length of stay, treatment costs, and central line associated infections [17]. Our results should trigger research to examine the influence of this switch on the selection of antimicrobial resistance. A recent investigation in Switzerland has shown that in acute care practice such a switch, leads to a two-step broad spectrum selection pressure, with an oral exposure of predominantly amoxicillin clavulanic acid, and to a lesser extent fluoroquinolones or clindamycine [4]. This impact on resistance in pathogens and commensals thus is substantial and we therefor plea to examine this in defined case control settings and larger at the population level. Infection control intervention studies likewise should include antimicrobial resistance data of pathogens, preferably over consecutive years [18]. Of notice, the IV/PO switch rationale is also fundamentally contradictory to the general mutation prevention theory. This theory states that a short high (loading) dose, followed by regular dosing intervals during an as short as possible time period is able to minimizes the resistance selection pressure while maintaining clinical efficacy [6, 19, 20]. Our study was conducted to assess such dynamics and persistence for E. coli retrieved from urine samples in the older adults (retired population). We assume many of these patients were suspected or confirmed to have a urinary tract infection. For urinary tract infections in women, a Cochrane review published in 2002 has shown that a reduction of treatment duration is feasible without impairing clinical efficacy and therefore should be encouraged to minimize the development and spread of resistance [21]. This is in line with our observations when using the number of week courses as a proxy for treatment duration and should further be stimulated in general and specialized practice.

The urinary tract mostly gets infected with E. coli by retrograde infection from commensal faecal bacteria. Each time an inappropriate antimicrobial therapy is initiated in the individual patient resistant genes can be selected. Other risk factors for developing drug resistant UTI include previous antimicrobial exposure, long-term care residence, older age and comorbidities such as diabetes [2]. Dutch investigators have also identified other medication and diet, including animal derived food, to be a risk factor for resistance in bacteria involved in UTI [22]. Bacteria can obtain antimicrobial resistant genes either by mutation or by acquisition f romneighboring bacteria (horizontal transfer). This has formerly been investigated and well documented for E. coli, both as a commensal [10, 23] and an invasive pathogen organism (e.g. EARS-net). This resistance selection process and maintenance after withdrawal of antibiotic pressure (i.e. persistence) can further be stimulated or driven by unrelated antimicrobial agents (co-selection) [23]. Despite that minimal inhibitory concentration determinations

are the golden standard, under routine laboratory conditions, in E. coli and many other fast growing organisms, disk diffusion tests have for long been the method to simultaneously determine susceptibility profiles for a wide variety of antimicrobial agents. For these reasons, the antimicrobial resistance index (ARI, [10, 24]) was used as primary outcome variable. It can theoretically even take subtle changes in the antibiogram into account, and merges selection pressure effects of virtually all antimicrobial agents used including co-selection by unrelated organisms. It has been shown to be strongly correlated with treatment incidences expressed as prescribed or administered daily dosages (PDD & DDD) at different population levels and settings [24–26]. Causal relationships between DDD and antimicrobial resistance have been found in single center longitudinal studies [27].

It was observed that patients who died during the study period were on average, more likely to have strains that were resistant to antibiotics. This is in line with similar observations in other bacteria [8]. The effect of number of days between the sample and the last prescription (log(time)) was significant and negative; indicating that probability of resistance is higher in the days after the treatment and decreases over time, confirming earlier findings in bacteria retrieved from the respiratory tract [28]. We further observed a high variability in ARI across participating laboratories and this demands further research in terms of validation of antimicrobial resistance surveillance.

Strengths and limitations

The study has several limitations, like the voluntary participation of the laboratories, the reliability of the(ir) disk diffusion tests, the lack of information on co-morbidities of the patients, the applied dosage assessment [25] and the absence of compliance information with regard to the prescribed antibiotics, and the unknown selection criteria related to patients that undergo laboratory examinations of the urinary tract. Selection bias due to inter-laboratory and gender driven differences in the panel of antimicrobial agents tested also could have influenced the analysis. Deviations in dosage regimens that might interfere with the resistance selection could not be identified with the applied methodology. Also patients not receiving antibiotics were excluded in the current study design. The latter information could be used to assess a baseline level of resistance as our study group earlier explored for the respiratory tract system [28]. Since also antimicrobial agents prescribed for indications other that urinary tract infections were included in the analysis it seems reasonable to conclude that resistance selection pressures are not restricted to one organ system, given the potential effect of antimicrobial agents on the digestive tract [14] and thereby indirectly on organisms shed by stool that can cause urinary tract infections. Also all prescriptions were considered in our analysis because of co-selection due to linked resistance genes as demonstrated for *E. coli* [23]. An additional confounder that potentially could have driven the selection between oral or injectable administrations is the difference between empirical, prophylactic and microbiologically directed regimes. In a European study in long term care facilities executed in 2009 [2], empirical treatments were most common (54.4%), followed by prophylactic (28.8%) and microbiologically documented (16.1%) regimes [2]. It is also recommended to repeat the analysis to confirm the finding by prospective randomized and controlled studies and in other study populations. Moreover, undesired effects of the switch of formulations, as recommended by several international guidelines on antimicrobial stewardship, should be considered in further studies.

Conclusion

In conclusion, this multicenter retrospective cohort study demonstrated a clear dose-effect of antimicrobial prescriptions on resistance in *E. coli* routinely isolated in urine samples from older adults. A substantial effect of route of administration, though subject to the number of preceding prescriptions, on the occurrence of antimicrobial resistance in uropathogens was demonstrated.

Additional files

Additional file 1: Table S1. Distribution of *Escherichia (E.) coli* isolates (*n* = 7379) per patient (retired, *n* = 5650) retrieved from 15 voluntary participating Belgian clinical laboratories (January 2005 – December 2005), for which an antimicrobial was prescribed (minimum 2 days before sampling) during the study period (July 2004–December 2005). **Table S2** Average number of defined daily dose (DDD) by gender prior to the isolation of uropathogens from retired patients (*n* = 5650) in Belgium (2004–2005). (DOCX 16 kb)

Additional file 2: Figure S1. Exhaustive distribution of antimicrobial susceptibilities stratified by patients' gender (left) and age (right) category, as reported for *Escherichia (E.) coli* isolates retrieved from urinary tract infections in Belgium (2005). (TIF 66 kb)

Abbreviations

AMR: antimicrobial resistance; ARI: Antimicrobial resistance index; ATC: Anatomic therapeutic chemical; CLSI: Clinical & Laboratory Standards Institute; CODA-CERVA: Veterinary & Agrochemical Research Centre (currently Sciensano); DDD: Defined daily dose; *E. coli*: *Escherichia coli*; EARS-Net: European Antimicrobial Resistance Surveillance-Network; GEE: Generalized estimating equations; IMA: Intermutualistic agency; Injectable%: The proportion of parenterally administered (non-oral) antimicrobials; IV/PO: Intravenously/per os; Lab ID: Laboratory identification code; N_prescriptions: The number of unique prescriptions; PDD: Prescribed daily dose; UTI: Urinary tract infection; WIV-ISP: Scientific Institute of Public Health (currently Sciensano)

Acknowledgements

This study was conducted on behalf of the Belgian National Council for Quality Promotion and concerned collaboration with the Intermutualistic Agency (IMA) (provided data on antimicrobial prescriptions and sociodemographic variables of patients). The project received the support from the Belgian Antibiotic Policy Coordination Committee (BAPCOC). Dr. Raf Mertens, Dr. Erik Hendrickx, and Dr. Carl Suetens, are acknowledged for their help during the execution of the study. Thanks also to the clinical laboratories that kindly volunteered to participate in the study (provide microbiological results). Preliminary results presented in this manuscript were part of the Master thesis Statistics, University Hasselt. Master Thesis Project of Camellia Diba (1335928), January 20, 2016.

Funding

This study (IARG) was supported by the Belgian National Council for the Promotion of Quality (Nationale Raad voor Kwaliteitspromotie; URL: http://www.riziv.fgov.be/nl/riziv/organen/Paginas/nrkp.aspx#.Wx9PtdUzapo). The funders had an initial advisory role in study design and data collection.

Authors' contributions

CD, CG and RB carried out the descriptive and statistical analysis. KL, BC and SC validated the data. BC and KL designed and coordinated the study and carried out the data management and drafted the article. RB and SC participated in the design, validation of the analysis, helped to coordinate the study, and helped to draft the manuscript. All authors read and approved the final manuscript.

Competing interests

The authors declare that they have no competing interests.

Author details

[1]Healthcare-associated infections & Antimicrobial resistance (https://www.nsih.be), Sciensano, Ruy Juliette Wytsmanstraat 14, Brussels 1050, Belgium. [2]Department of Public Health and Primary Care, KU Leuven - University of Leuven, Leuven, Belgium. [3]Interuniversity Institute for Biostatistics and statistical Bioinformatics (I-BIOSTAT), Hasselt University, Hasselt, Belgium. [4]Laboratory of Medical Microbiology, Vaccine & Infectious Disease Institute (VAXINFECTIO), University of Antwerp, Antwerp, Belgium.

References

1. Heytens S, Boelens J, Claeys G, De Sutter A, Christiaens T. Uropathogen distribution and antimicrobial susceptibility in uncomplicated cystitis in Belgium, a high antibiotics prescribing country: 20-year surveillance. Eur J Clin Microbiol Infect Dis. 2017;36:105–13.
2. Latour K, Catry B, Broex E, Vankerckhoven V, Muller A, Stroobants R, et al. Indications for antimicrobial prescribing in european nursing homes: results from a point prevalence survey. Pharmacoepidemiol Drug Saf. 2012;21:937–44.
3. Burke JP, Pombo DJ. Healthcare-associated urinary tract infections. In: Mayhall CG, editor. Hospital epidemiology and infection control. 4th ed: Wolters Kluwer/Lippincott Williams & Wilkins; 2012. p. 270–85.

4.   Beeler PE, Kuster SP, Eschmann E, Weber R, Blaser J. Earlier switching from intravenous to oral antibiotics owing to electronic reminders. Int J Antimicrob Agents. 2015;46:428–33.

5.   Catry B, Laevens H, Devriese LA, Opsomer G, De Kruif A. Antimicrobial resistance in livestock. J Vet Pharm Ther. 2003;26:81–93.

6.   Zhao X, Drlica K. A unified anti-mutant dosing strategy. J Antimicrob Chemother. 2008;62:434–6.

7.   Levy Hara G, Kanj SS, Pagani L, Abbo L, Endimiani A, Wertheim HF, et al. Ten key points for the appropriate use of antibiotics in hospitalised patients: a consensus from the antimicrobial stewardship and resistance working groups of the International Society of Chemotherapy. Int J Antimicrob Agents. 2016;48:239–48.

8.   Catry B, Latour K, Jans B, Vandendriessche S, Preal R, Mertens K, et al. Risk factors for methicillin resistant *Staphylococcus aureus*: a multi-laboratory study. PLoS One. 2014;9:e89579.

9.   WHO World Health Organisation. ATC classification. https://www.whocc.no/atc_ddd_index (2015). Accessed 24 Feb 2016.

10. Hinton M. The sub-species differentiation of *Escherichia coli* with particular reference to ecological studies in young animals including man. J Hyg (Lond). 1985;95:595–609.

11. Liang KY, Zeger SL. Longitudinal data analysis using generalized linear models. Biometrika. 1986;73:13–22.

12. Blommaert A, Hens N, Beutels P. Data mining for longitudinal data under multicollinearity and time dependence using penalized generalized estimating equations. Comp Stat Data Anal. 2014;71:667–80.

13. Molenberghs G, Verbeke G. Models for discrete longitudinal data. New York: Springer; 2005.

14. Zhang L, Huang Y, Zhou Y, Buckley T, Wang HH. Antibiotic administration routes significantly influence the levels of antibiotic resistance in gut microbiota. Antimicrob Agents Chemother. 2013;57:3659–66.

15. Checkley SL, Campbell JR, Chirino-Trejo M, Janzen ED, Waldner CL. Associations between antimicrobial use and the prevalence of antimicrobial resistance in fecal *Escherichia coli* from feedlot cattle in western Canada. Can Vet J. 2010;51:853–61.

16. Knudsen PK, Brandtzaeg P, Høiby EA, Bohlin J, Samuelsen Ø, Steinbakk M, et al. Impact of extensive antibiotic treatment on faecal carriage of antibiotic-resistant enterobacteria in children in a low resistance prevalence setting. PLoS One. 2017;12:e0187618.

17. Sevinç F, Prins JM, Koopmans RP, Langendijk PN, Bossuyt PM, Dankert J, et al. Early switch from intravenous to oral antibiotics: guidelines and implementation in a large teaching hospital. J Antimicrob Chemother. 1999;43:601–6.

18. Halaby T, al Naiemi N, Beishuizen B, Verkooijen R, Ferreira JA, Klont R, et al. Impact of single room design on the spread of multi-drug resistant bacteria in an intensive care unit. Antimicrob Resist Infect Control. 2017;6:117.

19. Thomas JK, Forrest A, Bhavnani SM, Hyatt JM, Cheng A, Ballow CH, et al. Pharmacodynamic evaluation of factors associated with the development of bacterial resistance in acutely ill patients during therapy. Antimicrob Agents Chemother. 1998;42:521–7.

20. Dryden M, Johnson AP, Ashiru-Oredope D, Sharland M. Using antibiotics responsibly: right drug, right time, right dose, right duration. J Antimicrob Chemother. 2011;66:2441–3.

21. Lutters M, Vogt-Ferrier NB. Antibiotic duration for treating uncomplicated, symptomatic lower urinary tract infections in elderly women. Cochrane Database Syst Rev. 2002;3:CD001535. https://doi.org/10.1002/14651858.CD001535.

22. Mulder M, Kiefte-de Jong JC, Goessens WH, de Visser H, Hofman A, Stricker BH, et al. Risk factors for resistance to ciprofloxacin in community-acquired urinary tract infections due to *Escherichia coli* in an elderly population. J Antimicrob Chemother. 2017;72:281–9.

23. Levy SB, Fitzgerald GB, Macone AB. Spread of antibioticresistant plasmids from chicken to chicken and from chicken to man. Nature. 1976;260:40–2.

24. Patrick DM, Chambers C, Purych D, Chong M, George D, Marra F. Value of an aggregate index in describing the impact of trends in antimicrobial resistance for *Escherichia coli*. Can J Infect Dis Med Microbial. 2015;26:33–8.

25. Bruyndonckx R, Hens N, Aerts M, Goossens H, Cortiñas Abrahantes J, Coenen S. Exploring the association between resistance and outpatient antibiotic use expressed as DDDs or packages. J Antimicrob Chemother. 2015;70:1241–4.

26. Catry B, Dewulf J, Maes D, Pardon B, Callens B, Vanrobaeys M, et al. Effect of antimicrobial consumption and production type on antibacterial resistance in the bovine respiratory and digestive tract. PLoS One. 2016;11:e0146488.

27. Lafaurie M, Porcher R, Donay JL, Touratier S, Molina JM. Reduction of fluoroquinolone use is associated with a decrease in methicillin-resistant *Staphylococcus aureus* and fluoroquinolone-resistant *Pseudomonas aeruginosa* isolation rates: a 10 year study. J Antimicrob Chemother. 2012;67:1010–5.

28. Bruyndonckx R, Hens N, Aerts M, Goossens H, Latour K, Catry B, et al. Persistence of antimicrobial resistance in respiratory streptococci. J Glob Antimicrob Resist. 2017;8:6–12.

20

Influence of weight gain, according to Institute of Medicine 2009 recommendation, on spontaneous preterm delivery in twin pregnancies

Paola Algeri[1][*], Francesca Pelizzoni[1], Davide Paolo Bernasconi[2], Francesca Russo[1], Maddalena Incerti[1], Sabrina Cozzolino[1], Salvatore Andrea Mastrolia[1] and Patrizia Vergani[1]

Abstract

Backgrounds: Maternal total weight gain during pregnancy influences adverse obstetric outcomes in singleton pregnancies. However, its impact in twin gestation is less understood. Our objective was to estimate the influence of total maternal weight gain on preterm delivery in twin pregnancies.

Methods: We conducted a retrospective cohort study including diamniotic twin pregnancies with spontaneous labor delivered at 28 + 0 weeks or later. We analyzed the influence of total weight gain according to Institute of Medicine (IOM) cut-offs on the development of preterm delivery (both less than 34 and 37 weeks). Outcome were compared between under and normal weight gain and between over and normal weight gain separately using Fisher's exact test with Holm-Bonferroni correction.

Results: One hundred seventy five women were included in the study and divided into three groups: under (52.0%), normal (41.7%) and overweight gain (6.3%). Normal weight gain was associated with a reduction in the rate of preterm delivery compared to under and over weight gain [less than 34 weeks: under vs. normal OR 4.97 (1.76–14.02), over vs. normal OR 4.53 (0.89–23.08); less than 37 weeks: OR 3.16 (1.66–6.04) and 6.51 (1.30–32.49), respectively].

Conclusions: Normal weight gain reduces spontaneous preterm delivery compared to over and underweight gain.

Keywords: Twin pregnancy, Preterm delivery, Preterm labor, Weight gain, Institute of medicine recommendation

Background

Pre-gestational body mass index (pBMI), gestational body mass index (gBMI) and total weight gain influence the incidence of preterm delivery and other adverse obstetric outcomes in singletons [1, 2] but their effect on twins is poorly understood, although multiple pregnancies appear to have similar associations between these outcomes, pBMI or weight gain compared to singletons [1, 2]. Indeed, studies evaluating the role of both total and weekly weight gain in twin pregnancies identified a strong correlation between low total weight gain during pregnancy and preterm

delivery (PD) [3, 4]. In 1990, the Institute of Medicine (IOM) proposed ranges of recommended total weight gain correlated to pBMI for singleton pregnancy and an optimal total weight gain between 15.9 and 20.5 kg not related to pBMI for twin pregnancy [5, 6].

In 2009, the IOM revised these guidelines and defined pBMI specific weight gain cut-off, also for twin pregnancies. Optimal ranges proposed for weight gain at term (≥ 37 weeks) are: 17–25 kg for normal weighted women (pBMI 18.5–24.9), 14–23 kg for over weighted women (pBMI 25–29.9) and 11–19 kg for obese women (pBMI 30 or more). No recommendations were given for underweighted women (pBMI less than 18.5) [7].

This is of higher importance due to the rise in the incidence of twin pregnancies in the last three decades because of the older age at childbearing and of the diffusion

* Correspondence: p.algeri@campus.unimib.it
[1]Department of Obstetrics and Gynecology, University of Milano-Bicocca, S. Gerardo Hospital, MBBM Foundation, Via Pergolesi 33, Monza, 20900 Monza, Monza e Brianza, Italy
Full list of author information is available at the end of the article

of assisted reproductive technology [8]. Today, approximately 1 of 80 pregnancies is a multiple gestation, corresponding to 2.6% of all newborns (1–3% in Italy) and they are more frequently diamniotic. Multiple pregnancies present a higher incidence of maternal and fetal adverse outcomes compared to singleton ones [3, 9–13]. Twin pregnancies account for 12.2% of preterm births and 15.4% of neonatal deaths [14–16].

In literature, both pBMI and total weight gain were reported as important influencing factors in pregnancies outcomes. However, the studies took into consideration only one of these parameters at a time. New cut-offs proposed by IOM allowed an easier evaluation of maternal weight influence on obstetrics outcomes, not only in singleton pregnancies but also in twins.

Few studies evaluated the role of the new IOM guidelines in influencing preterm delivery in twins, also considering that IOM gave cut-offs only for gestational age at delivery ≥ 37 weeks [17–19].

In 2010, Fox et al. conducted a study on a cohort of twins divided into subgroups considering pBMI. They show that patients whose weight gain during pregnancy met or exceeded the revised 2009 IOM guidelines had significantly improved pregnancy outcomes such as longer gestation, less overall PD, less spontaneous PD and larger neonates compared to lower weight gain [18]. In 2012, also Quintero et al. found that a weight gain below recommended guidelines was associated with higher rates of spontaneous PD at less than 35 weeks in twin pregnancies [19].

A recent review tried to define the role of absolute total weight gain in the development of adverse pregnancy outcomes. The authors suggested that a higher incidence of PD was correlated with underweight gain and underlined a positive correlation between total weight gain and gestation length [20].

Gestational gain weight and pBMI have been proven to influence not only the risk of PD but also other obstetric outcomes, such as birth weight, hypertensive disorders, gestational diabetes and neonatal adverse outcomes [17].

Contrasting results were instead reported about hypertensive disorders: while some authors described higher incidence of gestational hypertension and preeclampsia in women with excessive weight gain, others showed no differences among different weight gain groups in a series of twin pregnancies delivering at term [5, 17, 20].

In light of the above and due to the scarcity of data available in the literature about this topic, we designed a study with the aim to estimate the influence of total weight gain according to the 2009 IOM recommendations on preterm delivery before 37 and 34 weeks in twin pregnancies with spontaneous onset of labor. Secondary outcomes were the possible correlation with small for gestational age (SGA) and large for gestational age (LGA), pregnancy hypertensive disorders, gestational diabetes, and neonatal adverse outcomes.

Methods

We performed a retrospective cohort study on diamniotic twin pregnancies delivered at more or equal 28 + 0 weeks after spontaneous onset of labor at our Institution (Fondazione MBBM, San Gerardo Hospital, University of Milano Bicocca, Monza, Italy), between January 2010 and December 2013.

Exclusion criteria of our study were induction of labor (15% of all twin pregnancies at our Institution), elective cesarean section (4% of all twin pregnancies at our Institution), monoamniotic twins, intrauterine demise, fetal malformations, twin-to-twin transfusion syndrome, and gestational age at delivery < 28 weeks. We decided to set a gestational age < 28 weeks at delivery as an exclusion criteria in order to have a better definition of the weight gain trend for each patient. A shorter pregnancy duration could be a confounding factor in defining the maternal weight gain.

Patients with pBMI < 18.5 were also excluded since there are no IOM recommendations for underweight patients in case of multiple pregnancies.

All twin gestations were followed according to national guidelines for management of twin pregnancy [21]. The protocol included maternal clinical assessment and ultrasound monitoring every 2 weeks, from 16 weeks, for monochorionic diamniotic pregnancies and every 4 weeks, starting from 20 weeks, for dichorionic diamniotic gestations.

At our Maternal-Fetal Unit, women undergo their first access at obstetric booking that is usually performed during the first trimester after a positive pregnancy test (<8 weeks of gestation). At the first visit we collect patient's medical and obstetric history, define gestational age (calculated based on the last menstrual period and confirmed by ultrasound assessment), as well as chorionicity. Baseline characteristics and pregnancy outcomes were entered into our database by an assigned physician at every patient's access and periodically reviewed by a senior consultant. pBMI was recorded at the first visit, and maternal weight was measured at each obstetric control until delivery.

Since self-report of pBMI can be affected by recall bias, we attempted to reduce the risk of bias with an early assessment of pregnant women as described above.

Total weight gain was calculated as the difference between maternal weight at delivery and pre-gestational weight. This parameter was used to classify women who delivered at 37 weeks or more according to IOM guidelines [7]. In case of preterm delivery (between 28 and 36 + 6 weeks), we calculated a weekly weight gain cut-off as total weight gain during pregnancy in kg/gestational weeks at delivery. We compared this weekly weight gain to a hypothesized weekly IOM cut-off, calculated as IOM cut-off at term/37 weeks, as previously reported, represented for normal-weight women, this was 1.0 lb. per week (37 lbs. over 37 weeks); for overweight women, this was 0.84 lb. per week (31 lbs. over 37 weeks); for obese women, this was 0.68 lb. per week (25 lbs. over 37 weeks) [18].

The data used for the analysis were already available for every patient as part of the clinical report of the Obstetric Department.

SGA and LGA were defined, respectively, as neonatal weight at birth < 10° centile and > 90° centile compared to Italian Neonatal Study (INeS) charts [22]. We considered as separate outcomes the occurrence of at least one twin SGA/LGA and both twins SGA/LGA.

We defined "gestational hypertensive disorders" as the presence of at least one among gestational hypertension, preeclampsia or eclampsia, diagnosed according to American Congress of Obstetricians and Gynecologists (ACOG) criteria [23].

Gestational diabetes was defined as any degree of glucose intolerance with onset or first recognition during pregnancy [24].

We defined composite adverse neonatal outcome as the presence of at least one among: need for neonatal resuscitation, respiratory distress syndrome, disseminated intravascular coagulation, intra-ventricular hemorrhage, leucomalacia, sepsis, necrotizing enteritis, retinopathy of prematurity and neonatal death.

The present work was exempt from IRB approval as per Institutional policy on retrospective studies. At our medical center, women provide a written consent to the use of their clinical anonymized and de-identified data upon admission.

Statistical analysis

Population characteristics were compared among IOM weight gain groups using Chi Square test (categorical variables) or One Way ANOVA (continuous variables). Primary and secondary outcomes rates were compared between under and normal gain and between over and normal gain separately using Fisher's exact test with Holm-Bonferroni correction. Logistic regression analysis was carried out in order to evaluate the independent effect of weight gain adjusted for pBMI on the outcomes. A separate model was built for each primary and secondary outcome. All the analyses were performed using the R software, version 3.0.2. A p value of less than 0.05 was considered significant.

Results

The incidence of twin pregnancies at our Institution was 2.5–3% during the study period.

A cohort of 175 diamniotic twin pregnancies was included in our study, considering exclusion criteria: 91 (52.0%) presented underweight gain, 73 (41.7%) normal

weight gain and 11 (6.3%) over weight gain, according to IOM recommendations.

Table 1 shows general population characteristics in the three study groups, considering the IOM classification for total weight gain. The normal weight gain group had a higher mean gestational age at delivery compared with the under and over gain weight ones (respectively 36.5 ± 2.0, 35.3 ± 3.0, 35.3 ± 2.0 weeks). Normal and overweight gain patients presented higher neonatal weight at birth for both twins compared to the under gain ones (respectively 2494.11, 2974.55, 2196.54 g). The over weight gain group presented a higher incidence of pre–gestational over weighted patients (45.5%). The study groups did not differ for other characteristics.

The incidence of primary and secondary adverse outcomes was compared among the three groups, and the results are presented in Tables 2 and 3.

We found that the normal weight gain group presented a significant lower incidence of spontaneous PD compared to both under and over weight gain groups [respectively 39.7% vs 67.0% (p: 0.002); 39.7% vs 81.8% (p: 0.04)]. Underweight gain women presented significantly higher rates of early preterm spontaneous delivery compared to normal weight gain ones; a trend was also reported when overweight gain was compared to normal weight gain group [respectively 25.3% vs. 6.8% (p: 0.005); 27.3% vs. 6.8% (p: 0.13)].

No differences in the occurrence of SGA in one or both twins were observed among the three study groups. In addition, no cases of LGA were recorded. Gestational hypertensive disorders occurred in our population included 1 case of gestational hypertension and seven cases of preeclampsia in the underweight group, five and eight respectively in the normal weight, and one and six in the overweight one. No cases of eclampsia were reported. In the normal weight gain group, women presented a trend toward a higher incidence of hypertensive gestational diseases compared to underweight gain patients, even if not significant (17.8% vs. 7.7%, $p = 0.06$). This complication was significantly less frequent in the normal weight gain group compared with the over weight gain one (17.8% vs. 63.6%, $p = 0.006$). No difference in the incidence of gestational diabetes mellitus and neonatal adverse composite outcomes were reported in the three study groups, and we had no neonatal deaths.

The results of the bivariate analysis on both primary and secondary outcomes were confirmed in the multivariate logistic regression analysis, adjusting for the effect of pBMI (Tables 4 and 5, respectively). Both under and over weight gain increased the risk of PD compared to normal weight gain: ORs were 4.97 (1.76–14.02) and 4.53 (0.89–23.08) for early preterm and 3.16 (1.66–6.04) and 6.51 (1.30–32.49) for PD at less than 37 weeks

Table 1 Population general characteristics, according to weight gain groups

	Under (91)	Normal (73)	Over (11)	P value
Maternal age	34 ± 5.55	34 ± 5.86	34 ± 5.03	0.99
Nulliparity	52 (57.1%)	44 (60.3%)	8 (72.7%)	0.32
Smoker	3 (3.9%)	5 (6.8%)	1 (9.1%)	0.38
Chronic Hypertension	1 (1.1%)	1 (1.4%)	0	0.93
pBMI[a]	22.75 ± 4.44	23.00 ± 3.29	23.97 ± 2.50	0.70
18.5 ≤ pBMI[a] ≤ 24.9	74 (81.3%)	54 (74.0%)	6 (54.5%)	0.11
25 ≤ pBMI[a] ≤ 29.9	10 (11.0%)	15 (20.5%)	5 (45.5%)	*0.01*
pBMI[a] ≥ 30	7 (7.7%)	4 (5.5%)	0	0.57
Medically assisted procreation	16 (17.6%)	18 (24.7%)	4 (36.4%)	0.26
Mono- Chorionicity	13 (14.3%)	11 (15.1%)	2 (18.2%)	0.94
Clinical chorionamnionitis	1 (1.1%)	0	0	0.63
Preterm rupture of membranes[b]	30 (33.0%)	13 (17.8%)	3 (27.3%)	0.09
Gestational age at delivery (weeks)	35.3 ± 3.0	36.5 ± 2.0	35.3 ± 2.0	*0.002*
Vaginal delivery	34 (37.4%)	23 (31.5%)	4 (36.4%)	0.73
1st twin birth weight (gr)	2196.54 ± 592.16	2494.11 ± 426.87	2374.55 ± 471.63	*0.002*
2nd twin birth weight (gr)	2154.89 ± 499.41	2392.95 ± 413.94	2443.50 ± 334.47	*0.002*

Results are reported as means and standard deviations (continuous factors) or numbers and percentages (categorical factors). The *p*-value of an overall test comparing the three groups is also provided (One-way ANOVA for continuous factors and Chi-square test for categorical factors)
Italic data are statistically significant
[a]pBMI = pre-gestational Body Mass Index; [b]Preterm rupture of membrane = rupture before 37 weeks

(Table 4). Women in the underweight gain group had a lower risk of developing hypertensive gestational disorders compared to the women of the normal weight gain group, even if it was not significant, but only a trend (OR = 0.39, 0.15–1.05). The over weight gain group, instead, presented a significantly higher risk of hypertensive gestational disorders compared to the normal weight gain group (OR = 7.69, 1.94–30.47).

Discussion
Principal findings of the study
In this study, we evaluated the influence of total maternal weight gain, according to the revised IOM recommendations, on the development of spontaneous PD in diamniotic twin gestations [7]. Our results show that 1) normal weight gain is associated with a significant reduction in preterm parturition; and 2) when taking into consideration gestational age at delivery, both under and overweight gain groups presented an increased risk of early

preterm parturition compared to normal weight gain women; and 3) a significantly increased risk for preterm parturition before 37 weeks (three and six times respectively) was present in underweight and overweight women respectively, compared with normal weight gain women.

IOM recommendations for weight gain in twin pregnancies
The important novelty of 2009 IOM recommendations was to give pBMI correlated cut-offs in twin pregnancies. On the other side, a limitation on the clinical use of these guidelines was to refer only to term twin pregnancies, excluding a twin group that delivered before 37 weeks [7, 17]. Therefore, just because IOM guidelines may be used limitedly to term twin pregnancies, we wanted to value how to apply them also in preterm gestations. Thus, we used a weekly gain weight cut-off (IOM cut-off at term/37 weeks), as already done by Fox et al. in a previous study [18].

Table 2 Incidence of the primary outcomes in the weight gain groups

	Under (n. 91)	Normal (n. 73)	*p*-value§	Over (n. 11)	Normal (n. 73)	*p*-value§
Preterm delivery < 37 weeks	61 (67.0%)	29 (39.7%)	*P = .002*	9 (81.8%)	29 (39.7%)	*P = .04*
Early preterm delivery < 34 weeks	23 (25.3%)	5 (6.8%)	*P = .005*	3 (27.3%)	5 (6.8%)	P = .13

Results are reported as numbers and percentages. The *p*-value of an overall test (Chi-square test) correlating the three groups for the two by two comparison
Italic data are statistically significant
§Fisher' exact test with Holm-Bonferroni correction

Table 3 Incidence of the secondary outcomes in the weight gain groups

	Under (n. 91)	Normal (n. 73)	Over (n. 11)	P value[c]
At least one twin SGA[a]	16 (17.6%)	13 (17.8%)	0 (0%)	0.31
Both twins SGA[a]	4 (4.4%)	1 (1.4%)	0 (0%)	0.43
Hypertensive disorders	7 (7.7%)	13 (17.8%)	7 (63.6%)	*< 0.001*
Gestational diabetes	15 (16.5%)	7 (9.6%)	0	0.18
1st twin adverse outcomes[b]	20 (22.0%)	6 (8.2%)	2 (18.2%)	0.06
2nd twin adverse outcomes[b]	20 (22.0%)	8 (11.0%)	2 (18.2%)	0.18

Results are reported as numbers and percentages
Italic data are statistically significant
[a]SGA = small for gestational age; [b]Adverse outcomes = neonatal resuscitation, respiratory distress syndrome, disseminated intravascular coagulation, intra-ventricular hemorrhage, leucomalacia, sepsis, necrotic enteritis, retinopathy of prematurity; [c]Fisher's exact test with Holm-Bonferroni correction, for all comparison; ns, not significant

Available literature assessing the influence of weight gain on pregnancy outcomes, in twin gestations

Several studies [17–19] analyzed the influence of IOM recommendations on pregnancy outcomes in twin pregnancies. The available literature on the topic is presented herein: 1) Fox et al. [18] collected 297 twin women divided into four groups based on their pBMI (underweight, normal weight, overweight, and obese). They compared pregnancy outcomes for women whose weight gain per week equaled or exceeded the IOM recommendations to women whose weight gain per week was lower than IOM cut-off, in three pBMI-based subgroups (underweight patients were excluded). They found that weight gain was associated with the gestational age at delivery and birth weight of the larger and smaller twin. Specifically, their study showed that, in women with a normal pBMI, patients whose weight gain met or exceeded the IOM recommendations had significantly improved outcomes, such as increment in birthweight of the larger twin and a lower rate of PD before 32 weeks (3.4% vs. 11.5%). In women with an overweight pBMI, if the weight gain met or exceeded the IOM recommendations, they reported higher gestational age at delivery, larger birth weight, and less preterm birth. In pre-gestational obese women, no statistically significant differences were noted; 2) The same authors [17] retrospectively studied a cohort of 170 women restricted to

twin pregnancies at 37 weeks or more. Their analysis valued pregnancy outcomes in three groups based on IOM recommendations defined as poor, normal, and excessive weight gain. The rate of newborns weighing more than 2500 g was 40%, 60.5% and 79.5% in the three groups, respectively. No differences in gestational hypertension, pre-eclampsia, gestational diabetes or neonatal intensive care unit admission across groups were observed; 3) Gonzalez-Quintero et al. [19], aimed to determine the validity of IOM recommendations for weight gain in twin pregnancies in terms of impact on perinatal outcomes comparing women with mean weight gain per week meeting or exceeding recommendations versus patients who did not meet the suggested weight gain. There was a significantly higher number of both infants weighing > 2500 g or > 1500 g for women gaining weight at or above guidelines. Of interest, women whose gain was below recommended guidelines were 50% more likely to deliver spontaneously at < 35 weeks.

What do our study adds compared to the available literature

Our study follows, in line with the available literature, the idea of assessing whether changes in weight gain during pregnancy in twin gestations, may have an impact on maternal and perinatal outcomes. Moreover, our study design shows several peculiarities, which differentiate it from the previous reports.

Specifically, 1) considering that IOM recommendations were already pBMI correlated, we simplified our analysis and divided our population considering if patients met, exceeded, or presented lower gain weight according to pBMI IOM cut-offs, without performing further stratification of the study groups. The rationale for it was to make the influence of weight gain on PD clearer and useful in clinical practice. Indeed, our analysis showed that a normal weight gain, was correlated with better perinatal and maternal outcomes; 2) Compared with the analysis by Fox et al. [17], our study population also included twins delivered preterm at 28 weeks or more. This was done in order not to lose the effect of prematurity on the analyzed outcomes, since prematurity is common in twin gestations and different outcomes such as preeclampsia and SGA are more frequent in women delivering preterm; 3) In line with Quintero et al., we found that a weight gain below the recommended guidelines was associated with higher rates of spontaneous PD. Moreover, we compared normal weight gain both with under and over gain weight and did not associate patients who met or exceeded IOM recommendations. Of interest, we hypothesized that, both lower and excessive weight gain were associated with worse outcomes; our results confirmed the idea that pregnant women whose weight gain was over recommendation, are at higher risk of hypertensive disorder and PD.

Table 4 Effect of weight gain on the primary outcomes estimated by logistic regression

	Early preterm delivery OR (95%CI)	Preterm delivery < 37 weeks OR (95%CI)
Under vs normal	4.97 (1.76; 14.02)	3.16 (1.66; 6.04)
Over vs normal	4.53 (0.89; 23.08)	6.51 (1.30; 32.49)

The models were adjusted for pre-pregnancy BMI

Table 5 Effect of weight gain on the secondary outcomes estimated by logistic regression

	At least one twin SGA[a] OR(95%CI)	Hypertensive gestational disorders OR(95%CI)	Gestational diabetes mellitus OR(95%CI)	Neonatal adverse outcomes[b] OR(95%CI)
Under vs. normal	1.01 (0.45; 2.28)	0.39 (0.15; 1.05)	1.98 (0.75; 5.22)	0.94 (0.29; 3.05)
Over vs. normal	–	7.69 (1.94; 30.47)	–	0.44 (0.05; 3.82)

The model for "neonatal adverse outcomes" was adjusted for pre-pregnancy BMI and gestational age. All the other models were adjusted only for pre-pregnancy BMI
[a]SGA = small for gestational age; [b]Adverse outcomes = neonatal resuscitation, respiratory distress syndrome, disseminated intravascular coagulation, intra-ventricular hemorrhage, leucomalacia, sepsis, necrotic enteritis, retinopathy of prematurity

Strengths and limitations of the study

The novelty of our work was to evaluate if there is an effect of IOM guidelines on the development of spontaneous PD in a cohort of twins at both term and preterm.

Moreover, our study has some limitations, mainly related to its retrospective design and to the small sample size as well as on the fact that it is built on a database registry.

Another possible weakness is the potential for missing data. To minimize this, at our hospital, data is reported by the obstetrician directly after delivery and skilled personnel routinely reviews the information before entering it into the database thereby minimizing recall bias. Coding was done after assessing the medical and prenatal care records together with the routine hospital documents. In addition, since there were no data regarding weekly weight gain cut-offs for twin pregnancies in IOM recommendations, we decided to apply linearity to weekly gain cut-offs as performed within IOM recommendations for single pregnancies [25].

Conclusions

Our findings suggest that normal weight gain, according to revised IOM recommendations, is associated with a reduction of spontaneous PD and, in a selected population, with better pregnancy course and better obstetrics outcomes. This information could be useful for early counseling in twin pregnancy.

Abbreviations
IOM: Institute of medicine; LGA: Large for gestational age; pBMI: Pre-gestational body mass index; PD: Preterm delivery; SGA: Small for gestational age

Acknowledgments
None.

Funding
None.

Authors contributions
PA Protocol/project development; manuscript writing/editing; data collection or management; data analysis. FP Protocol/project development; manuscript writing/editing; data collection or management. DPB data analysis; manuscript writing/editing. FR manuscript writing/editing. MI Protocol/ project development; manuscript writing/editing. SC manuscript writing/ editing. SAM/manuscript editing. PV Protocol/project development; manuscript writing/editing. All authors have read and approved the final version of the manuscript.

Competing interests
The authors declare that they have no competing interests.

Author details
[1]Department of Obstetrics and Gynecology, University of Milano-Bicocca, S. Gerardo Hospital, MBBM Foundation, Via Pergolesi 33, Monza, 20900 Monza, Monza e Brianza, Italy. [2]Department of Health Sciences, Center of Biostatistic for Clinical Epidemiology, University of Milan-Bicocca, Via Pergolesi 33, Monza, 20900 Monza, Monza e Brianza, Italy.

References
1. Abenhaim HA, Kinch RA, Morin L, Benjamin A, Usher R. Effect of prepregnancy body mass index categories on obstetrical and neonatal outcomes. Arch. Gynecol. Obstet. 2007;275(1):39–43.
2. Menacker F, Hamilton BE. Recent trends in cesarean delivery in the United States. NCHS Data Brief. 2010;35:1–8.
3. Brown JE, Carlson M. Nutrition and multifetal pregnancy. J Am Diet Assoc. 2000;100(3):343–8.
4. Kanadys WM, Oleszczuk J. Maternal weight gain during twin pregnancy. Its relationship to the incidence of preterm delivery. Ginekol Pol. 2000;71(11): 1355–9.
5. Yeh J, Shelton JA. Association of pre-pregnancy maternal body mass and maternal weight gain to newborn outcomes in twin pregnancies. Acta Obstet Gynecol Scand. 2007;86(9):1051–7.
6. Institute of Medicine. Subcommittee on nutritional status and weight gain during pregnancy. Washington, DC: National Academy Press; 1990.
7. Institute of Medicine. Weight gain during pregnancy: reexamining the guidelines. Washington, DC: National Academies Press; 2009.
8. Vayssiere C, Benoist G, Blondel B, Deruelle P, Favre R, Gallot D, Jabert P, Lemery D, Picone O, Pons JC, et al. Twin pregnancies: guidelines for clinical practice from the French College of Gynaecologists and Obstetricians (CNGOF). Eur J Obstet Gynecol Reprod Biol. 2011;156(1):12–7.
9. Luke B, Gillespie B, Min SJ, Avni M, Witter FR, O'Sullivan MJ. Critical periods of maternal weight gain: effect on twin birth weight. Am J Obstet Gynecol. 1997;177(5):1055–62.
10. Lantz ME, Chez RA, Rodriguez A, Porter KB. Maternal weight gain patterns and birth weight outcome in twin gestation. Obstet Gynecol. 1996;87(4):551–6.
11. Luke B, Minogue J, Witter FR, Keith LG, Johnson TR. The ideal twin pregnancy: patterns of weight gain, discordancy, and length of gestation. Am J Obstet Gynecol. 1993;169(3):588–97.
12. Luke B. The evidence linking maternal nutrition and prematurity. J Perinat Med. 2005;33(6):500–5.
13. Russo FM, Pozzi E, Pelizzoni F, Todyrenchuk L, Bernasconi DP, Cozzolino S, Vergani P. Stillbirths in singletons, dichorionic and monochorionic twins: a comparison of risks and causes. Eur J Obstet Gynecol Reprod Biol. 2013; 170(1):131–6.
14. Ghai V, Vidyasagar D. Morbidity and mortality factors in twins. An epidemiologic approach. Clin Perinatol. 1988;15(1):123–40.

15. Gardner MO, Goldenberg RL, Cliver SP, Tucker JM, Nelson KG, Copper RL. The origin and outcome of preterm twin pregnancies. Obstet Gynecol. 1995;85(4):553-7.

16. Lee CM, Yang SH, Lee SP, Hwang BC, Kim SY. Clinical factors affecting the timing of delivery in twin pregnancies. Obstet Gynecol Sci. 2014;57(6):436-41.

17. Fox NS, Saltzman DH, Kurtz H, Rebarber A. Excessive weight gain in term twin pregnancies: examining the 2009 Institute of Medicine definitions. Obstet Gynecol. 2011;118(5):1000-4.

18. Fox NS, Rebarber A, Roman AS, Klauser CK, Peress D, Saltzman DH. Weight gain in twin pregnancies and adverse outcomes: examining the 2009 Institute of Medicine guidelines. Obstet Gynecol. 2010;116(1):100-6.

19. Gonzalez-Quintero VH, Kathiresan AS, Tudela FJ, Rhea D, Desch C, Istwan N. The association of gestational weight gain per institute of medicine guidelines and prepregnancy body mass index on outcomes of twin pregnancies. Am J Perinatol. 2012;29(6):435-40.

20. Bodnar LM, Pugh SJ, Abrams B, Himes KP, Hutcheon JA. Gestational weight gain in twin pregnancies and maternal and child health: a systematic review. J Perinatol. 2014;34(4):252-63.

21. Nicola C, Mariarosaria DT, Giovanni BLS, Anna MM, Antonio R, Nicola R, Tamara S, Alessandro S, Bianiamino T, Patrizia V. In collaborations with: Pietro A, Maria EB, Giuseppe C, Giancarlo C, Marzia M, Stefano P, Giuliana S. Revised by: Paolo S, Vito T, Nicola C, Fabio S. Gestione della gravidanza multipla - Linee guida italiane, Fondazione Confalonieri Ragonese su mandato SIGO, AOGOI, AGUI. 2016. Online at http://www.sigo.it/wp-content/uploads/2016/03/Gestione-della-Gravidanza-Multipla.pdf.

22. Bertino E, Spada E, Occhi L, Coscia A, Giuliani F, Gagliardi L, Gilli G, Bona G, Fabris C, De Curtis M, et al. Neonatal anthropometric charts: the Italian neonatal study compared with other European studies. J Pediatr Gastroenterol Nutr. 2010;51(3):353-61.

23. ACOG Committee on Obstetric Practice. ACOG practice bulletin. Diagnosis and management of preeclampsia and eclampsia. Number 33, January 2002. American College of Obstetricians and Gynecologists. Int J Gynaecol Obstet. 2002;77(1):67-75.

24. American Diabetes Association (2004). Gestational diabetes mellitus. Diabetes Care. Jan;27 Suppl 1:S88-90.

25. Weight Gain During Pregnancy: Reexamining the guidelines. Editors Institute of Medicine (US) and National Research Council (US) committee to reexamine IOM pregnancy weight guidelines; Rasmussen KM, Yaktine AL, editors. Source Washington (DC): National Academies Press (US); 2009. The National Academies Collection: Reports funded by National Institutes of Health.

21

Temporal trends and risk factors for extended-spectrum beta-lactamase-producing *Escherichia coli* in adults with catheter-associated urinary tract infections

Joseph T Spadafino[1], Bevin Cohen[1,2]*, Jianfang Liu[2] and Elaine Larson[1,2]

Abstract

Background: Extended-spectrum beta-lactamase (ESBL)-producing *Escherichia coli* cause up to 10% of catheter-associated urinary tract infections (CAUTI). We report changes in ESBL prevalence among CAUTIs in an adult acute care hospital from 2006-2012 and describe factors associated ESBL-production among *E. coli* CAUTI.

Findings: Data on patients ≥18 years discharged from a 647-bed tertiary/quaternary care hospital (2006-2012), a 221-bed community hospital (2007-2012), and a 914-bed tertiary/quaternary care hospital (2008) were obtained retrospectively from an electronic database (N = 415,430 discharges). Infections were identified using a previously validated electronic algorithm. Information on medical conditions and treatments were collected from electronic health records and discharge billing codes. A case-control design was used to determine factors associated with having a CAUTI caused by an ESBL-producing *E. coli* versus a non-ESBL-producing *E. coli*. Changes in yearly proportion of ESBL *E. coli* CAUTI at the 647-bed tertiary/quaternary care hospital were evaluated. ESBL increased from 4% in 2006 to 14% in 2012, peaking at 18% in 2009. Prior antibiotic treatment and urinary tract disease significantly increased odds of ESBL.

Conclusions: This study provides evidence that treatment with beta-lactam and non-beta-lactam antibiotics is a risk factor for acquiring ESBL-producing *E. coli* CAUTI, and the prevalence of this organism may be increasing in acute care hospitals.

Keywords: Catheter-associated urinary tract infections, Extended-spectrum beta-lactamase-producing *Escherichia coli*, Antimicrobial resistance

Introduction

Escherichia coli is the most common causative agent of catheter-associated urinary tract infections (CAUTI; >20%) [1]. Extended-spectrum beta-lactamase (ESBL)-producing strains of *E. coli*, while representing a small percentage (<10%), are particularly concerning because they confer resistance to a myriad of antibiotics including penicillins and third generation cephalosporins, and because their prevalence has been increasing in community and hospital settings during recent years [2,3]. The purpose of this study is to describe changes in prevalence and factors associated with CAUTI caused by ESBL-producing *E. coli* in three adult acute care hospitals from 2006 through 2012.

Methods

Data on all patients ≥18 years discharged from three New York City hospitals within a single network were obtained retrospectively from a larger electronic database as part of an NIH-funded study (Distribution of the Costs of Antimicrobial Resistant Infections, NR010822). The study was approved by the Institutional Review Board of Columbia University Medical Center. Data were available from 2006-2012 for a 647-bed tertiary/quaternary care hospital, from 2007-2012 for a 221-bed

* Correspondence: bac2116@columbia.edu
[1]Department of Epidemiology, Columbia University Mailman School of Public Health, 722 West 168th Street, New York, NY 10032, USA
[2]Columbia University School of Nursing, 630 West 168th Street, New York, NY 10032, USA

community hospital, and from 2008 for a 914-bed tertiary/quaternary care hospital (N = 415,430 discharges). As described in detail in Apte et al. [4], the database contained information from a number of electronic sources, including patients' electronic health, discharge, laboratory, and medication administration records. The discharge data provided admission and discharge dates, International Classification of Diseases Ninth Revision Clinical Modification (ICD-9-CM) codes for primary and secondary diagnoses present on admission, age, gender, comorbidities, and surgical procedures. The clinical data sources provided time stamped information on catheterization and medications.

CAUTI were defined based on National Healthcare Safety Network (NHSN, http://www.cdc.gov/nhsn/about.html) guidelines (positive urine culture >48 hours after urinary catheterization) and identified using previously validated computerized algorithms [4,5]. If a patient had multiple CAUTIs during the study period, only the first was included. We performed a case-control study to determine factors associated with having a CAUTI caused by an ESBL-producing *E. coli* versus a non-ESBL-producing *E. coli*. First, we determined the bivariable associations between ESBL production and age, sex, comorbidities including diabetes mellitus, HIV, urinary tract disease, and malignancies, Charlson Comorbidity Index score (http://www.uroweb.org/fileadmin/livesurgery/Charlson_Comorbidity_Index.pdf), urinary tract procedures, days of catheterization, and antibiotic treatment received during the patient's hospitalization prior to infection onset. All variables significantly associated (p ≤ 0.05) with ESBL production were included in a multivariable logistic regression model. We evaluated changes in yearly proportion of ESBL *E. coli* CAUTI at the 647-bed tertiary/quaternary care hospital, for which data were available from 2006-2012, using the Cochran-Armitage test for trend. All statistical analyses were performed using SAS version 9.2 (SAS Institute Inc., Cary, NC).

Results

During the seven-year study period a total of 2,164 patients (1,616 women, 74.7%, and 548 men, 25.3%) developed a CAUTI with *E. coli* as the primary infecting pathogen, and 271 (12.5%) were ESBL-producing. The proportion of *E. coli* CAUTI that were ESBL-producers in the 647-bed tertiary/quaternary care hospital increased from 4% in 2006 to 14% in 2012, peaking at 18% in 2009 (p < 0.0001; Figure 1). Over half of patients with CAUTI were diagnosed within 4 days of catheter insertion, over three-quarters within 8 days, and over 98% (n = 2,123) within 30 days. Descriptive characteristics and antibiotics administered prior to CAUTI onset are summarized for cases and controls in Table 1.

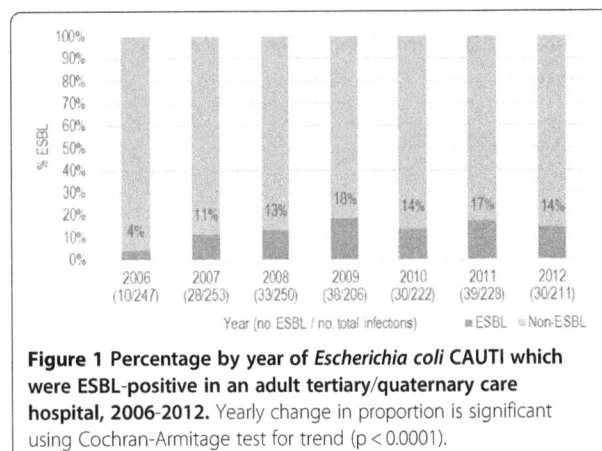

Figure 1 Percentage by year of *Escherichia coli* CAUTI which were ESBL-positive in an adult tertiary/quaternary care hospital, 2006-2012. Yearly change in proportion is significant using Cochran-Armitage test for trend (p < 0.0001).

Results of the case control study are presented in Table 1. In the crude analyses, cases were significantly older than controls (70.4 and 67.5 years, respectively) and had greater Charlson Comorbidity scores (7.06 and 6.44, respectively). Male sex, preexisting urinary tract disease, having a urinary tract procedure, and longer duration of catheterization prior to CAUTI onset were also associated with increased odds of ESBL production. Receiving any antibiotic prior to CAUTI onset was significantly associated with ESBL production, and six antibiotics specifically were administered significantly more often in cases than in controls: aminoglycosides, first-generation cephalosporins, third-generation cephalosporins, macrolides, fourth-generation penicillins, and vancomycin. In the multivariable model, age, urinary tract disease, and receipt of aminoglycosides, first-generation cephalosporins, macrolides, fourth-generation penicillins, and vancomycin were significantly associated with ESBL production.

Discussion

Though several studies have examined risk factors for ESBL emergence in hospitalized and non-hospitalized patients with urinary tract infections (UTI), these studies were community-based and not focused on catheterized patients [2,3,6-8]. Since CAUTI may result in antibiotic susceptibility patterns different from those of non-catheter-related UTI, understanding the prevalence trends and risk factors for ESBL emergence unique to this population is important for the development and implementation of effective prevention efforts [9]. The prevalence of ESBL-producing strains in this sample (12.2%) was slightly higher than reported in previous studies which included both catheterized and non-catheterized patients (7-10.9%) [6,7,10], but the overall increase in ESBL prevalence over time is consistent with other reports [2,3,10]. An analysis of trends in gram-negative bacterial resistance among patients with UTI from a nationally representative sample of US hospitals between 2000 and 2009 found a

Table 1 Factors associated with catheter-associated urinary tract infections caused by extended-spectrum beta-lactamase (ESBL)-producing Escherichia coli versus non-ESBL-producing E. coli

Variable	ESBL-producing E. coli isolates (N = 271)	Non-ESBL-producing E. coli isolates (N = 1893)	Total (N = 2164)	Bivariable analysis p-value[a]	Multivariable analysis Odds Ratio (95% CI)
Mean (range) age, in years	70.4 (24-98)	67.5 (18-103)	67.9 (18-103)	*0.003[b]	1.01 (1.00, 1.02)
Gender (reference, female)				0.01	1.22 (0.91, 1.65)
Male (n (%))	86 (31.7%)	462 (24.4%)	548 (25.3%)		
Female (n (%))	185 (68.3%)	1431 (75.6%)	1616 (74.7%)		
HIV Positive	5 (1.9%)	12 (0.6%)	17 (0.8%)	0.052[c]	2.09 (0.66, 6.55)
Diabetes	89 (32.8%)	522 (27.6%)	611 (28.2%)	0.07	NA
Urinary Tract Disease	226 (83.4%)	1420 (75.0%)	1646 (76.1%)	0.003	1.43 (1.01, 2.03)
Malignancy	59 (21.8%)	363 (19.2%)	422 (19.5%)	0.31	NA
Mean (range) Duration of Catheterization Prior to CAUTI Onset, in days (Mean)	7.74 (0-78)	6.32 (0-124)	6.50 (0-124)	*0.03[b]	0.99 (0.98, 1.01)
Urinary Tract Procedure	26 (9.59%)	113 (5.97%)	139 (6.42%)	0.02	1.43 (0.88, 2.32)
Mean (range) Charlson Comorbidity Score	7.73 (0-35)	6.76 (0-51)	6.88 (0-51)	0.001[d]	1.03 (0.99, 1.06)
Antibiotics Received Prior to CAUTI Onset	174 (64.2%)	804 (42.5%)	978 (45.2%)	<0.0001	NA
Antibiotic received**					
Aminoglycoside	27 (9.9%)	73 (3.9%)	100 (4.6%)	<0.0001	5.42 (1.77, 16.55)
Cephalosporin, 1st Gen.	66 (24.4%)	346 (18.3%)	412 (19.0%)	0.02	2.34 (1.63, 3.36)
Cephalosporin, 3rd Gen.	23 (8.5%)	29 (1.5%)	52 (2.4%)	<0.0001	2.89 (0.79, 10.67)
Macrolide	22 (8.1%)	69 (3.7%)	91 (4.2%)	0.001	2.39 (1.12, 5.08)
Penicillin, 2nd Gen.	17 (6.3%)	91 (4.8%)	108 (5.0%)	0.30	NA
Penicillin, 4th Gen.	50 (18.5%)	173 (9.1%)	223 (10.3%)	<0.0001	2.65 (1.48, 4.76)
Vancomycin	59 (21.8%)	203 (10.7%)	262 (12.1%)	<0.0001	3.40 (2.26, 5.12)

CAUTI, catheter-associated urinary tract infection; ESBL, extended-spectrum beta-lactamase; NA, not included in multivariable model.
[a]Chi-Square test unless otherwise denoted; [b]T-test; [c]Fisher's Exact Test; [d]Wilcoxon-Mann-Whitney Test.
*F-Test for Equality of Variances indicated unequal variance and appropriate p-value was used.
** In the multivariable model, antibiotics were examined as a seven-level categorical variable. Reference category: No antibiotics prior to CAUTI onset.

threefold increase in cases of ESBL-producing E. coli, similar to our results [3].

Our findings regarding risk factors for ESBL production are also similar to those reported in previous studies that included community-acquired UTIs and/or non-catheter-associated hospital-acquired UTIs. In our sample of hospitalized, catheterized patients, we found a strong positive association between prior treatment with beta-lactam and non-beta-lactam antibiotics and ESBL production, consistent with other studies of UTI caused by E. coli [2,6,8]. Like most other studies, we failed to detect significant differences in odds of ESBL by age, gender, comorbid conditions, and overall severity of illness; however we did find a significant positive association with urinary tract disease [6-8,10]. Patients who undergo a urinary tract procedure or surgery may be at greater risk for the emergence of resistance due in part to longer catheterization periods and increased antibiotic use. Nevertheless, urinary tract disease remained significant even after adjustment for length of catheterization

and treatment with antibiotics, suggesting that it may have an independent association with ESBL.

While this is one of the largest studies to focus on CAUTI with ESBL-producing E. coli and document trends in resistance over time, the research does have some limitations. First, this study makes use of electronically available data to identify infections, as well as to determine patients' clinical risk factors and comorbid health conditions. Information on preexisting health conditions was garnered from medical billing data, which are not collected for the purposes of research and may have low sensitivity and/or specificity. Aside from potential misclassification, using electronic data also prohibited us from reporting detailed information on the resistance patterns exhibited by the isolates. In addition, data on antimicrobial use was limited to those prescribed during the patients' hospitalizations. The case-control study was restricted to three hospitals within a single, geographically narrow network, possibly limiting generalizability. Additionally, we were only able to investigate trends over time at one hospital due to limited data availability. Lastly, although our definition of CAUTI is consistent with NHSN guidelines of UTI onset >48 hours after catheterization, it is possible that some patients were bacteriuric prior to catheter insertion.

This study provides further evidence that treatment with beta-lactam and non-beta-lactam antibiotics is a risk factor for acquiring ESBL-producing *E. coli* CAUTI. Urinary tract disease is also identified as a risk factor, independent of antibiotic treatment and length of catheterization. Consistent with other reports, this study found an increase in ESBL prevalence among CAUTI in recent years. Risk factors for ESBL emergence may be different in CAUTI than in non-catheter-associated UTI.

Competing interests

The authors declare that they have no competing interests.

Authors' contributions

JTS performed the data analysis and drafted the manuscript. BC contributed to the data analysis and manuscript development. JL programmed the database and contributed to data analysis. EL contributed to the conception and design of the study and manuscript development. All authors reviewed, revised, and approved of the final manuscript.

References

1. Hidron AI, Edwards JR, Patel J, Horan TC, Sievert DM, Pollock DA, Fridkin SK: NHSN annual update: Antimicrobial-resistant pathogens associated with healthcare-associated infections: Annual summary of data reported to the national healthcare safety network at the centers for disease control and prevention, 2006-2007. *Infect Control Hosp Epidemiol* 2008, 29:996–1011.
2. Ena J, Arjona F, Martinez-Peinado C, Lopez-Perezagua Mdel M, Amador C: Epidemiology of urinary tract infections caused by extended-spectrum beta-lactamase-producing Escherichia coli. *Urology* 2006, 68:1169–1174.
3. Zilberberg MD, Shorr AF: Secular trends in gram-negative resistance among urinary tract infection hospitalizations in the United States, 2000-2009. *Infect Control Hosp Epidemiol* 2013, 34:940–946.
4. Apte M, Neidell M, Furuya EY, Caplan D, Glied S, Larson E: Using Electronically Available Inpatient Hospital Data for Research. *Clin Transl Sci* 2011, 4:338–345.
5. Landers T, Apte M, Hyman S, Furuya Y, Glied S, Larson E: A comparison of methods to detect urinary tract infections using electronic data. *Jt Comm J Qual Patient Saf* 2010, 36:411–417.
6. Azap OK, Arslan H, Serefhanoqlu K, Colakoğlu S, Erdoğan H, Timurkaynak F, Senger SS: Risk factors for extended-spectrum b-lactamase positivity in uropathogenic Escherichia coli isolated from community-acquired urinary tract infections. *Clin Microbiol Infect* 2010, 16:147–151.
7. Arslan H, Azap OK, Ergönül O, Colakoğlu S, Erdoğan H, Timurkaynak F, Senger SS: Risk factors for ciprofloxacin resistance among Escherichia coli strains isolated from community-acquired urinary tract infections in Turkey. *J Antimicrob Chemother* 2005, 56:914–918.
8. Calbo E, Romaní V, Xercavins M, Gómez L, Vidal CG, Quintana S, Vila J, Garau J: Risk factors for community-onset urinary tract infections due to Escherichia coli harbouring extended-spectrum b-lactamases. *J Antimicrob Chemother* 2006, 57:780–783.
9. Yamamichi F, Shigemura K, Matsumoto M, Nakano Y, Tanaka K, Arakawa S, Fujisawa M: Relationship between Urinary Tract Infection Categorization and Pathogens' Antimicrobial Susceptibilities. *Urol Int* 2012, 88:198–208.
10. Briongos-Figuero LS, Gómez-Traveso T, Bachiller-Luque P, Domínguez-Gil González M, Gómez-Nieto A, Palacios-Martín T, González-Sagrado M, Dueñas-Laita A, Pérez-Castrillón JL: Epidemiology, risk factors, and comorbidity for urinary tract infections caused by extended-spectrum beta-lactamase (ESBL)-producing Enterobacteria. *Int J Clin Pract* 2012, 66:891–896.

22

Multidrug resistant and carbapenemase producing Enterobacteriaceae among patients with urinary tract infection at referral Hospital, Northwest Ethiopia

Setegn Eshetie[1], Chandrashekhar Unakal[2], Aschalew Gelaw[2], Birhanu Ayelign[3], Mengistu Endris[2] and Feleke Moges[2*]

Abstract

Background: Updates on the epidemiology of antibiotic resistance bacterial pathogens is important. This is because the spread of multidrug resistant enterobacteriaceae (MDRE) and recently carbapenemase producing enterobacteriaceae (CPE) have emerged as a major public health concern in patients with urinary tract infections (UTIs). This study is therefore, aimed to assess the prevalence and associated risk factors of MDR and CPE among patients with UTIs.

Methods: A cross sectional study was conducted among 442 symptomatic UTI suspected patients. Data on socio-demographic characteristics, clinical information and possible risk factors were collected using structured questionnaire. Early morning mid-stream urine samples were collected and processed to characterize bacterial isolates. Disk diffusion method was used to determine the antibiotic susceptibility patterns of isolates. Carbapenemase producing strains were detected using CHROMagar KPC medium. Data were entered and analyzed using SPSS version 20. P-value <0.05 was considered as statistical significant.

Results: Among 442 patients enrolled a total of 183 Enterobacteriaceae were recovered. Of these isolates; 160 (87.4%) were MDRE; the most common isolates were *K. pneumoniae* and *E.coli*. Five (2.73%) of the isolates were found to be carbapenemase producers and all of CPE strains were 100% ESBL producers. Significant drug resistances were observed among CPE compared to other MDRE, low resistance rates were noted to ciprofloxacin (20%). Being female (OR 4.46; P = 0.018), age (OR 1.08; P = 0.001), hospitalization (OR 5.23; P = 0.006), and prior antibiotic use (OR 3.98; P = 0.04) were associated risk factors for MDRE.

Conclusion and recommendation: High rates of MDR (87.4%) were observed among enterobacteriaceae uropathogens; *K. pneumoniae* and *E.coli* were the principal MDR isolates. Overall prevalence of CPE was 2.73% and all of these strains were 100% ESBL producer. Attributing risk factors for MDR UTIs were found to be sex (female), age, hospitalization, and history of antibiotic therapy. Therefore, efforts should be made to reduce patient hospital stay and maximize rational use of drugs. Additional and vigorous investigation especially on CPE should be encouraged.

Keywords: Carbapenemase, Enterobacteriaceae, Multidrug resistant, Urinary tract infection

* Correspondence: mogesfeleke@gmail.com
[2]Department of Microbiology, University of Gondar, Gondar, Ethiopia
Full list of author information is available at the end of the article

Background

Urinary tract infections (UTIs) are one of the most common infectious diseases ranking next to upper respiratory tract infection. Urinary tract infections are often associated with significant morbidity and mortality. Worldwide, about 150 million people are diagnosed with UTI each year, costing the global economy in excess of 6 billion dollars [1]. In developing countries, including Ethiopia, the facilities for urine culture and antimicrobial susceptibility testing are still not sufficiently available, leading to improper diagnosis and irrational antibiotic treatment of UTI, which expedites the emergence of multidrug resistant (MDR) strains [2]. Gram negative bacteria, especially the family enterobacteriaceae are the common cause of both community and hospital acquired UTIs. *Escherichia coli* and *Klebsiella pneumoniae* are most commonly implicated among patients with UTI [3,4].

Previously, the emergences of MDR among enterobacteriaceae were mainly due to the production of enzymes, such as pencillinases, cephalosorinases, and extended spectrum β-lactamase (ESBL). However, recently carbapenemase production is one of the main mechanisms in the occurrence of drug resistance in the family of enterobacteriaceae. Carbapenemase producing enterobacteriaceae (CPE) are difficult to treat because they have high levels of resistance to antibiotics, which capable of break down all β-lactam agents including carbapenems and make it ineffective. Carbapenem such as imipenem, meropenem, ertapenem, & doripenem are considered as the last resort antibiotics to treat ESBL producing enterobacteriaceae [5,6].

Currently, increased burden of MDRE causing UTI compounded by harboring carbapenem resistance genes mainly among E. *coli* and K. *pneumonia*. These strains become a serious threat to public health, associated with high mortality rates and have the potential to spread widely. Infections are difficult, and in some cases impossible to treat and have been associated with mortality rates up to 50%. Due to the movement of patients throughout the health care system, if CPE is a problem in one facility, then typically they are a problem in other facilities in the region as well. Carbapenemase producing enterobacteriaceae are mostly endemic in specific geographical regions, but reports of their spread into other geographical locations are point of grave concern these days [5,7].

The aetiology of UTI and the antibiotic resistance of uropathogens have been changing over the past years, both in community and health care associated infections. Current knowledge on the burden and antimicrobial susceptibility pattern of the enterobacteriaceae isolates is essential for appropriate therapy, since those groups of bacteria are the main cause of UTIs and possess several mechanisms to dismantle currently available antibiotics including carbapenems and the condition in Ethiopia is not yet assessed. Therefore, the objective of this study was aimed to determine the prevalence and risk factors of MDR and CPE producing strains among patients with UTI at the University of Gondar Hospital, Ethiopia.

Materials and methods

Study area

The study was conducted at the University of Gondar Hospital. It is referral hospital that provides services to over 5 million inhabitants in the Northwest, Ethiopia. The hospital has an accredited referral level laboratory with 7 sections and a separate reception room. Microbiology section is one of the principal area, it is estimated that 9,600 samples delivered per annum to this working area. In this section, culturing is one of the main activities, mainly applicable for bacterial isolation and identification.

Study design, participants and data collection

A cross-sectional study was conducted from February to May 2014. A total of 442 patients with symptomatic UTI were selected from both in and out-patients using systematic random sampling technique. Socio-demographic characteristics such as gender, age, residence, educational status and history of travel were gathered from eligible patients. Clinical features such as history of hospitalization, ICU admission, prior antibiotic use, prior UTI and chronic diseases, pregnancy status, presence of urinary catheter and mechanical ventilation were also collected. Moreover, after instructing how to collect urine specimen, about 20 ml of a clean catch morning mid-stream urine was collected from each patient [8] using a sterile screw-capped, wide-mouth container and labeled with the unique sample number, date and time of collection.

Isolation and identification of enterobacteriaceae

Urine specimens were directly inoculated on 5% Sheep blood agar and incubated at 37°C for 24 hours. Urine culture was considered as positive, if it contains $\geq 10^5$ cfu/ml. Enterobacteriaceae from positive urine cultures were identified by their characteristic appearance on the media, gram staining reaction, by the pattern of biochemical profiles using standard procedures. Biochemical tests such as indole production, sugar fermentation, H_2S and gas production, citrate utilization, motility test, urease test, oxidase, were used to identify enterobacteriaceae isolates [8].

Susceptibility and carbapenemase testing

Antibiotic susceptibility was performed by employing Kirby Bauer disk diffusion method using Mueller Hinton agar (Oxoid) in accordance with the guidelines of clinical and laboratory standards institute [9]. Enterobacteriaceae were tested against the following antibiotic disks (Oxoid): cefotaxime (CTX; 30 µg), ceftriaxone (CTR; 30 µg), cefepime (CPM; 30 µg), ceftazidime (CAZ; 30 µg), cefpodoxime

(CPD: 30 μg), ciprofloxacin (CIP; 5 μg), tetracycline (TE; 30 μg), chloramphenicol (C; 30 μg), amoxicillin-calvulanic acid (AMC; 30 μg), naldixic acid (NA; 30 μg), gentamycin (GEN; 10 μg), ampicillin (AMP; 10 μg) and trimethoprim-sulfamethoxazole (SXT; 25 μg). After incubation of plates at 37°C for 24 hours, diameters of zone of inhibition were measured. Bacteria classified as susceptible, intermediate and resistant strains according to the criteria of the clinical and laboratory standards institute [9].

After antimicrobial susceptibility testing, all MDRE (resistance to 2 or more classes of antibiotics) isolates were collected and sub-cultured on CHROMagar ^{TM} KPC agar to determine carbapenemase production. After overnight incubation (24 hr), carbapenemase producing isolates were assessed by visualizing colonies with typical coloring characteristics. Carbapenemase producing E. coli developed dark pink to reddish colony features, while other enterobacteriaceae isolates produced metallic blue colonies [10]. Those Carbapenemase producing colonies with metallic blue color were further identified following different classical biochemical tests (. Besides, all CPE strains were tested whether they are extended spectrum beta- lactamase (ESBL) producer or not using CHROM agar ESBL medium.

Quality control

All materials, equipment and procedures were adequately controlled. Culture media were tested for sterility and performance. Pre-analytical, analytical and post-analytical stages of quality assurance that are incorporated in standard operating procedures of the microbiology laboratory were strictly followed. Standard strains of E.coli® ATCC 25922 (positive control) and S. aureus ATCC® 25923 (negative control) were used to control the performance of CHROMagar ^{TM} KPC medium and other media. To standardize the inoculum density of bacterial suspension for a susceptibility test, 0.5 McFarland standards was used [9,10].

Ethical consideration

This study was approved by research and ethics committee of School of Biomedical Laboratory Sciences, University of Gondar, Ethiopia. Informed written consent was also obtained from patients and/or guardians after explaining the objective of the study. The laboratory results were communicated with the physicians for better management of the patients.

Data analysis and interpretation

Data were collected, summarized and analyzed using SPSS version 20 software and results were presented through tables, pie charts and graphs. Associations were measured using chi-square test, binary logistic regression. P-values < 0.05 were considered as statistically significant.

Results

Socio-demographic characteristics

A total of 442 patients with symptomatic UTI were enrolled in this study to investigate prevalence and associated risk factors of MDRE and CPE. Majority of the participants were females 282 (63.8%). The mean age of patients was 37.05 ± 10.5 years, 86 (19.5%) of the patients were younger than 16 years, and 73 (16.5%) were older than 60 years. Two hundred fifty two (57.0%) of patients were rural residents, and majority, 286 (64.7%) of study participants had educational level of elementary school and below (Table 1).

Multidrug resistance and carbapenemase producing enterobacteriaceae in UTI suspected patients

Among study participants, 183 (41.4%) patients had positive urine culture with a single non-duplicate isolates of enterobacteriaceae. The most common isolates were E.coli 112 (61.2%) followed by K. pneumoniae 29 (15.8%) and E. aerogenes 13(7.1%) (Table 2). The isolates were tested for antimicrobial susceptibility, 160 (87.4%, 95% CI; 82—92.3%) of them showed resistance to two or more classes of antibiotics. Among MDR strains, only 1 (0.6%) isolate was resistant to 2 classes of antibiotics, the rest 159 (99.4%) were resistant to three or more classes of antibiotics. Result of drug resistance patterns compared within species showed that, 28 (95.6%) of K. pneumoniae and 104(92.9%) of E. coli were MDR isolates (Table 2).

Of the 183 enterobacteriaceae isolates, 160 (87.4%) were MDR strains, and these strains were tested for carbapenemase production by using phenotypic methods

Table 1 Socio-demographic characteristics of UTI suspected patients at the University of Gondar Hospital, February to May 2014 (N = 442)

Variables		Frequency	Percentage
Sex	Male	160	36.2
	Female	282	63.8
Age (Years)	≤15	86	19.5
	16-30	84	19
	31-45	101	22.9
	46-60	98	22.2
	≥61	73	16.3
Residence	Rural	252	57
	Urban	190	43
Educational status	Illiterate	196	44.3
	Primary school	90	20.4
	Secondary school	69	15.6
	Diploma and Above	87	19.7
Sender of the patient	Outpatient	212	48
	Inpatient	230	52

Table 2 Multidrug resistance pattern of enterobacteriaceae among UTI suspects at the University of Gondar Hospital, February to May 2014

Isolates	Degree of resistance										Total MDR isolates (≥R2)
	R0	R1	R2	R3	R4	R5	R6	R7	R8	≥R9	
E. coli (N = 112)	2 (1.8)	6 (5.4)	—	5 (4.5)	28 (25)	24 (21.4)	32 (28.6)	9 (8.0)	4 (3.6)	2 (1.8)	104 (92.9)
K. pneumoniae (N = 29)	—	1 (3.4)	—	3 (10.3)	5 (17.2)	6 (20.7)	4 (13.8)	3 (10.3)	4 (13.8)	3 (10.3)	28 (95.6)
Enterobacter spp. (N = 16)	2 (12.5)	1 (6.3)	—	1 (6.3)	2 (12.5)	3 (18.8)	5 (31.3)	1 (6.3)	—	1 (6.3)	13 (81.3)
Citrobacter spp. (N = 6)	1 (16.7)	—	1 (16.7)	—	1 (16.7)	—	2 (33.3)	—	1 (16.7)	—	5 (83.3)
Proteus spp. (N = 9)	5 (55.6)	3 (33.3)	—	—	—	1 (11.1)	—	—	—	—	1 (11.1)
Other Klebsiella spp. (N = 11)	—	2 (18.2)	—	—	—	3 (27.3)	3 (27.3)	1 (9.1)	1 (9.1)	1 (9.1)	9 (81.8)
Total (N = 183)	10 (5.5)	13 (7.1)	1 (0.5)	9 (4.9)	36 (19.7)	37 (20.2)	46 (25.1)	14 (7.7)	10 (5.5)	2 (1.1)	160 (87.4)

Note: Data are in number (%) unless otherwise indicated.R0: susceptible to all antibiotics, R1-8: resistance to 2, 3, 4, 5, 6, 7, and 8 antibiotics, ≥R9: resistance to 9 or more antibiotics, ≥R2: resistance to 2 or more antibiotics.

(CHROMagar KPC media). A total of 5 bacterial strains were found to be CPE producers, notably E.coli (2), K. pneumoniae (2) and E. aerogenes (1). All of the isolates were from hospital admitted patients. The overall prevalence of CPE was 2.73% (95%CI; 0.5-5.5%) among all isolates and 3.1% among MDRE isolates. Besides, all CPE strains were 100% ESBL producer, which were demonstrated by using phenotypic methods (CHROMagar ESBL media).

Rate of resistance for different antibiotics tested in MDRE and CPE Isolates

The overall resistance profile of MDRE isolates are shown in Table 3. High resistance rate were observed to ampicillin (97.5%) followed by cotrimoxazole (64.4%), and chloramphenicol (61.2%). Whereas, ciprofloxacin, cefepime, and ceftriaxone had an overall resistance rates of 2.5%, 10.6%, and 11.9%, respectively. Species specific antibiotic resistance rates revealed that more than 55%

of E.coli isolates were resistant to ceftazidime, gentamycin, chloramphenicol, cotrimoxazole, and ampicillin and low rates of resistance were observed in ciprofloxacin (1%), cefepime (8.7%) and ceftriaxone (11.5%). Over 60% of K. pneumoniae were exhibited resistance to amoxicillin-calvulanic acid, chloramphenicol, cefpodoxime, and ampicillin, relatively low resistance rates were observed to ciprofloxacin (10.7%), cefepime (14.3%), and ceftriaxone (17.9%).

The overall resistance pattern of CPE isolates are summarized in Figure 1. All isolates were 100% resistant to cefotaxime, cefpodoxime, cotrimoxazole, chloramphenicol, ampicillin, and amoxicillin-calvulanic acid. However, only 20% of strains were resistant to ciprofloxacin. The overall antibiotic resistance rates of CPE isolates were significantly higher than other MDRE strains for more than half of tested antibiotics including cefotaxime (100% versus 22.6%; P < 0.001), ceftriaxone (60% versus 10.3%; P = 0.001), cefpodoxime (100% versus 42.6%; P = 0.011). On the other hand

Table 3 Antibiotic resistance patterns of MDRE among study participants: University of Gondar Hospital, February to May 2014

MDR isolates	Antibiotics												
	CTX	CAZ	CTR	CPD	CPM	CIP	TE	SXT	C	AMP	NA	GEN	AMC
E.coli (N = 104)	25 (24.0)	58 (55.8)	12 (11.5)	43 (41.3)	9 (8.7)	1 (1)	49 (47.1)	72 (69.2)	61 (58.7)	103 (99)	19 (18.3)	59 (56.7)	47 (45.2)
K. pneumoniae (N = 28)	8 (28.6)	16 (57.1)	5 (17.9)	18 (64.3)	4 (14.3)	3 (10.7)	15 (53.6)	14 (50)	18 (64.3)	26 (92.9)	7 (25)	16 (57.1)	17 60.7)
K. ozaenae (N = 6)	1 (16.7)	4 (66.7)	0	3 (50)	0	0	4 (66.7)	5 (83.3)	5 (83.3)	6 (100)	2 (33.3)	4 (66.7)	5 (83.3)
E. aerogenes (N = 12)	4 (33.3)	7 (58.3)	2 (16.7)	5 (41.7)	3 (25)	0	5 (41.7)	5 (41.7)	7 (58.3)	12 (100)	2 (16.7)	7 (58.3)	9 (75)
Citrobacter spp (N = 5)	1 (20)	2 (40)	0	1 (20)	0	0	4 (80)	3 (60)	4 (80)	4 (80)	1 (20)	4 (80)	2 (40)
*Others (N = 5)	2 (40)	3 (60)	0	1(20)	1(20)	0	2(40)	4 (80)	3(60)	5(100)	1(20)	4(80)	1(20)
Total MDRE N = 160 (87.4%)	40 (25)	90 (56.2)	19 (11.9)	71 (44.4)	17 (10.6)	4 (2.5)	79 (49.4)	103 (64.4)	98 (61.2)	156 (97.5)	32 (20)	94 (58.8)	81 (50.6)

Note: Data are in number (%) unless otherwise indicated. *Others = K. oxytoca (N = 3); E. cloacae (N = 1); P. vulgaris (N = 1).
CTX: Cefotaxime, CAZ: Ceftazidime, CTR: Ceftriaxone, CPD: Cefpodoxime, CPM: Cefepime, CIP: Ciprofloxacin, TE: Tetracycline, SXT: Cotrimoxazole, C: Chloramphenicol, NA: Naldixic acid, GEN: Gentamycin, AMC: Amoxicillin-Calvulanic acid.

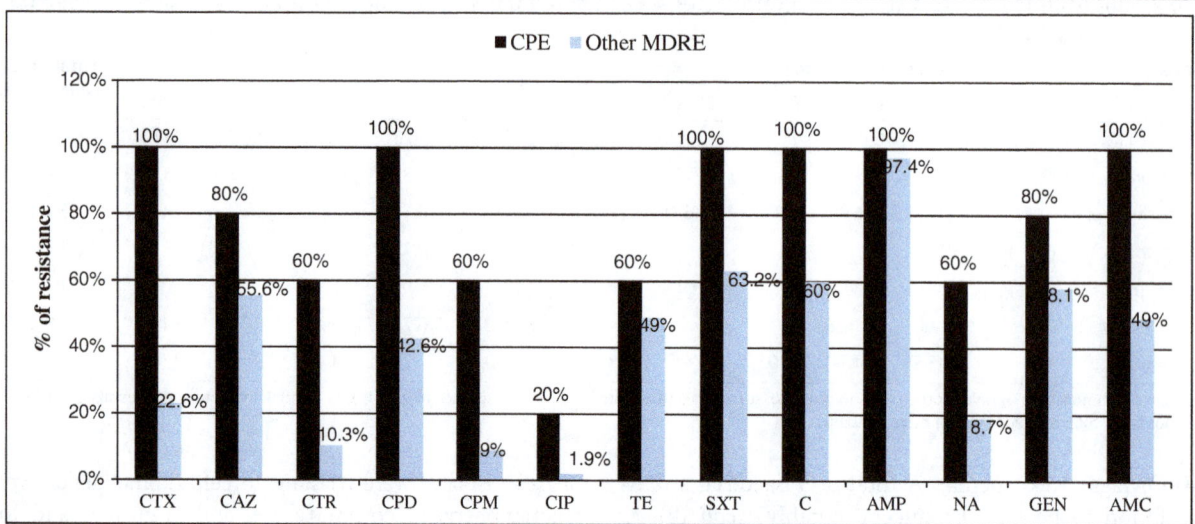

	Antibiotics												
	CTX	CAZ	CTR	CPD	CPM	CIP	TE	SXT	C	AMP	NA	GEN	AMC
P-value [a]	**<0.001**	0.277	**0.001**	**0.011**	**<0.001**	**0.011**	0.629	0.091	0.071	0.716	**0.023**	0.327	**0.025**

Note that: a: compared between CPE and other MDRE

CTX: Cefotaxime, CAZ: Ceftazidime, CTR: Ceftriaxone, CPD: Cefpodoxime, CPM: Cefepime, CIP: Ciprofloxacin, TE: Tetracycline, SXT: Cotrimoxazole, C: Chloramphenicol, NA: Naldixic acid, GEN: Gentamycin, AMC: Amoxicillin-Calvulanic acid.

Figure 1 Antibiotic resistance rate of CPE isolates compared to other MDRE among study participants: University of Gondar Hospital, February to May 2014.

the difference in antibiotic resistance rate of CPE to ceftazidime, tetracycline, cotrimoxazole, chloramphenicol, ampicillin, and gentamycin were not statistically significant compared to other MDRE isolates.

Risk factors for MDRE and CPE among study participants

Risk factors associated with MDRE UTIs were analyzed by comparing patients with and without MDRE UTIs. Bivariate analysis showed that, age, hospitalization for the last 12 months, prior urinary tract infection for the past 12 months, prior antibiotic use for the past 6 months were associated with MDRE infections. In the analysis of multivariate logistic regression, independent risk factors for MDRE were prior antibiotic use, and hospitalization since the past 12 months, age, and sex (female) (Table 4).

Discussion

The overall prevalence of MDR among enterobacteriaceae isolates identified from patients with symptomatic UTI was 87.4% (95% CI; 82–92.3%), which is similar with the results from previous study in Gondar (85.5%) and Mozambique (88.2%) [11,12] while it was higher than reports from other study in Ethiopia: Gondar (68%), and Dessie (74.6%) [13,14] and many other countries, such as USA (19.1%), Belgium (62%), and Italy (62%), Nepal (40.1%, 64.04%) [15-19]. However, it was lower than reports from different parts of

Ethiopia such as Gondar (93.5%), Bahirdar (95.6%), and Jimma (100%) [20-22]. The variation in prevalence of MDRE isolates could be due to increase trend of MDR strains with time, difference in study period and study population.

The present study showed that, *K. pneumoniae* (95.6%) and *E.coli* (92.9%) were found to be the principal MDR isolates. Although the rate of proportion of MDR is different in different area similar group of bacteria were reported in Bahirdar, Ethiopia *E.coli* (94.6%) & *K. pneumoniae* (80%) [21] and Nepal, *E.coli* (74%) and *K. pneumoniae* (44%) and Dakar, *E. coli* and *K. pneumoniae* (89%) [23] were the predominant MDR uropathogens [19]. These pathogens are the most common isolates in both hospital and community acquired urinary tract infections. Besides, these bacteria are frequently difficult to treat because of both their intrinsic and acquired resistance to multiple groups of antimicrobial agents [3,4].

Among 183 enterobacteriaceae isolates, 5(2.73%) were found to be carbapenemase producers. Comparable result were reported in studies from Morocco (2.8%) [24], Bangladesh (4.8%) [25], Taiwan (2.5%) [26], Belgium (3.5%) [27], and India (5.4%) [28]. However, this was lower than from studies in Pakistan (8.6%) [29], Turkey (10.9%) [30], India (12.9%) [31], Nigeria (14%, 33.5%) [32,33], Iran (14.5%) [34], and USA (21%) [35]. The

Table 4 Risk factors associated with MDRE among UTI suspected patients at the University of Gondar Hospital, February to May 2014

Risk factors	MDRE		Bivariate analysis		Multivariable analysis	
	Yes (N = 160)	No (N = 23)	COR (95% CI)	P-value	AOR (95% CI)	P-value
Sex						
Female	106	12	1.79 (0.75 – 4.34)	0.191	4.46 (1.29 – 15.35)	**0.018**
Male	54	11	1		1	
Age (years)						
Mean age	38.5	13.2	1.08 (1.05 - 1.12)	**<0.001**	1.08 (1.03 – 1.13)	**0.001**
Hospitalization						
Yes	114	9	3.86 (1.56 – 9.53)	**0.003**	5.22 (1.59 – 17.17)	**0.006**
No	46	14	1		1	
Prior UTI						
Yes	65	4	3.25 (1.06 – 9.99)	**0.040**	2.41 (0.56 – 10.34)	0.239
No	95	19	1		1	
Prior antibiotic use						
Yes	129	7	9.51 (3.60 – 25.11)	**< 0.001**	3.98 (1.056 – 14.97)	**0.041**
No	31	16	1		1	

Note that: COR: crude odds ratio, AOR: adjusted odds ratio, CI: confidence interval.

difference in the prevalence of CPE in different studies may be due to trends in the utilization of carbapenems and other broad spectrum antibiotics, cultural/traditional relationships, cross boarder transfer of patients with other countries of high prevalence. Additionally, difference in target population, sample size and methodological variability could bring variation in the epidemiology of CPE.

Moreover, according to World Health Organization (WHO) 2014 report [36], the epidemiology of CPE has not well studied in developing countries, therefore the report insisted that integrated surveillance program and involvement of very active investigation have to be maximized in order to know the extent of resistant strains in these countries. Even though carbapenems drugs are not formally introduced in to Ethiopia, as the report claimed that increase international travel, globalization and migration might have contributing role in the dissemination of resistant strains from potentially risk countries [36]. Especially, in this study area; there is high tourist flow, and many of residences have relatives from abroad, which may have an impact on the emergence of carbapenemase producing strains in this locality, particularly.

All carbapenemase producing isolates were from hospital admitted patients. This was supported by the fact that inpatients admitted to critical care units for treatment of acute emergencies and chronic diseases are especially liable to get CRE infections because of the presence of highly resistant organisms available in an environment and selective pressure on them due to overuse of antibiotics [37].

In the present study *K. pneumoniae, E.coli,* and E. *aerogenes* were carbapenemase producers. This result

was supported by the reports from European Antimicrobial Resistance Surveillance Network (EARS-Net) that many of carbapenemase producers were *K. pneumoniae* followed by *E.coli* and *Enterobacter* spp., [38]. The same situations were also notified in finding from Turkey and Morocco indicated that *K. pneumoniae* were the principal isolate followed by *E.coli* and *K. oxytoca* [30,35]. On the other hand, a study from Nigeria demonstrated that *E.coli* was the main carbapenemase producer followed by *Proteus* spp. and *K. pneumoniae* [32]. The variation among studies with regard to the proportion of carbapenemase producing isolates; could be due to difference in geographical distribution of isolates, target population, sample size, and methodology used in each investigation.

In Bivariate analysis, age (years), hospitalization within the past 12 months, prior antibiotic therapy in the past 6 months, and prior UTI in the past 12 months were associated with MDRE UTI in this study. Likewise, in multivariable analysis, age, being female, hospitalization within the past 12 months, and prior antibiotic use in the past 6 months were the independent risk factors for MDRE UTIs. The same result was documented in a study done from USA [15]. However, additional risk factors like health care associated risks (use of urinary catheter, mechanical ventilation, and hemodialysis) were identified in the former study, which were not indicated in this study.

Conclusion and recommendation

High rates of multi-drug resistance were observed among enterobacteriaceae uropathogens, (87.4%). Very high resistance was reported to ampicillin, followed by cotrimoxazole and chloramphenicol. Isolates of *K. pneumonia* and *E. coli* were the principal MDR isolates. Overall prevalence of CPE was 2.73% and all CPE strains were 100% ESBL producer and completely resistant to ampicillin, cefotaxime, cefpodoxime, cotrimoxazole, chloramphenicol, and amoxicillin-calvulanic acid. The only drug that shows low resistance rate was ciprofloxacin. Being female, age, hospitalization, and prior antibiotic use were associated risk factors for MDRE. Therefore, efforts should be made to reduce patient hospital stay and maximize rational use of drugs. Additional and vigorous investigation especially on CPE should be encouraged.

Abbreviations

CPE: Carbapenemase producing enterobacteriaceae; ESBL: Extended spectrum β-Lactamase; ICU: Intensive Care Unit; IMP: Imipenemase; KPC: *Klebsiella pneumoniae* Carbapenemase; MDR: Multi-drug resistant; MDRE: Multi-drug resistant enterobacteriaceae; NDM- 1: New Delhi Metallo-beta-lactamase; OXA-48: Oxacillin-hydrolzying metallo-β-lactamases; UTI: Urinary tract infection; VIM: Verona integron encoded Metallo-beta-lactamase.

Competing interests

The authors declare that they have no competing interests.

Authors' contributions

SE: conception of research idea, study design, data collection, analysis and interpretation, and the drafting of manuscript; FM: conception of research idea, supervision, and reviewing manuscript. CU, AG: supervision and reviewing manuscript. ME: Support during laboratory work, reviewing manuscript. BA: Data collection especially part of laboratory work. All authors read the final manuscript. All authors read and approved the final manuscript.

Acknowledgments

We want to acknowledge; the study participants, Amhara health bureau for partial funding of the research, and University of Gondar laboratory for allowing us to use the laboratory facilities.

Author details

[1]Department of Medicine, Debre Markos University, Debre Markos, Ethiopia. [2]Department of Microbiology, University of Gondar, Gondar, Ethiopia. [3]University of Gondar Hospital, Gondar, Ethiopia.

References

1. Lee JB, Neild GH. Urinary tract infection. J Med. 2007;35(8):423–8.
2. Soraya Sgambatti de Andrade, Ana Cristina Galas, Helio Silva Sader. Antimicrobial Resistance in Gram-Negative Bacteria from Developing Countries. In A. de J. Sosa et al. (eds.), Antimicrobial resistance in developing countries. doi:10.1007/978-0-387-89370-9_14, Springer Science+ Business Media, LLC. 2010. New York 249–62.
3. Sharma I, Paul D. Prevalence of community acquired urinary tract infections in silchar medical college, Assam, India and its antimicrobial susceptibility profile. Indian J Med Sci. 2012;66(11–12):273–9.
4. Melaku S, Kibret M, Abera B, Gebre-Sellassie S. Antibiogram of nosocomial urinary tract infections in Felege Hiwot referral hospital, Ethiopia. Afr Health Sci. 2012;12(2):134–9.
5. Habte TM, Dube S, Ismail N, Hoosen AA. Hospital and community isolates of uropathogens at a tertiary hospital in South Africa. S Afr Med J. 2009;99(8):584–7.
6. Huttner A, Harbarth S, Carlet J, Cosgrove S, Goossens H, Holmes A, et al. Antimicrobial resistance: a global view from the 2013 World Healthcare-Associated Infections Forum. Antimicrob Resist Infect Control. 2013;2(1):31.
7. Nordmann P, Naas T, Poirel L. Global spread of Carbapenemase-producing Enterobacteriaceae. Emerg Infect Dis. 2011;17(10):1791–8.
8. Cheesbrough M. Manual of medical microbiology. Low price ed. Britain: Oxford Press; 2000. p. 251–60.
9. Clinical and Laboratory Standards Institute. Performance standards for antimicrobial susceptibility testing: twenty-first informational supplement M100-S21. Wayne, PA, USA: CLSI; 2013.
10. Microbiology chromagar kpc focus on carbapenem resistance. USA: CHROMagar; 2012 [cited 2014 January-9]. http://www.chromagar.com/clinical-microbiology-chromagar-kpc-focus-on-kpc-resistance-32.html#.VTZhadJVikp.
11. Tessema B, Kassu A, Mulu A, Yismaw G. Pridominant isolates of urinary tract pathogens and their antimicrobial susceptiblity patterns in Gondar University Teaching Hospital, nothwest Ethiopia. Ethiop Med J. 2007;45(1):61–7.
12. van der Meeren BT, Chhaganlal KD, Pfeiffer A, Gomez E, Ferro JJ, Hilbink M, et al. Extremely high prevalence of multi-resistance among uropathogens from hospitalised children in Beira, Mozambique. S Afr Med J. 2013;103(6):382–6.
13. Moges F, Genetu A, Mengistu G. Multi drug resistance in urinary pathogens at Gondar Hospital, Ethiopia. E Afr Med J. 2002;79(3):140–2.
14. Kibret M, Abera B. Antimicrobial susceptibility patterns of E. coli from clinical sources in Northeast Ethiopia. Afr Health Sci. 2011;11(3):40–5.
15. Khawcharoenporn T, Vasoo S, Singh K. Urinary tract infections due to multidrug-resistant Enterobacteriaceae: prevalence and risk factors in a Chicago Emergency Department. J Emerg Med. 2013;2013:258517.
16. Huang T-D, Berhin C, Bogaerts P, Glupczynski Y. In vitro susceptibility of multidrug-resistant Enterobacteriaceae clinical isolates to tigecycline. J Antimicrob Chemother. 2012;67(11):2696–9.
17. Luca A, Migliavacca R, Regattin L, Brusaferro S, Raglio A, Pagani L, et al. Prevalence of urinary colonization by extended spectrum-beta-lactamase Enterobacteriaceae among catheterised inpatients in Italian long term care facilities. BMC Infect Dis. 2013;13(1):124.
18. Baral P, Neupane S, Marasini BP, Ghimire KR, Lekhak B, Shrestha B. High prevalence of multidrug resistance in bacterial uropathogens from Kathmandu, Nepal. BMC Res Notes. 2012;5(1):38.
19. Thakur SPN, Sharma M. Prevalence of multidrug resistant Enterobacteriaceae and extended spectrum β lactamase producing *Escherichia Coli* in urinary tract infection. Res J Pharm Biol Chem Sci. 2013;4(2):1615.
20. Agersew AMD, Meseret A, Mucheye G. Uropathogenic bacterial isolates and their antimicrobial susceptibility patterns among HIV/AIDS patients attending Gondar University Specialized Hospital Gondar, Northwest Ethiopia. J Microb Res Rev. 2013;1(4):42–51.
21. Biadglegne F, Abera B. Antimicrobial resistance of bacterial isolates from urinary tract infections at Felge Hiwot Referral Hospital, Ethiopia. Ethiop J Health Dev. 2009;23:236–8.
22. Beyene G, Tsegaye W. Bacterial uropathogens in urinary tract infection and antibiotic susceptibility pattern in JimmaUniversity specialized hospital, Southwest Ethiopia. Ethiop J Health Sci. 2011;21(2):141–6.
23. Dromigny JA, Ndoye B, Macondo EA, Nabeth P, Siby T, Perrier-Gros-Claude JD. Increasing prevalence of antimicrobial resistance among Enterobacteriaceae uropathogens in Dakar, Senegal: a multicenter study. Diagn Microbiol Infect Dis. 2003;47(4):595–600.
24. Wartiti MAEL, Bahmani F-Z, Elouennass M, Benouda A. Prevalence of Carbapenemase-Producing Enterobacteriaceae in a University Hospital in Rabat, Morocco: a 19-months prospective study. Int Arab J Antimicrob Agents. 2012;2(3):1–6.
25. Hayder N, Hasan Z, Afrin S, Noor R. Determination of the frequency of carbapenemase producing Klebsiella pneumoniae isolates in Dhaka city, Bangladesh. Stam J Microbiol. 2013;2(1):28–30.
26. Lai CC, Wu UI, Wang JT, Chang SC. Prevalence of carbapenemase-producing Enterobacteriaceae and its impact on clinical outcomes at a teaching hospital in Taiwan. J Formos Med Assoc. 2013;112(8):492–6.
27. Huang TD, Berhin C, Bogaerts P, Glupczynski Y. Prevalence and mechanisms of resistance to carbapenems in Enterobacteriaceae isolates from 24 hospitals in Belgium. Antimicrob Agents Chemother. 2013;68(8):1832–7.
28. Agrawal GNSS. β-lactamase Production in Uropathogens. Indian J Bas Appl Med Res. 2013;3(1):206–8.
29. Day KM, Salman M, Kazi B, Sidjabat HE, Silvey A, Lanyon CV, et al. Prevalence of NDM-1 carbapenemase in patients with diarrhoea in Pakistan and evaluation of two chromogenic culture media. J Appl Microbiol. 2013;114(6):1810–6.
30. Nazik H, Ongen B, Ilktac M, Aydin S, Kuvat N, Sahin A, et al. Carbapenem resistance due to Bla(OXA-48) among ESBL-producing Escherichia coli and Klebsiella pneumoniae isolates in a univesity hospital, Turkey. Southeast Asian J Trop Med Pub Health. 2012;43(5):1178–85.
31. Dugal S, Purohit H. Antimicrobial susceptibility profile and detection of extended spectrum beta-lactamase production by gram negative uropathogens. Int J Pharm Pharml Sci. 2013;4(5):435–8.

32. Yusuf I, Magashi AM, Firdausi FS, Sharif AA, Getso MI, Bala JA, et al. Phenotypic detection of Carbapenemases in members of Enterobacteriacea. Int J Sci Technol. 2012;2(11):802–6.

33. Yusuf I, Yusha'u M, Sharif A, Getso M, Yahaya H, Bala J, et al. Detection of metallo betalactamases among gram negative bacterial isolates from Murtala Muhammad Specialist Hospital, Kano and Almadina Hospital Kaduna, Nigeria. Bayero J Pur Appli Sci. 2013;5(2):84–8.

34. Haji Hashemi BFM, Dolatyar A, Imani M, Farzami MR, Rahbar M, Hajia M. A study on prevalence of KPC producing from Klebsiella pneumoniae using Modified Hodge Test and CHROMagar in Iran. Ann Bio Res. 2012;3(12):5659–64.

35. Lascols C, Peirano G, Hackel M, Laupland KB, Pitout JD. Surveillance and molecular epidemiology of Klebsiella pneumoniae isolates that produce carbapenemases: first report of OXA-48-like enzymes in North America. Antimicrob Agents Chemother. 2013;57(1):130–6.

36. World Health Organization. Antimicrobial resistance. Geneva: WHO; 2014.

37. Hidron AI, Edwards JR, Patel J, Horan TC, Sievert DM, Pollock DA, et al. Antimicrobial-resistant pathogens associated with healthcare-associated infections: annual summary of data reported to the National Healthcare Safety Network at the Centers for Disease Control and Prevention, 2006–2007. Infect Control Hosp Epidemiol. 2008;29(11):996–1011.

38. Canton R, Akova M, Carmeli Y, Giske CG, Glupczynski Y, Gniadkowski M, et al. Rapid evolution and spread of carbapenemases among Enterobacteriaceae in Europe. J ClinI Microbiol. 2012;18(5):413–31.

23

Multidrug resistant Enterobacteriaceae and extended spectrum β-lactamase producing *Escherichia coli*: a cross-sectional study in National Kidney Center, Nepal

Kamlesh Kumar Yadav[1]*, Nabaraj Adhikari[1], Rama Khadka[1], Anil Dev Pant[2] and Bibha Shah[3]

Abstract

Background: Emergence of antibacterial resistance and production of Extended spectrum β-lactamases (ESBLs) are responsible for the frequently observed empirical therapy failures. Most countries have experienced rapid dissemination of ESBLs producing Enterobacteriaceae isolates, particularly *E. coli* and *Klebsiella pneumoniae*. ESBLs are clinically significant and when detected, indicate the need for the use of appropriate antibacterial agents. But antibacterial choice is often complicated by multi-resistance.

Methods: This study was carried from June to November 2014 to study the multidrug resistant (MDR) Enterobacteriaceae and ESBL producing *E. coli* among urine isolates in hospital setting. Isolates from urine samples were primarily screened for possible ESBL production followed by phenotypic confirmation. Antibiotic susceptibility testing (AST) was done by Kirby Bauer disk diffusion method following Clinical and Laboratory Standard Institute (CLSI) guidelines.

Results: Out of 450 urine samples processed, 141 significant growths were obtained including 95 Enterobacteriaceae isolates with 67 *E. coli*. Among Enterobacteriaceae, 92 (96.84 %) were recorded as MDR and 18 (26.87 %) *E. coli* were confirmed as ESBLs producers.

Conclusions: Using the phenotypic confirmatory test forwarded by the CLSI, relatively significant *E. coli* isolates tested were ESBL producers. Also high numbers of MDR organisms were isolated among Enterobacteriaceae. Isolates showed significant resistance to the commonly prescribed drugs. These findings suggest for further study in this field including the consequences of colonization with MDR and ESBL-producing bacteria both in the community and in the hospital setting.

Keywords: Antibiotic resistance, *E. coli*, Enterobacteriaceae, ESBL, Multidrug resistance, Nepal, Urine, UTI

Background

Urinary tract infection (UTI) is a common disease ailment among Nepalese population as well as one of the commonest nosocomial infection [1]. Because of the evolving and continuing antibiotic resistance phenomenon, regular monitoring of resistance patterns is necessary to improve guidelines for empirical antibiotic therapy [2]. Uropathogens have developed resistance to commonly prescribed antimicrobial agents; this severely limits the treatment options of an effective therapy. One of the important resistance mechanisms is production of enzymes destroying the drug β-lactam antibiotics. To date several types of β-lactamases have been characterized depending on the characteristic and hydrolytic activity. Extended spectrum β-lactamases (ESBLs) is one of the important groups of β-lactamases [3].

ESBLs are the enzymes that have the ability to hydrolyze and cause resistance to various types of newer β-lactam antibiotics, including the expanded-spectrum (or third generation) cephalosporins (eg. cefotaxime, ceftriaxone, ceftazidime) and monobactams (eg. aztreonam), but not the cephamycins (eg. cefoxitin

* Correspondence: nepkamlesh@gmail.com
[1]Department of Microbiology, Kantipur College of Medical Science, Sitapaila, Kathmandu, Nepal
Full list of author information is available at the end of the article

and cefotetan) and carbapenems (eg. imipenem, meropenem and etrapenem) [4]. These enzymes are sensitive to β-lactamase inhibitors (sulbactam, clavulanic acid, and tazobactam) [5].

A large number of outbreaks of the infections which are caused by ESBL producing organisms have been described in every continent of the globe [5]. There is ample evidence to suggest the spread of ESBL infections is higher in resource poor countries [6]. Major risk factors for colonization or infection with ESBL producing organisms are long term antibiotic exposure, prolonged intensive care unit (ICU) stay, nursing home residency, severe illness, residence in an institution with high rates of ceftazidime and other third generation cephalosporin use and instrumentation or catheterisation [7].

E. coli, that can produce ESBLs, has arisen and disseminated worldwide as an important cause of both nosocomial and community infections and nowadays represents a major threat. Early identification of potential ESBL carriers is the first step to withhold the dispersal of these microorganisms and to avoid possible complications [8]. Since, ESBL production is usually plasmid mediated, it is possible for one specimen to contain both ESBL producing and non ESBL producing cells of the same species. This suggests that for optimal detection, several colonies must be tested from a primary culture plate [7]. Adequate detection of ESBL-producing strains is crucial for appropriate choice of antimicrobial therapy and infection control measures [9].

MDR Enterobacteriaceae has been frequently reported from different parts of the world as an emergence of treatment problem. Antibiotics given empirically without proper antibiotic susceptibility testing are one of the major causes for the development of MDR. So, to ensure appropriate therapy, current knowledge of the organism that causes UTI and their antibiotic susceptibility is mandatory [10]. The dissemination of ESBL-producing Enterobacteriaceae in the hospital setting is a problem with major therapeutic and epidemiological consequences [11]. This study was aimed to investigate the current situation of ESBL-producing *Escherichia coli* among Enterobacteriaceae isolates and sensitivity pattern of isolates toward various chemotherapeutic agents.

Methods
Sample
This is a cross-sectional study conducted from June to November 2014 in National Kidney Center, Vanasthali, Kathmandu, Nepal. The study population included patients visiting the hospital suspected of UTIs and patients undergoing dialysis in the hospital.

Patients included in the study were given pre-labelled (date, time, identification code, age and sex), leak proof,

sterile, screw-capped container to collect the mid-stream urine (MSU) sample. Urine samples from all age group were included in the study. Samples those held for more than two hours at room temperature and those without proper labelling were excluded from the study.

Laboratory assessment
The collected urine specimens were processed in the Microbiology laboratory within 2 h of collection. Urine samples were streaked directly on MacConkey agar (MA) and Blood agar (BA) plates. These plates were incubated at 37 °C aerobically and after overnight incubation, they were checked for bacterial growth. The Gram negative isolates were identified by their colony morphology, Gram staining characteristics, catalase test, oxidase test, and other relevant biochemical tests as per standard laboratory methods of identification.

Antibiotic susceptibility testing of bacterial isolates was done by Kirby Bauer disk diffusion method following CLSI guidelines using Mueller Hilton Agar (MHA) [12]. The discs were taken from HiMedia Laboratories (India). The followings are the concentrations of drugs used for disc diffusion testing: amikacin (30 µg), cefalexin (30 µg), cefixime (5 µg), cefotaxime (30 µg), ceftazidime (30 µg), ceftriaxone (30 µg), ciprofloxacin (5 µg), cotrimoxazole (23.75 µg sulfamethoxazole/1.25 µg trimethoprim), doxycycline (30 µg), imipenem (10 µg), nalidixic acid (30 µg), nitrofurantoin (300 µg), Norfloxacin (10 µg), and ofloxacin (5 µg). An isolate was considered as MDR if it was resistant to three or more drugs of different classes/groups of antibiotics.

ESBL detection
All the *E. coli* isolates were subjected to the screening test for ESBL detection. Screening test for ESBL detection was done according to the CLSI guidelines [12]. Isolates showing inhibition zone size of ≤ 22 mm with ceftazidime (30 µg), ≤ 25 mm with ceftriaxone (30 µg), and ≤ 27 mm with cefotaxime (30 µg) were interpreted as screening test positive for ESBL production.

For the confirmatory test for ESBL, two or three colonies of organisms were suspended in 0.5 ml of sterile broth and the turbidity matched to 0.5 McFarland. Using a sterile cotton swab the broth culture was uniformly swabbed on MHA. All the *E. coli* isolates which were resistant to at least ceftazidime, ceftriaxone and/or cefotaxime were subjected to the ESBL confirmatory test using ceftazidime (30 µg) and ceftazidime-clavulanic acid (30 µg + 10 µg) and the cefotaxime (30 µg) and cefotaxime-clavulanic acid (30 µg + 10 µg) combination disks. The tests were interpreted according to CLSI guidelines and a difference of 5 mm between zone of inhibition of a single disk and in combination with clavulanic acid (inhibitor) was confirmed to be produced by an ESBL positive isolate.

Results

Out of 450 urine samples processed in the laboratory, growth on MA and/or BA was obtained in 141 (31.33 %) urine samples (Table 1). Highest number of isolates was from the sample of patients with age above 60 years.

Among the isolates (n = 141) 41 (29.08 %) were Gram positive organism and 100 (70.92 %) were Gram negative organisms (Table 2). S. aureus and E. coli were the most predominant organism among Gram positive and Gram negative respectively. Out of 100 Gram negative organisms, 95 (95 %) were of Enterobacteriaceae family. E. coli was the most predominant genera of Enterobacteriaceae followed by Klebsiella spp, Proteus spp and Citrobacter spp. E. coli was isolated in 67 (47.52 %) samples. Other Gram negative organisms isolated were Pseudomonas spp and Neisseria spp.

The resistance of Enterobacteriaceae isolates against a spectrum of 14 selected antimicrobial agents of different classes were analyzed (Table 3). Enterobacteriaceae isolates showed variable result in their antibiotic sensitivity pattern against commercial antibiotic discs tested. According to the susceptibility pattern imipenem (92.63 %) was the most effective antibiotics against Enterobacteriaceae followed by the amikacin (82.11 %) and nitrofurantoin (57.89 %). Out of 14 antibiotics tested, 11 were found effective only for less than half of the Enterobacteriaceae isolates. Among the 95 Enterobacteriaceae isolates none of them were sensitive to all antibiotics tested.

Seventy three varied patterns of the antibiotic susceptibility were observed among the enterobacteriaceae isolates against the 14 different antibiotics. Each of these patterns was common in one or up to eight isolates which were analyzed. Enterobacteriaceae isolates include 67 E. coli, 24 Klebsiella spp, 3 Proteus spp. and one Citrobacter spp. Out of 95 Enterobacteriaceae, 92 (96.84 %) isolates were MDR (Table 4). Sixty four (95.52 %) isolates of E. coli and all isolates of Klebsiella spp, Proteus spp and Citrobacter spp were detected as MDR.

Out of total 67 strains of E. coli, which were screened for ESBL production, 53 (79.10) isolates were positive. All the E. coli isolates which were resistant to at least ceftazidime, ceftriaxone and/or cefotaxime were considered as screening positive isolates. After performing phenotypic confirmation test 18 (26.87 %) E. coli isolates were confirmed as ESBL producers (Fig. 1).

ESBL positive E. coli showed high degree of resistance to the antibiotics tested. All 18 ESBL positive E. coli isolates were resistant (100 %) to cefotaxime, ceftazidime and ceftriaxone (Table 5). These isolates also showed high resistance to other antibiotics as well. More than 60 % of ESBL positive isolates were resistant to 11 antibiotics out 14 antibiotics used for test. Most effective drug for the ESBL positive isolates was amikacin, to which all (100 %) isolates were susceptible. Amikacin was followed by imipenem (94.44 %) and nitrofurantoin (72.22 %).

High degree of resistance was shown by ESBL producers than ESBL non producers (Fig. 2). Only in case of cotrimoxazole, nitrofurantoin, imipenem and amikacin ESBL non producers showed a bit higher resistance than ESBL producers. Most effective drug for the ESBL non producers was found to be imipenem which was susceptible to 45 (91.84 %) out of 49 isolates, followed by amikacin susceptible to 35 (71.43 %) isolates and nitrofurantoin susceptible to 34 (69.39 %) isolates.

Discussion

This study was aimed to investigate ESBL-producing E. coli among Enterobacteriaceae isolates and sensitivity pattern of isolates toward various chemotherapeutic agents. Organisms producing ESBLs are clinically relevant and remain an important cause of failure of therapy with cephalosporins. ESBLs are primarily produced by the Enterobacteriaceae family, in particular K. pneumoniae and E. coli. Bacteria harbouring ESBLs may also acquire and most often exhibit additional resistances to other antimicrobial classes such as the quinolones, tetracyclines, cotrimoxazole, trimethoprim, and aminoglycosides, which further limits therapeutic options and thus pose a therapeutic dilemma [13].

Significant growth was obtained in 31.33 % urine culture samples. The majority of urine specimens showed no growth (68.67 %). The possible cause of low rate of growth positivity might be due to urine samples obtained from patients on antibiotics therapy, infection due to slow growing organisms or due to those organisms that were not able to grow on the routine media used [1, 14]. Number of female patients requesting for urine culture was higher than the

Table 1 Age and gender wise distribution of isolates

Age group	Male		Female		Total	
	Sample	Growth (%)	Sample	Growth (%)	Sample	Growth (%)
≤ 20	13	1 (1.79)	13	8 (9.41)	26	9 (6.38)
21 – 40	45	16 (28.57)	89	24 (28.24)	134	40 (28.37)
41 – 60	79	18 (32.14)	81	22 (25.88)	160	40 (28.37)
≥61	68	21 (37.50)	62	31 (36.47)	130	52 (36.88)
Total	205	56 (100)	245	85 (100)	450	141 (100)

Table 2 Microbiological profile of urinary isolates

	Isolates	Number (%)
Gram positive	Coagulase-negative staphylococci	18 (12.77)
	S. aureus	15 (10.64)
	Enterococcus spp	8 (5.67)
Sub total		41 (29.08)
Gram negative	E. coli	67 (47.52)
	Klebsiella spp	24 (17.02)
	Proteus spp	3 (2.13)
	Citrobacter spp	1 (0.71)
	Pseudomonas spp	2 (1.42)
	Neisseria spp	3 (2.13)
Sub total		100 (70.92)
Total		141 (100)

male patients. Significant microbial growth was higher in case of female than in male. Urethral opening in females, short urethra and complicated physiology especially during pregnancy can be considered as reason [15]. Female patients requesting for urine culture was higher, than the male patients, in age group of 21–40 years this may be because this age group consists sexually active women. Frequent or recent sexual activity is the most important risk factor for UTIs in young women. Nearly 80 % of all UTIs in premenopausal women occur within 24 h of intercourse. UTIs are very rare in celibate women. Certain types of contraceptives can also increase the risk of UTIs [16].

Numbers of gram negative organisms isolated were much higher than the gram positive. Similar predominance of gram negative organism in urine sample has

Table 3 Antimicrobial resistance amongst Enterobacteriaceae (n = 95)

Antibiotics class	Antibiotics	Resistance no. (%)
Aminoglycoside	Amikacin	17 (17.89)
Beta-lactams	Imipenem	7 (7.37)
	Cefalexin	79 (83.16)
	Cefixime	72 (75.79)
	Cefotaxime	71 (74.74)
	Ceftazidime	79 (83.16)
	Ceftriaxone	65 (68.42)
Nitrofuran	Nitrofurantoin	40 (42.11)
Quinolones/ Fluoroquinolones	Ciprofloxacin	58 (61.05)
	Nalidixic Acid	77 (81.05)
	Norfloxacin	61 (64.21)
	Ofloxacin	59 (62.11)
Sulfonamide	Co-Trimoxazole	59 (62.11)
Tetracycline	Doxycycline	56 (58.95)

Table 4 MDR trend in Enterobacteriaceae family

Organisms	Total number	MDR strains (%)
E. coli	67	64 (95.52)
Klebsiella spp	24	24 (100.00)
Proteus spp	3	3 (100.00)
Citrobacter spp	1	1 (100.00)
Total	95	92 (96.84)

been observed by other researchers too [17, 18]. *Staphylococcus aureus,* Coagulase-negative staphylococci (CoNS) and *Enterococcus* spp. were the gram positive organisms isolated. *E. coli, Klebsiella* spp., *Proteus* spp., *Citrobacter spp., Pseudomonas* spp. and *Neisseria* spp. were the gram negative organisms isolated. Among the gram negative organisms, Enterobacteriaceae were most frequent, 95 out of 100 gram negative organisms. Members of Enterobacteriaceae are more likely to cause UTIs than other organisms. In various studies predominant organisms isolated in UTI cases is Enterobacteriaceae [17, 19, 20].

Antibiotic susceptibility pattern shown by the Enterobacteriaceae isolates were variable. Imipenem was the most effective antibiotic as 92.63 % of isolates were susceptible, followed by amikacin (82.11 %). Isolates were comparatively less susceptible to cephalosporins than other antibiotics. Resistance to β-lactams in Enterobacteriaceae is mainly due to the production of β-lactamases, which may be encoded either chromosomally or on

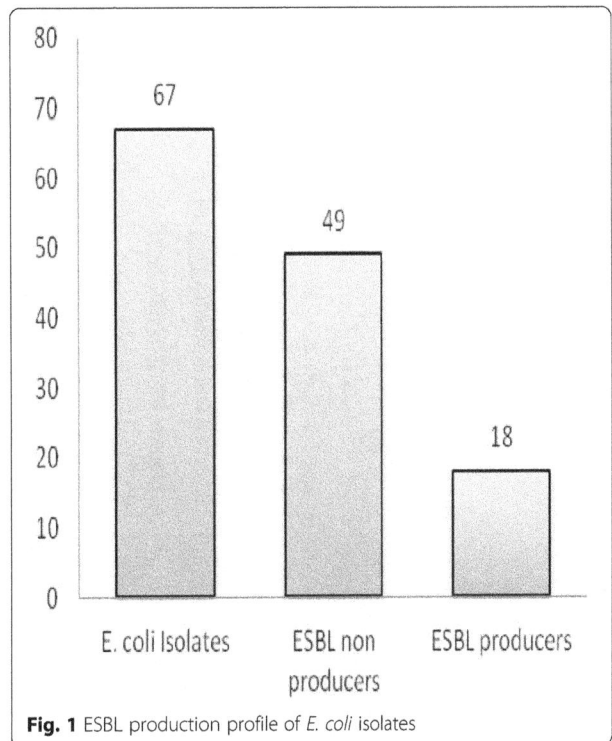

Fig. 1 ESBL production profile of E. coli isolates

Table 5 Antimicrobial resistance among ESBL producing *E. coli* (*n* = 18)

Antibiotics	Resistance no. (%)
Amikacin	0 (0.00)
Imipenem	1 (5.56)
Cefalexin	17 (94.44)
Cefixime	17 (94.44)
Cefotaxime	18 (100.00)
Ceftazidime	18 (100.00)
Ceftriaxone	18 (100.00)
Ciprofloxacin	16 (88.89)
Co-Trimoxazole	11 (61.11)
Doxycycline	13 (72.22)
Nalidixic Acid	17 (94.44)
Nitrofurantoin	5 (27.78)
Norfloxacin	17 (94.44)
Ofloxacin	16 (88.89)

plasmids [4]. Out of 14 antibiotics used, 11 were found effective to only less than half of the isolates. Majority (96.84 %) of Enterobacteriaceae isolates were found to be MDR. Thakur et al. [21] has observed 64.04 % MDR Enterobacteriaceae and 73.68 % MDR *E. coli* isolates. The widespread use of antibiotics could be associated with the selection of antibiotic resistance mechanisms in pathogenic and non pathogenic isolates of *E. coli* [22]. MDR isolates were more in females than in males and common in age group ≥ 61 years.

Over the past few years, the prevalence of ESBL producing strains among clinical isolates varies greatly with

different geographic regions and rapidly changing over time [23]. In this study, phenotypically 18 (26.87 %) isolates were confirmed as ESBL producers *E. coli* isolates. ESBL positive *E. coli* was distributed equally among male and female. Highest number of ESBL producers *E. coli* was obtained from the patients of age above 60 years. Other studies have also shown that ESBL isolates are encountered more frequently in the elderly, according to Roshan et al. [24], Shah et al. [25] and Rajan and Prabavathy [26] majority of isolates were from patients between 40 to 70 years, 50 to 60 years and 51 to 70 years respectively. The ESBLs-producing *E. coli* were most frequent in older age group in this study; it can be due to the reason that older patients are immunocompromised and more prone to infections by resistant organisms [27]. Nosocomial infections caused by ESBL producing pathogens are associated with risk factors such as elderly age, prolonged hospitalization, previous antibiotic use, and presence of invasive devices [28].

All ESBL positive *E. coli* strains were resistant to cefotaxime, ceftazidime and ceftriaxone. This outcome is in agreement with the study done by Islam et al. [29]. Similarly all *E. coli* isolates were resistant to cefotaxime and ceftriaxone in a study by Sompolinsky et al. [30] and to ceftazidime and ceftriaxone in a study by Chander and Shrestha [6]. High percentage of resistance to cefotaxime (99.2 %), ceftazidime (99.2 %) and ceftriaxone (99.5 %) was observed by Wani et al. [31]. ESBL positive isolates also showed high degree of resistance to other antibiotics like cefalexin, norfloxacin, cefixime, nalidixic acid, ciprofloxacin and ofloxacin. Aminoglycosides have good activity against clinically important gram negative bacilli [32]. Aminoglycosides are very important group of antibiotics with activity against many gram-negative rods

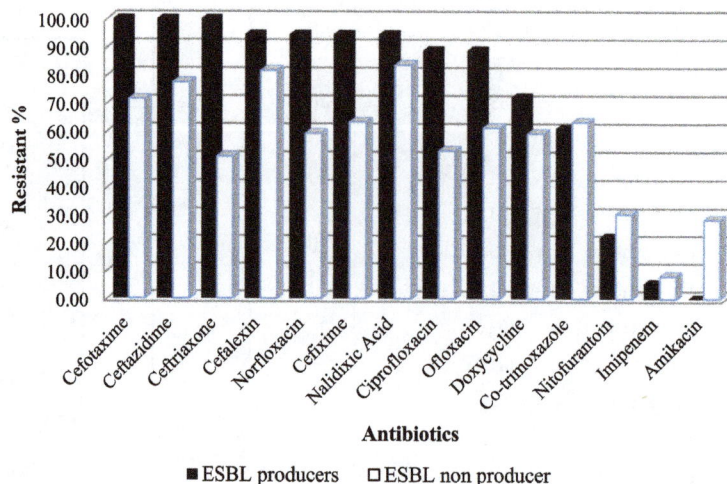

Fig. 2 Comparison of ESBL producers and non producers to the antibiotics tested

and the most common mechanism of aminoglycoside resistance is enzymatic modification of antibiotic molecule. All ESBL positive isolates were sensitive to the amikacin (100 %) followed by imipenem (94.44 %) and nitrofurantoin (72.22 %). Antimicrobial resistance surveillance done Nepal Public Health Laboratory (NPHL) found that ESBL *E. coli* were susceptible to imipenem (98.5 %), amikacin (96.1 %) followed by nitrofurantoin (89.2 %) and chloramphenicol (90.8 %) [33]. Amikacin and nitrofurantoin can therefore be used effectively against ESBL producing isolates but these antibiotics have many limitations. High percentage of isolates were susceptible to the carbapenem. The study done by Kader and Angamuthu [34] revealed more than 89 % of the ESBL producers were susceptible to imipenem and meropenem, whereas Mekki et al. [35] found 100 % isolates sensitive to the carbapenems. The production of β-lactamase may be of chromosomal or plasmid origin [4, 36]. Plasmid mediated production is often acquired by transfer of genetic information from one organism to another. Such transferable plasmid also codes for resistant determinants to antimicrobial agents other than β-lactams [37]. Hence multidrug resistance is expected to be more common in ESBL producing organisms.

The production of ESBL pathogens like *E. coli* has an important clinical importance. It has been well recognized that poor outcome occurs when patients with serious infections due to ESBL-producing organisms are treated with antibiotics like cephalosporins and penicillins to which the organisms are resistant. The mortality rate in such patients is significantly higher than in patients treated with antibiotics to which the organism is susceptible. All patients with antibiotics failure either die or have continued sign of infections, which necessitates change in antibiotic [38]. Microbiology laboratories can play an important role in detecting and promptly reporting the isolation of ESBL-positive bacteria, since drug susceptibility data are important for the clinical management of patients infected by these organisms [39]. Clinicians, whose laboratories do not perform tests for detection of ESBLs, and report ESBL producers as resistant to cephalosporins, risk poor outcome for their patients infected with ESBL producing organisms. The detection of ESBLs in any clinical isolate has great potential significance from the point of view of infection control [38].

This study also has some limitations; the study was carried out in a hospital. The picture of the study does not necessarily reveal the picture of the whole country, therefore systematic prospective surveillance should be carried covering wide geographical region in order to obtain information on seasonal, geographical and ethnic variation of pathogens and their antibiotic susceptibility profile. Moreover, characterization of ESBL strains should be performed genotypically, so that the information can be used in fighting with increasing resistance to antimicrobials.

Conclusion

The present study looked at the ESBL production in *E. coli* isolates in National Kidney Center in Kathmandu, Nepal. Using the phenotypic confirmatory test forwarded by the CLSI, relatively significant *E. coli* isolates tested were ESBL producers. Multidrug resistance to the antibiotics tested was also seen more among ESBL producer than the non-producers. In this study Enterobacteriaceae isolates showed significant resistance to the commonly prescribed drugs. In the present study 96.84 % Enterobacteriaceae were found to be multidrug resistant and 26.87 % *E. coli* were ESBL producers. These findings suggest for further study in this field including the consequences of colonization with multidrug resistant and ESBL-producing bacteria both in the community and in the hospital setting. These findings also suggest incorporating early detection mechanism of ESBL by clinical setting so that appropriate antibiotics can be used and this will also help in controlling increasing multidrug resistance due empirical therapy. With the spread of ESBL producing strains in hospitals all over the world, it is necessary to know the prevalence of ESBL positive strains in a hospital so as to formulate a policy of empirical therapy in high risk units where infections due to resistance organisms is higher.

Abbreviations
AST: Antibiotic susceptibility testing; BA: Blood agar; CLSI: Clinical and Laboratory Standard Institute; CoNS: Coagulase-negative staphylococci; ESBL: Extended spectrum β-lactamase; ICU: Intensive care unit; MA: MacConkey agar; MHA: Mueller Hilton agar; MDR: Multidrug resistant; MSU: Mid-stream urine; NPHL: Nepal Public Health Laboratory; UTI: Urinary tract infection.

Competing interests
The authors declare that they have no competing interests.

Authors' contributions
KKY performed the experiments. NA, RK and ADP guided the necessary laboratory tests. KKY and BS reviewed the published literatures. KKY wrote the manuscript and BS guided the manuscript preparation. All authors read and approved the final manuscript.

Acknowledgements
The authors would like to acknowledge Kantipur College of Medical Science and National Kidney Center.

Author details
[1]Department of Microbiology, Kantipur College of Medical Science, Sitapaila, Kathmandu, Nepal. [2]Consultant pathologist, National Kidney Center, Vanasthali, Kathmandu, Nepal. [3]Quality Control Department, Qmed Formulations Pvt. Ltd., Chhaling, Bhaktapur, Nepal.

References

1. Kattel HP, Acharya J, Mishra SK, Rijal BP, Pokhrel BM. Bacteriology of urinary tract infection among patients attending Tribhuvan University Teaching Hospital, Kathmandu, Nepal. J Nepal Assoc Med Lab Sci. 2008;9:25–9.

2. Nachimuthu R, Sumathi CS, Balasubramanian V, Palaniappan KR, Kannan VR. Urinary tract infection and antimicrobial susceptibility pattern of extended spectrum of beta lactamase producing clinical isolates. Adv Biol Res. 2008;2:78–82.

3. Thirapanmethee K. Extended spectrum β-lactamases: critical tools of bacterial resistance. Mahidol Univ J Pharm Sci. 2012;39:1–8.

4. Bradford PA. Extended-Spectrum β-Lactamases in the 21st Century: characterization, epidemiology, and detection of this important resistance threat. Clin Microbiol Rev. 2001;14:933–51.

5. Mukherjee M, Basu S, Mukherjee SK, Majumder M. Multidrug-resistance and extended spectrum beta-lactamase production in uropathogenic E. coli which were isolated from hospitalized patients in Kolkata, India. J Clin Diagn Res. 2013;7:449–53.

6. Chander A, Shrestha CD. Prevalence of extended spectrum beta lactamase producing Escherichia coli and Klebsiella pneumoniae urinary isolates in a tertiary care hospital in Kathmandu, Nepal. BMC Res Notes. 2013;6:487–92.

7. Chaudhary U, Aggarwal R. Extended spectrum β-lactamases (ESBL) - An emerging threat to clinical therapeutics. Indian J Med Microbiol. 2004;22:75–80.

8. Sahuquillo-Arce JM, Perpinan H, Armero C, Lopez-Quilez A, Selva M, Gonzalez F. Bayesian Approach to Urinary ESBL-Producing Escherichia coli. J Pharmacovigilance. 2014;2:133.

9. Cohen Stuart J, Dierikx C, Al Naiemi N, Karczmarek A, Van Hoek AHAM, Vos P, et al. Rapid detection of TEM, SHV and CTX-M extended-spectrum β-lactamases in Enterobacteriaceae using ligation-mediated amplification with microarray analysis. J Antimicrob Chemother. 2010;65:1377–81.

10. Tambekar DH, Dhanorkar DV, Gulhane SR, Khandelwal VK, Dudhane MN. Antibacterial susceptibility of some urinary tract pathogens to commonly used antibiotics. Afr J Biotechnol. 2006;5:1562–65.

11. Mena A, Plasencia V, García L, Hidalgo O, Ayestarán JI, Alberti S, et al. Characterization of a Large Outbreak by CTX-M-1-Producing Klebsiella pneumoniae and Mechanisms Leading to In Vivo Carbapenem Resistance Development. J Clin Microbiol. 2006;44:2831.

12. Clinical and Laboratory Standards Institute (CLSI). Performance Standards for Antimicrobial Susceptibility Testing. USA: CLSI: M100-S25; 2015. Wayne, PA.

13. Maina D, Makau P, Nyerere A, Revathi G. Antimicrobial resistance patterns in extended-spectrum β-lactamase producing Escherichia coli and Klebsiella pneumoniae isolates in a private tertiary hospital, Kenya. Microb Discov. 2013;1:5.

14. Sharma AR, Bhatta DR, Shrestha J, Banjara MR. Antimicrobial Susceptibility Pattern of Escherichia coli isolated from Urinary Tract Infected Patients Attending Bir Hospital. Nepal J Sci Technol. 2013;14:177–84.

15. Moyo SJ, Aboud S, Kasubi M, Lyamuya EF, Maselle SY. Antimicrobial resistance among producers and non-producers of extended spectrum beta-lactamases in urinary isolates at a tertiary Hospital in Tanzania. BMC Res Notes. 2010;3:348–52.

16. Simon H. Urinary Tract Infection. 2015. http://pennstatehershey.adam.com/content.aspx?productId=10&pid=10&gid=000036. Accessed 05 Sep 2015.

17. Dhakal S, Manandhar S, Shrestha B, Dhakal R, Pudasaini M. Extended spectrum β-lactamase producing multidrug resistant urinary isolates from children visiting Kathmandu Model Hospital. Nepal Med Coll J. 2012;14:136–41.

18. Ahmed OB, Omar AO, Asghar AH, Elhassan MM. Increasing prevalence of ESBL-producing Enterobacteriaceae in Sudan community patients with UTIs. Egypt Acad J Biolog Sci. 2013;5:17–24.

19. Acharya A, Gautam R, Subedee L. Uropathogens and their antimicrobial susceptibility pattern in Bharatpur, Nepal. Nepal Med Coll J. 2011;13:30–3.

20. Khawcharoenporn T, Vasoo S, Singh K. Urinary Tract Infections due to Multidrug-Resistant Enterobacteriaceae: Prevalence and Risk Factors in a Chicago Emergency Department. Hindawi Publishing Corporation Emergency Medicine International. 2013; doi:10.1155/2013/258517

21. Thakur S, Pokhrel N, Sharma N. Prevalence of Multidrug Resistant Enterobacteriaceae and Extended Spectrum β Lactamase Producing Escherichia Coli in Urinary Tract Infection. RJPBCS. 2013;4:1615–24.

22. Sorum H, Sunde M. Resistance to antibiotics in the normal flora of animals. Vet Res. 2001;32:227–41.

23. Kandeel A. Prevalence and risk factors of extended-spectrum β-lactamses producing Enterobacteriaceae in a general hospital in Saudi Arabia. JMID. 2014;4:50–4.

24. Roshan M, Ikram A, Mirza IA, Malik N, Abbasi SA, Alizai SA. Susceptibility Pattern of Extended Spectrum ß-Lactamase Producing Isolates in Various Clinical Specimens. J Coll Physicians Surg Pak. 2011;21:342–6.

25. Shah AA, Hasan F, Ahmed S, Hameed A. Extended-spectrum beta-lactamases in Enterobacteriaceae: related to age and gender. New Microbiol. 2002;25:363–6.

26. Rajan S, Prabavathy J. Antibiotic Sensitivity and Phenotypic Detection of ESBL producing E. coli Strains Causing Urinary Tract Infection In a Community Hospital, Chennai, Tamil Nadu, India. WebmedCentral. Pharm Sci. 2012;3, WMC003840.

27. Mumtaz S, Ahmad M, Aftab I, Akhtar N, ul Hassan M, Hamid A. Extended spectrum β-lactamases in enteric gram-negative bacilli: related to age and gender. JAMC. 2007;19:107–11.

28. Khanfar HS, Bindayna KM, Senok AC, Botta GA. Extended spectrum beta-lactamases (ESBL) in Escherichia coli and Klebsiella pneumoniae: trends in the hospital and community settings. J Infect Dev Ctries. 2009;3:295–9.

29. Islam MS, Yusuf MA, Islam MB, Jahan WA. Frequency of ESBL in Surgical Site Infection at a Tertiary Care Hospital. J Curr Adv Med Res. 2014;1:25–9.

30. Sompolinsky D, Nitzan Y, Tetry S, Wolk M, Vulikh I, Kerrn MB, et al. Integron-mediated ESBL resistance in rare serotypes of Escherichia coli causing infections in an elderly population of Israel. J Antimicrob Chemother. 2005;55:119–22.

31. Wani KA, Thakur MA, Fayaz AS, Fomdia B, Gulnaz B, Maroof P. Extended Spectrum B-Lactamase Mediated Resistance in Escherichia Coli in a Tertiary Care Hospital. Int J Health Sci (Qassim). 2009;3:155–63.

32. Gonzalez US, Spencer JP. Aminoglycosides: a practical review. Am Fam Physician. 1998;58:1811–20.

33. Nepal Public Health Laboratory (NPHL). Dissemination of important findings of Anti Microbial Resistance Surveillance programme. http://www.nphl.gov.np/index.php?obj=content&id=161. Accessed 22 June 2014.

34. Kader AA, Angamuthu K. Extended-spectrum beta-lactamases in urinary isolates of Escherichia coli, Klebsiella pneumoniae and other gram-negative bacteria in a hospital in Eastern Province, Saudi Arabia. Saudi Med J. 2005;26:956–9.

35. Mekki AH, Hassan AN, Elsayed DEM. Extended spectrum beta lactamase among multi drug resistant E. coli and Klebsiella species causing urinary tract infections in Khartoum. J Bact Res. 2010;2:18–21.

36. Smet A, Martel A, Persoons D, Dewulf J, Heyndrickx M, Herman L, et al. Broad-spectrum β-lactamases among Enterobacteriaceae of animal origin: molecular aspects, mobility and impact on public health. FEMS Microbiol Rev. 2010;34:295–316.

37. Paterson DL. Resistance in gram-negative bacteria: Enterobacteriaceae. Am J Med. 2006;119:S20–8.

38. Paterson DL, Ko WC, Gottberg AV, Casellas JM, Mulazimoglu L, Klugman KP, et al. Outcome of cephalosporin treatment for serious infections due to apparently susceptible organisms producing extended spectrum β-lactamases: implications for the clinical microbiology laboratory. J Clin Microbiol. 2001;39:2206–12.

39. Shah AA, Hasan F, Ahmed S, Hameed A. Prevalence of extended spectrum β-lactamases in nosocomial and outpatients (ambulatory). Pak J Med Sci. 2003;19:187–91.

24

Changing epidemiology of infections due to extended spectrum beta-lactamase producing bacteria

Steven Z Kassakian[1] and Leonard A Mermel[1,2,3]*

Abstract

Background: Community-associated infections caused by extended-spectrum beta-lactamase (ESBL) producing bacteria are a growing concern.

Methods: Retrospective cohort study of clinical infections due to ESBL-producing bacteria requiring admission from 2006-2011 at a tertiary care academic medical center in Providence, RI.

Results: A total of 321 infections due to ESBL-producing bacteria occurred during the study period. Fifty-eight cases (18%) were community-acquired, 170 (53%) were healthcare–associated, and 93 (29%) were hospital-acquired. The incidence of ESBL infections per 10,000 discharges increased during the study period for both healthcare-associated infections, 1.9 per year (95% CI 1-2.8), and for community-acquired infections, 0.85 per year (95% CI 0.3-1.4) but the rate remained unchanged for hospital-acquired infections. For ESBL-producing *E. coli* isolates, resistance to both ciprofloxacin and trimethoprim-sulfamethoxazole was 95% and 65%, respectively but 94% of isolates were susceptible to nitrofurantoin.

Conclusions: Community-acquired and healthcare-associated infections due to ESBL-producing bacteria are increasing in our community, particularly urinary tract infections due to ESBL-producing *E. coli*. Most isolates are resistant to oral antibiotics commonly used to treat urinary tract infections. Thus, our findings have important implications for outpatient management of such infections.

Keywords: Extended-spectrum beta-lactamase, Urinary tract infection, Antimicrobial resistance, Community-acquired infections, Ciprofloxacin

Background

ESBL-producing bacteria cause infections in hospitalized patients [1-3], patients housed in long-term care facilities [4,5], and they are gaining a foothold in community settings [6,7]. Human fecal carriage with these microorganisms is increasing, as well as their ubiquity in non-human species [8]. The increasing prevalence of infections due to ESBL-producing bacteria creates a challenge regarding appropriate antimicrobial therapy, especially in the community setting where oral antibiotics are used.

Most ESBLs are found in *Escherichia coli* and *Klebsiella pneumoniae*, frequently harboring resistance to other classes of antibiotics [9,10]. The majority of infections caused by these pathogens are urinary tract infections with occasional secondary bloodstream infections. In general, the preferred antibiotic class for management of infections due to ESBL-producing bacteria are carbapenems [11]. The purpose of this study was to better understand the changing epidemiology of ESBL-producing bacteria.

Methods

Study population

This study was conducted at Rhode Island Hospital, a tertiary care hospital licensed for 719 beds in Providence, RI.

* Correspondence: lmermel@lifespan.org
[1]Department of Medicine, Warren Alpert Medical School of Brown University, Providence, RI, USA
[2]Department of Epidemiology and Infection Control, Rhode Island Hospital, 593 Eddy Street, Providence RI 02903, USA
Full list of author information is available at the end of the article

Study design

This was an IRB-approved, retrospective cohort study of all adult patients hospitalized between January 2006 through December 2011 who had a positive clinical culture for an ESBL-producing microorganism.

Microbiology

Clinical cultures were identified and tested for antimicrobial susceptibility utilizing the Vitek 2 System (bioMérieux, Inc. Durham, NC). The detection of ESBL in *E. coli* and *K. pneumoniae* was done as previously described [12]. The phenotype confirmatory test for ESBL production was performed with use of ceftazidime (30 µg) and cefotaxime (30 µg), with and without clavulanic acid, against the isolates. The discs were placed on pre-inoculated Mueller-Hinton agar and incubated at 37°C. A difference of ≥5 mm between the zone diameters of either of the cephalosporin disks and their respective cephalosporin/clavulanate disk was considered phenotypic confirmation of ESBL production.

Demographic and clinical data

Cases were identified using infection control software (Theradoc, Hospira Inc. Lake Forest, IL). Cases were included if all three of the following were documented: an ESBL-producing microorganism was grown from a patient's clinical specimen; the treating physician noted that the patient had an infection in the medical record; and the physician treated the patient with antibiotics. All charts were reviewed by one of the study authors (SK) to determine the infection acquisition type (i.e., community-acquired, healthcare-associated or hospital-acquired) using the Centers for Disease Control and Prevention definitions [13]. The antibiogram was obtained from the electronic medical record.

Definitions

The site of infection was defined according to CDC definitions [14]. If a culture was obtained more than 48 hours after hospital admission, it was classified as hospital-acquired. If a culture was obtained within 48 hours after admission, it was classified as a healthcare-associated infection if a) within the prior 90 days the patient resided in a long-term care facility or, had a prior admission to an acute-care facility in our hospital system, or an outside hospital as mentioned in the admission note; b) or had undergone hemodialysis or received an intravenous medications or c) if they underwent an invasive procedure within the last 30 days prior to admission. Otherwise, a patient was considered to have a community-acquired infection.

Statistical analysis

Age comparisons between the three groups were analyzed using a two-tailed t test. Sex differences among the three groups were analyzed using chi-square testing. Linear regression was performed to determine whether changes in the incidence of infection were statistically significant (SPSS, Chicago, IL). This analysis was repeated including only the first occurrence of an infection in a given patient. Differences in antibiotic resistance between acquisition groups were analyzed using either a chi-square test or a Fischer exact test when appropriate. Use of a two-tailed test of significance with a P-value <0.05 was employed to determine statistical significance.

Results

During the study period, there were 321 incident infections due to ESBL-producing bacteria. Twenty-six patients experienced more than one infection. One patient had two different ESBL-producing bacteria in the same clinical sample at one time. The number of infections due to these pathogens increased consistently from 23 infections in 2006 to 81 in 2011 (Figure 1). Overall, 58 cases (18%) were community-acquired, 170 (53%) healthcare–associated, and 93 (29%) hospital-acquired. The incidence of infection due to ESBL-producing bacteria per 10,000 discharges increased significantly during the study period for healthcare associated infections, 1.9 per year (95% CI 1-2.8; p = .003) and for community-acquired infections, 0.85 per year (95% CI 0.3-1.4; p = .01). There was no significant change in the hospital-acquired infection group. When this analysis was repeated after removing 26 recurrent episodes of infections, none of the significant changes over time became non-significant (data not shown).

The mean age among the three groups was 69, 70 and 65 years in the community, healthcare and hospital-acquired infection groups, respectively. The difference in age between the healthcare-associated and the hospital-acquired infection groups was significant (p = 0.04). There were fewer males (26%) in the community-acquired group compared with healthcare-associated (42%) and hospital-acquired groups (41%; p = 0.1).

Urinary tract infection predominated (80%), followed by bloodstream infection (10%), skin and soft-tissue infection (5%), pneumonia (3%) and intra-abdominal infection (2%). There was a marked shift in the predominant organism in all three acquisition types from *K. pneumoniae* to *E. coli* (Figure 2). For the entire study period, *E. coli* accounted for 78%, 66% and 65% of the community, healthcare-associated, and hospital-acquired groups, respectively.

Resistance to trimethoprim-sulfamethoxazole (TMP-SMZ) and ciprofloxacin was commonly observed among *E. coli* isolates (Table 1); however, 94% of *E. coli* isolates were susceptible to nitrofurantoin with no difference

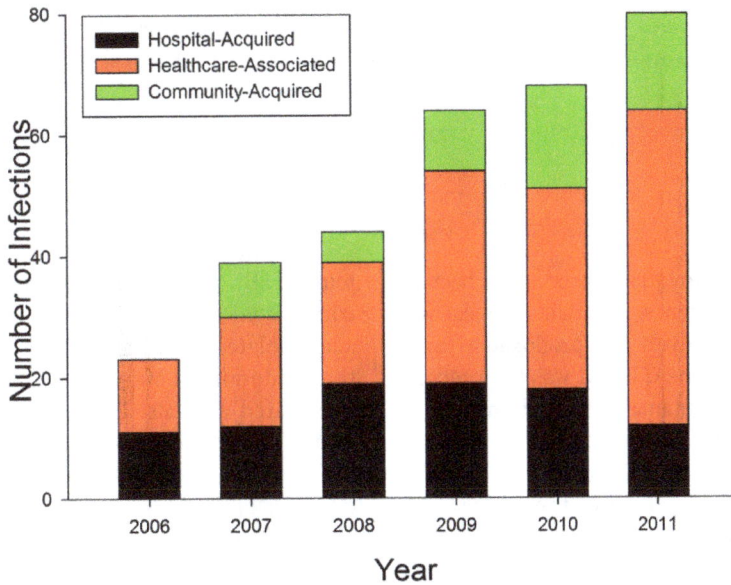

Figure 1 Origin of infection due to ESBL-producing bacteria. Incidence of infections due to ESBL-producing bacteria by classification of origin over the study period.

between acquisition groups (p = 0.8). In contrast, 76% of all *K. pneumoniae* isolates were resistant to nitrofurantoin.

Discussion

The number of infections due to ESBL-producing bacteria are increasing, especially community or non-hospital healthcare-associated infections as demonstrated by others [15,16]. Although the focus of infection control measures has been on transmission of such pathogens within hospitals, many of the infections due to ESBL-producing bacteria appear to arise outside of the acute-care setting where there is limited infection control resources [17].

We found high levels of resistance to TMP-SMZ and ciprofloxacin in all acquisition types. *E. coli* resistance to TMP-SMZ was similar to other studies [18]; however, ciprofloxacin resistance among *E. coli* in our study (95%) is higher than found in other reports [10,15,16,19-21]. The level of ciprofloxacin resistance we documented in our community-acquired ESBL-producing *E. coli* (92%) is also higher than the level of resistance among all *E. coli* isolates tested at our hospital in 2011 (31%) [22].

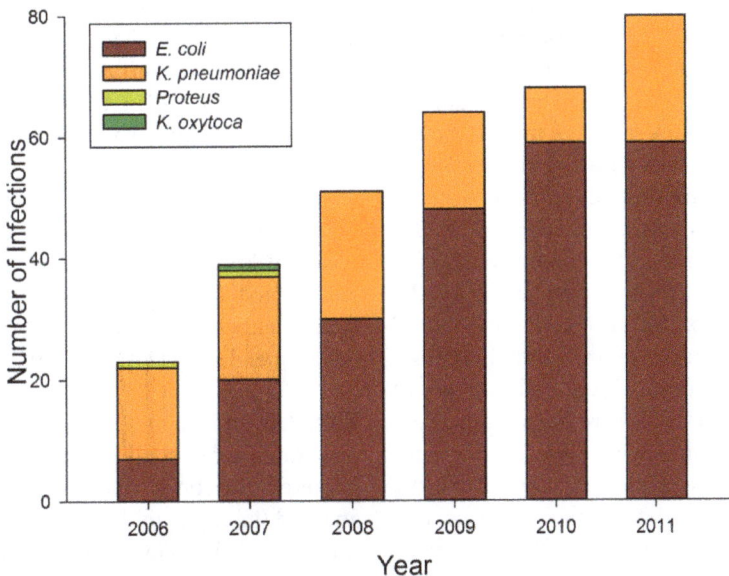

Figure 2 ESBL-producing bacteria. ESBL-producing bacteria identified during the study period.

Table 1 Antimicrobial resistance of ESBL-producing *E. coli*

Antimicrobial	Community acquired		Healthcare associated		Hospital acquired		Total		P value
	Bacteria	n(%) Resistant	Bacteria	n(%) Resistant	Bacteria	n(%) Resistant	Bacteria	n(%) Resistant	
TMP-SMZ*	51	32 (69)	111	75 (68)	57	45 (79)	219	152 (69)	0.2
Ciprofloxacin	52	48 (92)	111	109 (98)	57	53 (92)	220	210 (95)	0.1
Nitrofurantoin	50	3 (6)	85	7 (8)	43	1 (2)	178	11 (6)	0.5

Legend: *Trimethoprim-sulfamethoxazole.

While it is known that many ESBL-producing bacteria harbor additional resistance genes, it remains unclear why our isolates had such high levels of ciprofloxacin resistance. One possibility is that the CTX-M was the predominant gene regulating beta-lactamase production in most of our isolates. While we did not investigate the molecular mechanisms of resistance in our study, we wonder whether our isolates which showed the persistently increasing predominance of *E. coli* may indeed be the advance of CTX-M in our region, as has been found in rectal colonizers in other patients admitted to our hospital (L.A. Mermel, unpublished data, February 2013). Of note, a US multi-centered study documented 99% ciprofloxacin resistance among CTX-M-containing *E. coli* [23] and a recent US multi-centered study of community-acquired *E. coli* ESBL infections found the majority contained CTX-M genes [15]. This finding raises concern for treatment failure in the community setting given the levels of resistance to antimicrobial agents commonly used for cystitis, namely TMP-SMZ and ciprofloxacin. We found a low level of nitrofurantoin resistance in our *E. coli* isolates. As such, patients in our study with community-acquired infections may have been outpatient treatment failures owing to initial empiric therapy with either ciprofloxacin or TMP-SMZ, prompting hospital admission. While we did not have susceptibility data to fosfomycin, a recent study found no resistance among community-acquired ESBL-producing *E. coli* [16]. Thus, it seems prudent to consider the use of nitrofurantoin or fosfomycin as empiric therapy for acute uncomplicated cystitis in those at risk for, or with a history of infection or colonization with an ESBL-producing *E. coli*.

What accounts for the increasing numbers of ESBL-producing *E. coli* and the increase in community-acquired infections? Traditionally, *K. pneumoniae* made up the majority of infections due to ESBL-producing pathogens and the majority of those occurred in hospital settings. However, 88% of our community-acquired isolates of ESBL-producing bacteria in 2011 were *E. coli*, a marked shift from four years earlier when it was 55%. The presence of ESBL-producing *E. coli* as commensal flora in healthy livestock has been documented throughout Europe and Asia with as many as 40% of poultry populations colonized with these bacteria and their presence has been identified in retail meats [8,24,25]. Additionally, several studies have found ESBL-producing *E. coli* in the fecal flora of healthy companion animals, namely cats and dogs, and recently such isolates have been detected in US animals, where the predominant strain was CTX-M [8,26]. Beyond domesticated animals, ESBL-producing *E. coli* have been found in wildlife in several continents and many such isolates have been shown to be genotypically-related to human isolates [27].

Regarding limitations in our study, it is possible that patients were misclassified as community-acquired given the lack of available documentation in the medical record. Given the lack of admission screening, it is possible that some cases deemed hospital-acquired infections were community-acquired. Our community-acquired cohort is likely a biased subset as they required hospital admission, thus indicating that they likely were more ill than those whom developed such infections and remained in the community. Additionally, our antibiotic resistance patterns for the community-acquired and healthcare-associated organisms likely present a biased sample as only those patients ill enough to require admission are represented. Use of the Vitek 2 system alone for identification of ESBL-producing *Enterobacteriacae* is insufficient [28]. As such, our laboratory used confirmatory testing as noted in the Methods section. Lastly, our laboratory uses CLSI breakpoints for susceptibilty testing. The CLSI has updated recommendations for interpretation of antibiotic susceptibility testing results in the 2010 and 2011 CLSI guidelines, in part adopting European Committee for Antimicrobial Susceptibility Testing (EUCAST) strategies. The CLSI now recommends higher zone diameter susceptibility breakpoints for 3rd generation cephalosporins and carbapenems; fluoroquinolone breakpoints were unchanged. Thus, our data must be interpreted in context, based on previously used CLSI breakpoints rather than revised CLSI breakpoints or those recommended by EUCAST [29].

Conclusion

In summary, our study noted the emergence of community-acquired infections due to ESBL-producing bacteria, a marked increase in healthcare-associated infections, as well *E. coli* becoming the predominant pathogen in all three acquisition groups. We found high levels of TMP-SMZ and ciprofloxacin resistance. This has implications regarding empiric therapy for urinary tract infections since these frequently utilized antibiotics in the outpatient setting are ineffective for such pathogens. Another important finding is the susceptibility of ESBL-producing *E. coli* to nitrofurantoin. Further elucidation of underlying genetic makeup of ESBL-producing pathogens will assist in better understanding the epidemiology of these emerging infections.

Abbreviations
ESBL: Extended-spectrum beta-lactamase; TMP-SMZ: Trimethoprim-sulfamethoxazole.

Competing interests
The authors declare that they have no competing interests.

Authors' contributions
SZK and LAM are both fully responsible for the entirety of the study from conception through critical revisions of the manuscript. Both SZK and LAM had full access to all the data in the study and take responsibility for the integrity of the data and the accuracy of the data analysis. Both authors approved the final manuscript.

Acknowledgements
Stephen Parenteau, MS, Department of Infection Control and Epidemiology, Rhode Island Hospital, Providence, RI, provided assistance with data extraction from the infection control database. Kimberle Chapin, MD, Director of Microbiology, Rhode Island Hospital, Providence, RI, provided the on line data in reference [22].

Author details
[1]Department of Medicine, Warren Alpert Medical School of Brown University, Providence, RI, USA. [2]Department of Epidemiology and Infection Control, Rhode Island Hospital, 593 Eddy Street, Providence RI 02903, USA. [3]Division of Infectious Diseases, Rhode Island Hospital, 593 Eddy Street, Providence, RI 02903, USA.

References
1. Meyer KS, Urban C, Eagan JA, Berger BJ, Rahal JJ: **Nosocomial outbreak of Klebsiella infection resistant to late-generation cephalosporins.** *Ann Intern Med* 1993, **119**(5):353–358.
2. Paterson DL, Ko WC, Von Gottberg A, Mohapatra S, Casellas JM, Goossens H, Mulazimoglu L, Trenholme G, Klugman KP, Bonomo RA, Rice LB, Wagener MM, McCormack JG, Yu VL: **International prospective study of Klebsiella pneumoniae bacteremia: implications of extended-spectrum beta-lactamase production in nosocomial Infections.** *Ann Intern Med* 2004, **140**(1):26–32.
3. Alcantar-Curiel D, Tinoco JC, Gavosso C, Carlos A, Daza C, Perez-Prado MC, Salcido L, Santos JI, Alpuche-Aranda CM: **Nosocomial bacteremia and urinary tract infections caused by extended-spectrum beta -lactamase-producing Klebsiella pneumoniae with plasmids carrying both SHV-5 and TLA-1 genes.** *Clin Infect Dis* 2004, **38**(8):1067–1074.
4. Trick WE, Weinstein RA, DeMarais PL, Kuehnert MJ, Tomaska W, Nathan C, Rice TW, McAllister SK, Carson LA, Jarvis WR: **Colonization of skilled-care facility residents with antimicrobial-resistant pathogens.** *J Am Geriatr Soc* 2001, **49**(3):270–276.
5. Wiener J, Quinn JP, Bradford PA, Goering RV, Nathan C, Bush K, Weinstein RA: **Multiple antibiotic-resistant Klebsiella and Escherichia coli in nursing homes.** *JAMA* 1999, **281**(6):517–523.
6. Pitout JD, Nordmann P, Laupland KB, Poirel L: **Emergence of Enterobacteriaceae producing extended-spectrum beta-lactamases (ESBLs) in the community.** *J Antimicrob Chemother* 2005, **56**(1):52–59.
7. Ben-Ami R, Rodriguez-Bano J, Arslan H, Pitout JD, Quentin C, Calbo ES, Azap OK, Arpin C, Pascual A, Livermore DM, Garau J, Carmeli Y: **A multinational survey of risk factors for infection with extended-spectrum beta-lactamase-producing enterobacteriaceae in nonhospitalized patients.** *Clin Infect Dis* 2009, **49**(5):682–690.
8. Smet A, Martel A, Persoons D, Dewulf J, Heyndrickx M, Herman L, Haesebrouck F, Butaye P: **Broad-spectrum beta-lactamases among Enterobacteriaceae of animal origin: molecular aspects, mobility and impact on public health.** *FEMS Microbiol Rev* 2010, **34**(3):295–316.
9. Ben-Ami R, Schwaber MJ, Navon-Venezia S, Schwartz D, Giladi M, Chmelnitsky I, Leavitt A, Carmeli Y: **Influx of extended-spectrum beta-lactamase-producing enterobacteriaceae into the hospital.** *Clin Infect Dis* 2006, **42**(7):925–934.
10. Rodriguez-Bano J, Navarro MD, Romero L, Muniain MA, deCueto M, Rios MJ, Hernandez JR, Pascual A: **Bacteremia due to extended-spectrum beta -lactamase-producing Escherichia coli in the CTX-M era: a new clinical challenge.** *Clin Infect Dis* 2006, **43**(11):1407–1414.
11. Pitout JD, Laupland KB: **Extended-spectrum beta-lactamase-producing Enterobacteriaceae: an emerging public-health concern.** *Lancet Infect Dis* 2008, **8**(3):159–166.
12. Institute, C.a.L.S: *Performance Standards for Antimicrobial Susceptibility Testing.* Wayne, PA: Clinical and Laboratory Standards Institute; 2008.
13. Garner JS, Jarvis WR, Emori TG, Horan TC, Hughes JM: **CDC definitions for nosocomial infections, 1988.** *Am J Infect Control* 1988, **16**(3):128–140.
14. Prevention, C.f.D.C.a: *CDC/NHSN Surveillance Definition of Healthcare-Associated Infection and Criteria for Specific Types of Infections in the Acute Care Setting;* 2013. Available from: http://www.cdc.gov/nhsn/pdfs/pscmanual/17pscnosinfdef_current.pdf.
15. Doi Y, Park YS, Rivera JI, Adams-Haduch JM, Hingwe A, Sordillo EM, Lewis JS 2nd, Howard WJ, Johnson LE, Polsky B, Jorgensen JH, Richter SS, Shutt KA, Paterson DL: **Community-associated extended-spectrum beta-lactamase-producing Escherichia coli infection in the United States.** *Clin Infect Dis* 2013, **56**(5):641–648.
16. Meier S, Weber R, Zbinden R, Ruef C, Hasse B: **Extended-spectrum beta-lactamase-producing Gram-negative pathogens in community-acquired urinary tract infections: an increasing challenge for antimicrobial therapy.** *Infection* 2011, **39**(4):333–340.
17. Tschudin-Sutter S, Frei R, Dangel M, Stranden A, Widmer AF: **Rate of transmission of extended-spectrum Beta-lactamase-producing enterobacteriaceae without contact isolation.** *Clin Infect Dis* 2012, **55**(11):1505–1511.
18. Lewis JS 2nd, Herrera M, Wickes B, Patterson JE, Jorgensen JH: **First report of the emergence of CTX-M-type extended-spectrum beta-lactamases (ESBLs) as the predominant ESBL isolated in a U.S. health care system.** *Antimicrob Agents Chemother* 2007, **51**(11):4015–4021.
19. Pitout JD, Church DL, Gregson DB, Chow BL, McCracken M, Mulvey MR, Laupland KB: **Molecular epidemiology of CTX-M-producing Escherichia coli in the Calgary Health Region: emergence of CTX-M-15-producing isolates.** *Antimicrob Agents Chemother* 2007, **51**(4):1281–1286.
20. Bonkat G, Müller G, Braissant O, Frei R, Tschudin-Sutter S, Rieken M, Wyler S, Gasser TC, Bachmann A, Widmer AF: **Increasing prevalence of ciprofloxacin resistance in extended-spectrum-b-lactamase-producing Escherichia coli urinary isolates.** *World J Urol* 2013, **31**(6):1427–1432.
21. Tinelli M, Cataldo MA, Mantengoli E, Cadeddu C, Cunietti E, Luzzaro F, Rossolini GM, Tacconelli E: **Epidemiology and genetic characteristics of extended-spectrum beta-lactamase-producing Gram-negative bacteria causing urinary tract infections in long-term care facilities.** *J Antimicrob Chemother* 2012, **67**(12):2982–2987.
22. *2011 Rhode Island Hospital Clinical Microbiology Laboratory Antimicrobial Statistics Data.* [cited 2012 28 November 2012]; Available from: http://intra.lifespan.org/rih/microbiology/documents/2011RIHInpt.pdf.
23. Johnson JR, Urban C, Weissman SJ, Jorgensen JH, Lewis JS 2nd, Hansen G, Edelstein PH, Robicsek A, Cleary T, Adachi J, Paterson D, Quinn J, Hanson ND, Johnston BD, Clabots C, Kuskowski MA, AMERECUS Investigators: **Molecular epidemiological analysis of Escherichia coli sequence type ST131 (O25:H4) and blaCTX-M-15 among extended-spectrum-beta-lactamase-producing E. coli from the United States, 2000 to 2009.** *Antimicrob Agents Chemother* 2012, **56**(5):2364–2370.
24. Leverstein-van Hall MA, Dierikx CM, Cohen Stuart J, Voets GM, van den Munckhof MP, van Essen-Zandbergen A, Platteel T, Fluit AC, van de Sande-Bruinsma N, Scharinga J, Bonten MJ, Mevius DJ, National ESBL surveillance group: **Dutch patients, retail chicken meat and poultry share the same ESBL genes, plasmids and strains.** *Clin Microbiol Infect* 2011, **17**(6):873–880.
25. Kluytmans JA, Overdevest IT, Willemsen I, Kluytmans-van den Bergh MF, van der Zwaluw K, Heck M, Rijnsburger M, Vandenbroucke-Grauls CM, Savelkoul PH,

Johnston BD, Gordon D, Johnson JR: **Extended-spectrum beta-lactamase-producing Escherichia coli from retail chicken meat and humans: comparison of strains, plasmids, resistance genes, and virulence factors.** *Clin Infect Dis* 2013, **56**(4):478–487.

26. O'Keefe A, Hutton TA, Schifferli DM, Rankin SC: **First detection of CTX-M and SHV extended-spectrum beta-lactamases in Escherichia coli urinary tract isolates from dogs and cats in the United States.** *Antimicrob Agents Chemother* 2010, **54**(8):3489–3492.

27. Guenther S, Ewers C, Wieler LH: **Extended-spectrum beta-lactamases producing E. coli in wildlife, yet another form of environmental pollution?** *Front Microbiol* 2011, **2**:1–13.

28. Espinar MJ, Rocha R, Ribeiro M, Goncalves Rodrigues A, Pina-Vaz C: **Extended-spectrum beta-lactamases of Escherichia coli and Klebsiella pneumoniae screened by the VITEK 2 system.** *J Med Microbiol* 2011, **60**(Pt 6):756–760.

29. Hombach M, Mouttet B, Bloemberg GV: **Consequences of revised CLSI and EUCAST guidelines for antibiotic susceptibility patterns of ESBL- and AmpC beta-lactamase-producing clinical Enterobacteriaceae isolates.** *J Antimicrob Chemother* 2013, **68**(9):2092–2098.

25

Difficult-to-detect carbapenem-resistant IMP13-producing *P. aeruginosa*: experience feedback concerning a cluster of urinary tract infections at a surgical clinic in France

Odile Milan[1], Laurent Debroize[2], Xavier Bertrand[3,4], Patrick Plesiat[5], Anne-Sophie Valentin[6], Roland Quentin[6] and Nathalie Van der Mee-Marquet[6,7*]

Abstract

Background: We report a carbapenem-resistant *P. aeruginosa* clone responsible for a cluster of urinary tract infections in elderly surgery patients, diagnosed during a three-month period in a 59-bed surgical clinic.

Findings: The clonal nature of the cluster was established by molecular study of the *P. aeruginosa* isolates (PFGE and MLST). Despite an MIC of imipenem in the susceptibility range for two isolates, all were metallo-β-lactamase-producers (IMP13-type, clone ST621). We conducted a review of the medical and surgical procedures. We tested water delivered into the clinic and urological devices for the presence of the epidemic strain. The hygiene nurse observed hygiene practices. A week after the implementation of barrier precautions around the fourth infected patient, we studied the extent to which the patients hospitalised were colonised to assess whether the spread of the epidemic strain had been controlled.

Conclusions: 1/ Our findings indicate the difficulties in the detection of the metallo-β-lactamase in this clone, that resulted in the alert being delayed. 2/ Unlike most investigations of UTI outbreaks described in urology wards, we did not detect any contaminated urological devices or water colonisation. 3/ Consistent with outbreaks involving the IMP-13 clone in critical care units, the observation of inadequate application of standard precautions argued for patient-to-patient transmission during urinary management of the urology patients. 4/ The implementation of barrier precautions around infected patients resulted in control of the spread of the epidemic clone. This report serves as an alert concerning a difficult-to-detect multidrug-resistant *P. aeruginosa* clone in elderly urology patients.

Introduction

IMP-type enzymes, the first acquired metallo-β-lactamases (MBLs) to be detected in Gram-negative pathogens in the early 1990s, remain among the most prevalent and widely distributed MBLs. The *P. aeruginosa* clone ST621, producing IMP-13 [1], has been responsible for outbreaks in Italian critical care settings, and has recently been identified in other European countries and in South America [1-3].

Patient-to-patient transmission of *Pseudomonas aeruginosa* is frequent in high-risk patients. Numerous outbreaks of multi-drug resistant *P. aeruginosa* have been described in neonatal and adult intensive care units, burns units, oncohaematology units and transplantation units [4]. Outside critical care settings, nosocomial outbreaks of *P. aeruginosa* are mostly associated with contaminated water supplies or inadequately disinfected medical or surgical devices [5]. In urology wards, *P. aeruginosa* has been found to be associated with urinary tract infection (UTI) outbreaks linked to contaminated urodynamic systems, cystoscopes or urometers [6], or tap water colonisation [7].

We report a cluster of UTIs associated with a carbapenem-resistant IMP13-producing *P. aeruginosa*

* Correspondence: n.vandermee@chu-tours.fr
[6]Service de Bactériologie et Hygiène, Tours, France
[7]Réseau des Hygiénistes du Centre, Hôpital Trousseau, Centre Hospitalier Universitaire, Tours, France
Full list of author information is available at the end of the article

strain in a French small surgical clinic. This report serves as an alert concerning a difficult-to-detect and multidrug-resistant *P. aeruginosa* clone in elderly urology patients.

Methods

The *P. aeruginosa* isolates from the UTI cases were identified with Vitek 2 Gram-Negative Identification Cards (bioMerieux, France). Antibiotic susceptibility was tested by an agar disk diffusion method. The combined meropenem +/– dipicolinic acid disk test (Rosco, France) was used for the phenotypic detection of MBL in isolates displaying decreased susceptibility to imipenem according to CLSI and EUCAST breakpoints (MIC > 4 mg/L). The metallo-β-lactamase gene, *bla*IMP-13, was identified in the epidemic strain as previously described [2]. The isolates were also characterised by O-serotyping, pulsed-field gel electrophoresis (PFGE) and MLST as previously described [8]. We also studied three unrelated IMP-13-producing *P. aeruginosa* recently isolated in distant French regions (named R1 of ST 621, R2 of ST 308 and R3 of ST111).

During the outbreak investigation, we tested water delivered into the clinic and urological devices for the presence of the epidemic strain. Environmental samples (n=26) were taken from water fittings in each medical and surgical unit. Samples of 200 mL of cold water taken directly from the tap immediately after activating were filtered and the filters cultured on plates containing cetrimide medium. Environmental samples were also taken from the four cystoscopes of the clinic. Plates were incubated at 37°C for 48 hours, and all bacterial colonies likely to be *P. aeruginosa* were identified and studied as described above.

The hygiene nurse observed hygiene practices (materials and techniques used) in the clinic, to assess if the standard precautions (for all patients) and the barrier precautions (around IMP-13-producing *P. aeruginosa*-infected patients) were being followed by healthcare workers.

A week after the implementation of barrier precautions around the fourth infected patient, we studied the extent to which the patients hospitalised in the clinic were colonised with the epidemic strain to assess if its spread had been controlled. Rectal swabs were taken from each patient for screening. Swabs were immediately suspended in 0.5 mL of sterile water and 0.1 mL of the suspension was streaked on a plate containing cetrimide medium.

This study was run in accordance with the French Healthcare recommendations for the prevention of infection. Ethical approval was obtained at the national level from the Réseau Alerte Investigation Surveillance des Infections Nosocomiales (RAISIN). The study was managed jointly with the director of the clinic, the hygiene nurse, surgeons and physicians responsible for caring for the patients, and the regional infection-control practitioner. Patients and their relatives were enrolled after an individual interview for consent to allow access to medical records and to culture a faecal sample.

Results

The four clinical cases of UTI

The first case involved a 74-y-old man diagnosed on the 28th of October with a multidrug-resistant imipenem-intermediate *P. aeruginosa* UTI, 45 days after prostatectomy, and following imipenem treatment administered for multidrug-resistant imipenem-susceptible *P. aeruginosa* UTI identified one week earlier. The second case was a 90-y-old man diagnosed on the 19th of December with a multidrug-resistant imipenem-susceptible *P. aeruginosa* UTI, 15 days after nephrostomy. Patient 3 (80 y) was diagnosed on the 6th of January with a multidrug-resistant imipenem-susceptible *P. aeruginosa* UTI, one day after cystography and during a period when he was undergoing numerous urological surgical interventions. The fourth patient was a woman (89 y) diagnosed on the 16th of January with a multidrug-resistant imipenem-intermediate *P. aeruginosa* UTI, one month after nephrostomy. In all cases, UTIs were defined on the basis of clinical signs of infection and biological criteria (significant leukocyturia and bacteriuria).

Detection of the IMP-13-producing P. aeruginosa

The MICs of imipenem were 8 mg/L for isolates from patients 1 and 4. The *P. aeruginosa* isolates associated with these UTIs exhibited a high level of resistance to ceftazidime (>256 mg/L). Following the French Healthcare recommendations, the two isolates showing a decreased susceptibility to imipenem (MIC=8 mg/L) were screened for MBL. Both isolates were found to be MBL-producers. The clonal nature of the two isolates was established from the PFGE patterns of the isolates. As a consequence of these findings, a retrospective study of *P. aeruginosa* UTIs was conducted. Two UTIs associated with ceftazidime-resistant *P. aeruginosa* isolates were identified in patients 2 and 3; the MICs of imipenem were 4 mg/L for both isolates. We studied the two ceftazidime-resistant imipenem-susceptible *P. aeruginosa* isolates recovered from patients 2 and 3, even though their susceptibility to imipenem was not below the threshold value. These isolates were also MBL-producers. The clonal nature of the UTI cluster was then established from the PFGE patterns of the four isolates (Figure 1). All belonged to serogroup O:4, and were identified as being IMP13-type and members of clone ST621, also called the Italian clone. These investigations therefore established a cluster of four UTIs associated with an IMP-13-producing epidemic strain, diagnosed during a three-month period in a 59-bed surgical clinic in Chartres, France.

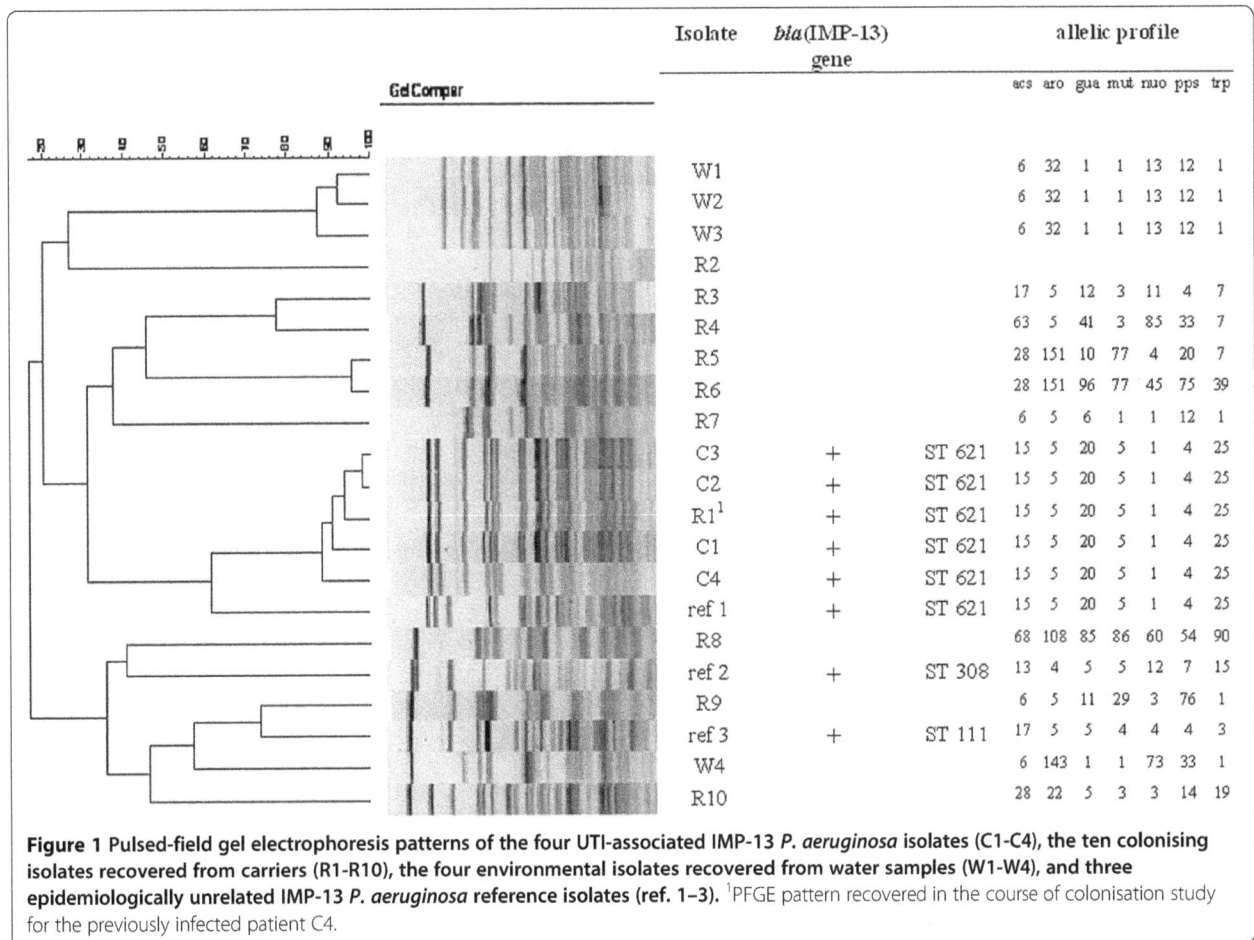

	Isolate	bla(IMP-13) gene		acs	aro	gua	mut	nuo	pps	trp
	W1			6	32	1	1	13	12	1
	W2			6	32	1	1	13	12	1
	W3			6	32	1	1	13	12	1
	R2									
	R3			17	5	12	3	11	4	7
	R4			63	5	41	3	85	33	7
	R5			28	151	10	77	4	20	7
	R6			28	151	96	77	45	75	39
	R7			6	5	6	1	1	12	1
	C3	+	ST 621	15	5	20	5	1	4	25
	C2	+	ST 621	15	5	20	5	1	4	25
	R1[1]	+	ST 621	15	5	20	5	1	4	25
	C1	+	ST 621	15	5	20	5	1	4	25
	C4	+	ST 621	15	5	20	5	1	4	25
	ref 1	+	ST 621	15	5	20	5	1	4	25
	R8			68	108	85	86	60	54	90
	ref 2	+	ST 308	13	4	5	5	12	7	15
	R9			6	5	11	29	3	76	1
	ref 3	+	ST 111	17	5	5	4	4	4	3
	W4			6	143	1	1	73	33	1
	R10			28	22	5	3	3	14	19

Figure 1 Pulsed-field gel electrophoresis patterns of the four UTI-associated IMP-13 P. aeruginosa isolates (C1-C4), the ten colonising isolates recovered from carriers (R1-R10), the four environmental isolates recovered from water samples (W1-W4), and three epidemiologically unrelated IMP-13 P. aeruginosa reference isolates (ref. 1-3). [1]PFGE pattern recovered in the course of colonisation study for the previously infected patient C4.

Review of procedures and techniques, and analysis of environmental samples and hygiene practices

A review of the medical and surgical procedures, and other techniques performed by the medical staff, did not reveal any factor common to the infected patients. P. aeruginosa isolates were recovered from four water samples collected from water fittings in the urological surgical unit, but none of these isolates exhibited high levels of resistance to any of the antibiotics tested. In addition, PFGE and MLST demonstrated that these environmental isolates were genetically distant from the epidemic IMP-13 strain (Figure 1). None of the environmental samples from the cystoscopes was positive for P. aeruginosa. Observations by the hygiene nurse revealed that the barrier precautions around IMP-13-producing P. aeruginosa-infected patient 4 were being followed by healthcare workers. By contrast, the application of standard precautions was not optimal, as hand hygiene practices were inadequate, especially for urinary management and/or the manipulation of urinary catheters, and before cystography. Overall, these observations suggest that transmission between patients was not likely to have been associated with surgery, invasive acts or contaminated water supplies, but with urinary managment.

Nosocomial acquisition of the IMP-13 P. aeruginosa after implementation of barrier precautions

On the 23th of January, all patients hospitalised in the clinic, were screened for the epidemic strain. Nine of the 55 patients (16%), all urology patients, were positive for P. aeruginosa carriage. PFGE and MLST showed genetically diverse colonising isolates and that none presented the IMP13-type (Figure 1). Note that the colonising isolate (R1) of ST 621 and presenting the PFGE IMP13 pattern, was recovered from patient 4, who was still hospitalised at the time of the colonisation study. In addition, no epidemic strain was recovered from any patient at the clinic during the following six months, suggesting that the spread of the epidemic isolate in the clinic had been controlled.

Discussion

Our results document the spread of the IMP13-producing clone in a small private surgical clinic, rather than in an intensive care unit of a university hospital as previously described for this clone.

For two of the four isolates, the MIC of carbapenem drugs was in the susceptibility range. Consequently, the detection of the cluster of UTIs was delayed for several weeks. Our findings confirm the previously described heterogeneous carbapenem-resistance phenotype of the IMP13-producing clone [9] and suggest that the spread of the clone may be, at least partially, facilitated by difficulties in its detection.

Despite extensive investigations prompted by this cluster of UTIs associated with the IMP-13 *P. aeruginosa*, no evidence was found for the involvement of the water supplies or contaminated medical or surgical devices. It is possible that the delay between the time of contamination of the patients and our investigations hindered the identification of a contaminated source. However, in all but one case, the time separating surgery and invasive acts from the onset of clinical signs of UTI was long. These observations do not argue for contamination of the patients during surgery or invasive acts.

By contrast, the temporal superposition of hospitalisation for the infected patients, and the observation of insufficiently strict application of hygiene practices in the urology unit and before cystography suggest that the UTI cases may have resulted from cross-transmission during post-surgery hospitalisation. The rate of faecal carriage of *P. aeruginosa* among elderly urology patients is frequently high, confirming the ability of this bacterium to colonise the urinary tract of such patients [10]. In view of the frequent and invasive nature of urinary care acts following surgery, and the well-described epidemic potential of the IMP-13 clone [1,3,11], we suggest that elderly urology patients should be considered to be at high risk of patient-to-patient cross-transmission of IMP-13-producing *P. aeruginosa*.

Concordant with MLST results, the recent sequence analysis of the *bla*IMP13 gene in numerous IMP-13-*P. aeruginosa* isolates from distant French regions showed that our epidemic isolates and the Italian clone have very similar characteristics [12]. Nevertheless, no link with countries experiencing IMP-13-*P. aeruginosa* outbreaks was identified in the index case history, and the origin of the IMP-13 clone involved in this outbreak remains unclear. Further studies are needed to improve our knowledge of the epidemiology of this highly resistant clone.

Because of the association between the use of broad-spectrum antibiotics and multidrug resistance, a campaign has been run to promote systematic microbiological documentation of UTI: this should favour the use of specific rather than broad-spectrum antibiotics. The early implementation of barrier precautions around infected patients successfully prevented the further spread of the carbapenem-resistant clone in the clinic. We suggest that, when facing a limited cluster of infections, such precautions may be sufficient for infection control, without the need for more extreme measures, such as cohorting, for example.

Competing interest
The authors declare that they have no competing interest.

Authors'contributions
NVDM conceived the study and wrote the manuscript. OD observed hygiene practices. LD isolated the epidemic strain and conducted the environmental study. Molecular characterization (PFGE) of the isolates was conducted by XB. ASV conducted MLST. XB, RQ and PP helped draft the manuscript. All authors read and approved the final manuscript.

Acknowledgments
This work was supported by the Centre de Coordination de la Lutte contre les Infections Nosocomiales de l'Ouest de la France (CCLIN Ouest), the Agence Régionale de Santé du Centre, and the Centre Hospitalier Universitaire de Tours, France. None of the authors has a competing interest.

Author details
¹Clinique Notre dame de Bon Secours, Chartres, France. ²Laboratoire d'Analyses Médicales, Luisant, France. ³Service d'Hygiène, Centre Hospitalier Universitaire, Besançon, France. ⁴UMR 6249 Chrono-environnement, Université de Franche-Comté, Besançon, France. ⁵Centre National de référence, Centre Hospitalier Universitaire, Université de Franche-Comté, Besançon, France. ⁶Service de Bactériologie et Hygiène, Tours, France. ⁷Réseau des Hygiénistes du Centre, Hôpital Trousseau, Centre Hospitalier Universitaire, Tours, France.

References
1. Naas T, Bogaerts P, Kostyanev T, Cuzon G, Huang TD, Ozsu S, Nordmann P, Glupczynski Y: Silent spread of IMP-13-producing *P. aeruginosa* belonging to sequence type 621 in Belgium. *J Antimicrob Chemother* 2011, 66:2178–9.
2. Toleman MA, Biedenbach D, Bennett D, Jones RN, Walsh TR: Genetic characterization of a novel metallo-B-lactamase gene, $bla_{IMP-13,}$ harboured by a novel Tn5051-type transposon disseminating carbapenemases genes in Europe: report from the SENTRY worldwide antimicrobial surveillance programme. *J Antimicrobial Chemoth* 2003, 52:583–590.
3. Santella G, Pollini S, Docquier JD, Mereuta AI, Gutkind G, Rossolini GM, Radice M: Intercontinental dissemination of IMP-13-producing *P. aeruginosa* belonging in sequence type 621. *J Clin Microbiol* 2010, 48:4342–4343.
4. Kohlenberg A, Weitzel-Kage D, van der Linden P, Sohr D, Vögeler S, Kola A, Halle E, Rüden H, Weist K: Outbreak of carbapenem-resistant *P. aeruginosa* infection in a surgical intensive care unit. *J Hosp Infect* 2010, 74:350–357.
5. Tosh PK, Disbot M, Duffy JM, Boom ML, Heseltine G, Srinivasan A, Gould CV, Berríos-Torres SI: Outbreak of *P. aeruginosa* surgical site infections after arthroscopic procedures. *Infect Control Hosp Epidemiol* 2011, 32:1179–86.
6. Wendelboe AM, Baumbach J, Blossom DB, Frank P, Srinivasan A, Sewell CM: Outbreak of cystoscopy related infections with *P. aeruginosa*: New mexico, 2007. *J Urol* 2008, 180:588–592.
7. Ferroni A, Nguyen L, Pron B, Quesne G, Brusset MC, Berche P: Outbreak of nosocomial urinary tract infections due to *P. aeruginosa* in a paediatric surgical unit associated with tap-water contamination. *J Hosp Infect* 1998, 39:301–307.
8. Kidd TJ, Grimwood K, Ramsay KA, Rainey PB, Bell SC: Comparison of three molecular techniques for typing *P. aeruginosa* isolates in sputum samples from patients with cystic fibrosis. *J Clin Microbiol* 2011, 49:263–268.
9. Pollini S, Fiscarelli E, Mugnaioli C, Di Pilato V, Ricciotti G, Neri AS, Rossolini GM: *P. aeruginosa* infection in cystic fibrosis caused by an epidemic metallo-B-lactamase-producing clone with a hetergoeneous carbapenem reistance phenotype. *Clin Microbiol Infect* 2011, 17:1272–1275.
10. Djeribi R, Bouchloukh W, Jouenne T, Menaa B: Characterization of bacterial biofilms formed on urinary catheters. *Am J Infect Control* 2012, 40:854–859.

26

High proportion of healthcare-associated urinary tract infection in the absence of prior exposure to urinary catheter: a cross-sectional study

Ilker Uçkay[1,2,3], Hugo Sax[1,11], Angèle Gayet-Ageron[1], Christian Ruef[4,12], Kathrin Mühlemann[5^], Nicolas Troillet[6], Christiane Petignat[7], Enos Bernasconi[8], Carlo Balmelli[7], Andreas Widmer[9], Karim Boubaker[10,13], Didier Pittet[1,3*] for the Swiss-NOSO network

Abstract

Background: Exposure to urinary catheters is considered the most important risk factor for healthcare-associated urinary tract infection (UTI) and is associated with significant morbidity and substantial extra-costs. In this study, we assessed the impact of urinary catheterisation (UC) on symptomatic healthcare-associated UTI among hospitalized patients.

Methods: A nationwide period prevalence survey of healthcare-associated infections was conducted during 1 May to 30 June 2004 in 49 Swiss hospitals and included 8169 adult patients (4313 female; 52.8%) hospitalised in medical, surgical, intermediate, and intensive care wards. Additional data were collected on exposure to UC to investigate factors associated with UTI among hospitalised adult patients exposed and non-exposed to UC.

Results: 1917 (23.5%) patients were exposed to UC within the week prior to survey day; 126 (126/8169; 1.5%) developed UTI. Exposure to UC preceded UTI only in 73 cases (58%). By multivariate logistic regression analysis, UTI was independently associated with exposure to UC (odds ratio [OR], 3.9 [95% CI, 2.6-5.9]), female gender (OR, 2.1 [95% CI, 1.4-3.1]), an American Society of Anesthesiologists' score > 2 points (OR, 3.2 [95% CI, 1.1-9.4], and prolonged hospital stay >20 days (OR, 1.9 [95% CI, 1.4-3.2]. Further analysis showed that the only significant factor for UTI with exposure to UC use was prolonged hospital stay >40 days (OR, 2.9 [95% CI, 1.3-6.1], while female gender only showed a tendency (OR, 1.6 [95% CI, 1.0-2.7]). In the absence of exposure to UC, the only significant risk factor for UTI was female gender (OR, 3.3 [95% CI, 1.7-6.5]).

Conclusions: Exposure to UC was the most important risk factor for symptomatic healthcare-associated UTI, but only concerned about half of all patients with UTI. Further investigation is warranted to improve overall infection control strategies for UTI.

Keywords: Prevalence, Urinary catheter, Acute care, Urinary tract infection, Nosocomial, Risk factors

* Correspondence: didier.pittet@hcuge.ch
^Deceased
[1]Infection Control Programme and WHO Collaborating Centre on Patient Safety, University of Geneva Hospitals and Faculty of Medicine, 4 Rue Gabrielle Perret-Gentil, 1211, Geneva 14, Switzerland
[3]Department of Infectious Diseases, University of Geneva Hospitals and Faculty of Medicine, Geneva, Switzerland
Full list of author information is available at the end of the article

Background

Indwelling urinary catheters (UC) are an integral part of medicine today [1,2], and as many as one-quarter of all patients require their placement during hospital stay [3]. Exposure to UC is currently considered the most important risk factor for healthcare-associated urinary tract infection (UTI) and is associated with significant morbidity [3-5] and substantial extra-costs [6,7]. The literature suggests that the rate of UTI acquisition is 5% per day of UC use [3]. Despite the harm potential and the existence of educational programmes to prevent unnecessary catheterisation, UC continues to be frequently used or maintained without clear indications [3,4,8].

In Switzerland, nationwide period prevalence surveys of healthcare-associated infections have been regularly conducted for the past 15 years and provide a unique opportunity to gain insight into their epidemiology [9-12]. During the 2004 survey, we collected additional data on exposure to UC and evaluated factors associated with UTI among hospitalised adult patients exposed and non-exposed to UC.

Methods

Setting and study organization

Five nationwide period prevalence surveys of healthcare-associated infections have been conducted since 1996 in Switzerland in over 100 acute care hospitals [9-12]. These were coordinated by *SwissNOSO*, an independent panel of experts in infectious diseases and hospital epidemiology representing all Swiss university-affiliated hospitals. Hospital participation was voluntary. Observers were infection control practitioners who attended at least three one-day training sessions during which detailed documentation was provided in their native language, including the study protocol, standardised case report form, written definitions for all study variables, practical exercises, and code lists [9]. The prevalence study was scheduled to assess all healthcare-associated infections. All nurses and physicians performing the study were trained to distinguish between community and healthcare-associated infections; the latter was defined as symptomatic infection occurring after 48 h of hospital admission. Infection control practitioners from centres with and without experience in prevalence studies were grouped as study teams and supervised by an infection control physician at each centre [9,12].

Study population and methodology

All patients hospitalised for at least 24 h during the survey conducted in May-June 2004 were assessed using a standardised case report form. Dermatological, ophthalmological, paediatric, and psychiatric wards were excluded, as well as long-term care sectors, defined as wards with a median hospital stay >30 days. In each hospital, one or several teams of two trained observers with experience in infection

control reviewed simultaneously all medical and nursing charts and evaluated patients for the presence of healthcare-associated infections and potential risk factors within a fixed time window, defined as the survey day plus the six previous days. Observers rated their interpretation of chart data on a six-point Likert scale (1 = strongly disagree; 6 = strongly agree). All results were checked by the data manager and physicians in the study centre for plausibility and completeness, and corrected if necessary. The following variables were assessed for each patient: gender; age; immune suppression; hemiplegia; surgery; antibiotic use; hospital size; ward type; and length of hospital stay at time of survey. All non-surgical wards, e.g., neurology, rheumatology, were classified as medical wards. Acuity and severity of the underlying illness were assessed by the American Association of Anesthesiologists' (ASA) score [13], McCabe and Jackson classification [14], Charlson comorbidity index [15], and nursing workload on survey day [16].

Definitions

Definitions for healthcare-associated infections were adapted from those of the United States Centers for Disease Control and Prevention (CDC) [17] as previously described [9,11]. UTI was the primary outcome and defined as an infection occurring after 48 h of hospitalisation, unless the patient was transferred from another hospital and cumulative hospital stay reached 48 h. Clinical (dysuria, pollakisuria, fever or shivering), laboratory (urine sedimentation profiles, urinary tract cultures), medical and/or radiological data (ultrasound or computed tomography scans) were required for the confirmation of infection in the absence of other signs or explications. Only the first episode of symptomatic UTI for each patient was recorded. Asymptomatic urinary tract colonization (CDC code, UTI-ASB) was not considered as UTI [9,10]. Previous exposure to UC was the secondary outcome. Exposure to UC, intensive care, and antibiotics were only considered when they lasted for at least 24 h. A condom collection system was not considered as UC. Duration of exposure to UC was censored at 30 days. Surgery was defined as any procedure performed in the operating room within 30 days prior to survey day.

Statistical analysis

The primary outcome was the occurrence of symptomatic UTI. First, we compared patients with and without UTI by using Chi-2 or Fisher's exact tests for categorical variables. We used Student's *t*-test or the non-parametric Mann–Whitney test to compare continuous variables. To take into account hospital clustering, we used a logistic regression model with a random effect at the hospital level (cluster effect) to assess the independent association between the main predictor (previous exposure to UC) and UTI after adjustment for the main confounders (gender, age, severity scores [McCabe, ASA], length of hospital stay,

Table 1 Patient characteristics according to the presence of healthcare-associated urinary tract infection (UTI) (n = 8169), *Swiss-NOSO* Nationwide Prevalence Study, 2004

	UTI (n = 126)	No UTI (n = 8043)	P value
Urinary catheter exposure (%)			<0.001
Yes	73 (57.9)	1912 (23.8)	
No	53 (42.1)	6131 (76.2)	
Gender, female (%)	85 (67.5)	4228 (52.6)	0.001
Mean age (±SD)	71.8 (15.6)	62.4 (19.0)	<0.001
Age groups (%)			<0.001
<40 years	7 (5.7)	1395 (17.9)	
41-70 years	37 (30.3)	3208 (41.2)	
> = 71 years	78 (63.9)	3184 (40.9)	
Hospital size			0.09
<200 acute care beds	23 (18.3)	1994 (24.8)	
200-500 beds	40 (31.8)	2748 (34.2)	
> = 501 beds	63 (50.0)	3301 (41.0)	
Mean length of stay (±SD)	20.5(22.2)	11.4 (41.0)	<0.001*
Length of stay			<0.001
<20 days	89 (70.6)	6990 (86.9)	
21-40 days	22 (17.5)	677 (8.4)	
> = 41 days	15 (11.9)	374 (4.7)	
Recent stay in intensive care (%)	34 (27.0)	1030 (12.8)	<0.001
Hospitalisation ward (%)			0.003*
Medical ward	45 (35.7)	3192 (39.7)	
Surgical ward	50 (39.7)	3219 (40.0)	
Gynaecology/obstetrics	5 (4.0)	778 (9.7)	
Intensive care unit	7 (5.6)	285 (3.5)	
Medico-surgical	19 (15.1)	569 (7.1)	
Recent surgery (%)	61 (48.4)	3292 (40.9)	0.09
Mean ASA score (±SD)	2.81 (0.67)	2.33 (0.89)	<0.001*
ASA (%)			<0.001*
1 pt	4 (3.2)	1587 (19.8)	
2-3 pts	109 (87.2)	5802 (72.3)	
4-5 pts	12 (9.6)	634 (7.9)	
McCabe/Jackson (%)			0.01*
Non fatal	82 (65.1)	6143 (76.4)	
Fatal within 5 years	36 (28.6)	1455 (18.1)	
Fatal within 6 months	8 (6.4)	445 (5.5)	
Mean nursing workload (±SD)	204.0 (161.4)	168.3 (162.8)	0.008*
Mean Charlson index (±SD)	1.8 (2.1)	1.2 (1.8)	<0.001*
Charlson group (%)			0.02
0-3 pts	106 (84.1)	7267 (90.4)	
> = 4 pts	20 (15.9)	776 (9.7)	
Co-morbidities (%)			
Diabetes mellitus	19 (15.1)	1074 (13.4)	0.57

Table 1 Patient characteristics according to the presence of healthcare-associated urinary tract infection (UTI) (n = 8169), *Swiss-NOSO* Nationwide Prevalence Study, 2004 *(Continued)*

Immune suppression°	26 (20.6)	1047 (13.0)	**0.01**
Hemiplegia	24 (19.1)	777 (9.7)	**<0.001**
Dementia	9 (7.1)	290 (3.6)	**0.04**

ASA, American Society of Anesthesiologists; (%) = proportion of all surveyed patients according to number of the variable of interest among the study population; *SD* = standard deviation; °autoimmune disease, transplantation, hepatopathy, nephropathy, neoplasia.

co-morbidities). We used the same regression model to assess the independent association between the secondary outcome (use of UC) and various risk factors. For both models, we used a backward stepwise procedure by selecting all variables associated with a p <0.20 at univariate and kept in the model all those significantly associated with the outcome (p <0.05). As we suspected that the pathophysiology of UTI differed according to gender and those exposed/not exposed to UC, we tested for an interaction between both variables and provided a stratified model on urinary catheter exposure/gender. We tested also for all interactions that were biologically plausible. Finally, we assessed the independent association between prior exposure to UC (secondary outcome) and the main confounders (gender, age, severity scores [McCabe, ASA], hospital length of stay, co-morbidities). The significance level was 0.05 (two-tailed). Statistical testing was performed, using SAS statistical software, version 9.2 (SAS Institute).

Results

A total of 8169 patients from 49 hospitals participated in the survey, representing a nationwide estimate of at least 30% of all hospitalised patients; 4313 (52.8%) were female [12]. Among these, 1917 (23.5%) were exposed to UC with an overall median duration of use of 4 days (interquartile range, 2–9 days). Of 126 patients overall who developed UTI (1.5%; 85 female; median age, 77 years), 73 (58%) had been exposed to UC within the week preceding UTI onset, while 53 (42%) had no exposure. Sixty-two percent of all case report forms for UTI patients were maximally rated (6/6 points on the Likert scale) by observers and a further 25% with almost complete agreement (5/6 points). Females were at higher risk for UTI (odds ratio [OR], 2.1 [95% confidence interval (CI), 1.4-3.1]). Four UTI episodes were classified as upper UTI or abscesses, and six were bacteraemic. We identified a total of 14 different causative pathogens, of which the most frequent in descending order were *Escherichia coli*, *Proteus* spp, *Klebsiella* spp, *Enterobacter* spp, and *Enterococcus* spp. On average, UTI was diagnosed 16 days after admission (range, 2 to 124 d). Patient population characteristics stratified according to the occurrence of UTI are shown in Table 1. The 38 episodes of asymptomatic urinary tract bacterial colonization were excluded according to our study protocol.

Multivariate adjustment
Overall UTI
By multivariate logistic regression analysis with a random effect at the hospital level, independent factors associated with higher odds for UTI were prior exposure to UC (odds ratio, OR, 3.9 [95% CI, 2.6-5.9]), female gender (OR, 2.1 [95% CI, 1.4-3.1]), ASA score of > 2 points (OR, 3.2 [95% CI, 1.1-9.4], and prolonged hospital stay > 20 days (OR, 1.9 [95% CI, 1.4-3.2]. When female gender and prior exposure were combined with UC as one risk factor, the likelihood of UTI increased by 10.4-fold compared to the combination of male gender and no prior exposure to UC. Women not exposed to UC had a 3.4-fold risk of UTI compared to men not exposed to UC. The likelihood of UTI increased independently with age, ASA group, and the length of hospital stay, after adjustment on the main other confounders (Tables 2 & 3).

UTI with and without prior UC exposure
In the model assessing the likelihood of UTI stratified on prior exposure to UC (Table 2), the only factor significantly associated was a prolonged hospital stay > 40 days, while female gender showed only a tendency for association. In the model stratified on no prior exposure to UC, female gender, hemiplegia, and a recent stay in intensive care all increased significantly the odds for UTI.

UTI stratified by gender
In the model assessing the likelihood of UTI stratified by gender (Table 3), prior exposure to UC was significantly associated with UTI for both, whereas the length of hospital stay was significantly associated with UTI for women, but not for men.

Exposure to UC
We investigated the variables associated with the use of UC after stratification by gender. There were no differences between genders according to exposure to UC. The following factors were independently associated with a higher odds for the use of UC: age >70 years; recent surgical intervention; ASA score > 4 points; Charlson index > 4 points; high McCabe classification; recent stay in intensive care; and hemiplegia.

Discussion
In this large study of patients hospitalised in Swiss acute care facilities, 25% were exposed to UC and 1.5% developed symptomatic UTI. Congruent with our results and other national and regional prevalence studies, a European report

estimated a prevalence of nosocomial UTI of 1.65% (Table 4). Our findings mirror reports revealing a prevalence of UC use of 20.3% in emergency departments [8], 32% to 36% in acute care wards [5], and similar rates in most surveys conducted elsewhere (Table 4). The median duration of exposure to UC was also congruent with the literature, i.e., 2–4 days [18-41].

By contrast, we are not able to compare healthcare-associated UTI prevalence with prevalence encountered in the community. Scientific data on the incidence or prevalence of UTI in the Swiss general population are non-existent, while the literature provides only data in predefined populations, such as elderly men or diabetic patients. Moreover, different survey studies define UTI differently, e.g., by excluding or including asymptomatic colonization. However, according to rough data, the overall life-long incidence of UTI could be around 2-4% for young males [42], 6.3% for older Scandinavian males [43], and up to 20% for females. Among Saudi diabetic males, the prevalence might be as high as 7%, whereas asymptomatic urinary tract colonization might be as high as 41% in diabetic women [44].

We found a significant association between UTI and UC use. However, the relation between prior exposure to UC and subsequent UTI was much less systematic than expected, and UC use preceded UTI in only 58% of cases. This does not appear to be unique to our study. In a European study reviewing 4.4 million admissions in 1999, 37.2% of all UTI episodes did not reveal prior exposure to UC [4]. A proportion of 41% UTI without prior exposure to UC has been similarly evidenced in Italian hospitals [31], while Jespen et al. found 56.7% of patients with healthcare-associated UTI attributed to prior UC use [19]. These reports did not further explore the relative low frequency of UC use prior to UTI.

In our study population, the low rate of UTI may reflect the low UC utilization rates. This is not surprising. One explanation might be recent surgery and/or a short ICU stay as these patients are often exposed to UC and acquire UTI more frequently than those hospitalised on medical wards. According to survey definitions, UC use was only recorded when it lasted > 24 h, but some patients undergoing surgery could have been exposed to UC for a shorter time, at least during surgery or ICU stay. Although it cannot be excluded that short duration catheterisation might predispose to subsequent UTI, this is unlikely given the low UTI incidence of only 2% [45] to 2.5% [46] at 24 h of UC use. Moreover, at least in the largest institution involved in the current study, this assumption would not be true [47]. Since 2001, UC during surgery is restricted to patients with a foreseen duration of more than 5 h or for arthroplasty surgery if the patient meets one of the following conditions:

Table 2 Multivariate logistic regression models clustered on hospitals presenting independent factors associated with urinary tract infection stratified on prior exposure to urinary catheter, *Swiss-NOSO* Nationwide Prevalence Study, 2004

Variables	Prior exposure to urinary catheter (n = 1917)			No prior exposure to urinary catheter (n = 5957)		
	Odds ratio	95% CI	P value	OR	95% CI	P value
Age groups (%)			0.62			**0.03***
<40 years	1.00	-	-	1.00	-	-
41-70 years	1.77	0.51-6.10	0.36	1.03	0.31-3.45	0.96
>= 71 years	1.84	0.54-6.26	0.33	2.53	0.81-7.94	0.11
Recent surgical intervention			0.75			0.59
No	1.00	-		1.00	-	
Yes	0.92	0.54-1.56		0.84	0.44-1.59	
ASA score (%)			**0.09***			0.39
1 pt	1.00	-	-	1.00	-	-
2-3 pts	7.21	0.96-54.35	0.06	1.99	0.54-7.28	0.30
4-5 pts	4.52	0.51-39.74	0.17	1.11	0.18-6.78	0.91
Charlson group			0.55			0.76
0-3 pts	1.00	-		1.00	-	
>= 4 pts	1.30	0.55-3.08		0.85	0.30-2.40	
Length of stay			**0.01***			**0.09***
<20 days	1.00	-	-	1.00	-	-
21-40 days	1.88	0.92-3.85	0.08	2.01	0.95-4.22	0.07
>= 41 days	2.87	1.34-6.11	0.006	2.12	0.84-5.35	0.11
Recent stay in intensive care			0.99			**0.05***
No	1.00	-		1.00	-	
Yes	1.00	0.58-1.73		2.30	1.01-5.20	
McCabe/Jackson (%)			0.95			0.18
Non fatal	1.00	-	-	1.00	-	-
Fatal within 5 years	0.98	0.54-1.77	0.95	1.71	0.88-3.31	0.11
Fatal within 6 months	1.15	0.45-2.93	0.76	0.50	0.06-3.87	0.50
Gender			**0.06***			**0.001***
Male	1.00	-		1.00	-	
Female	1.61	0.98-2.65		3.27	1.65-6.48	
Hemiplegia			0.78			**0.03***
No	1.00	-		1.00	-	
Yes	1.10	0.55-2.20		2.10	1.07-4.11	
Immune suppression°			0.67			0.45
No	1.00	-		1.00	-	
Yes	1.18	0.54-2.58		1.42	0.57-3.51	

*Independent variables significantly (or slightly significantly) associated with urinary tract infection.
ASA = American Society of Anesthesiologists; autoimmune disease, transplantation, hepatopathy, nephropathy, neoplasia.

age >75 years; ASA class >3 points; presence of morbid obesity or urinary incontinence [43,48]. Thus, only 15.7% of all orthopaedic surgery is performed with a UC in place. For postanaesthesia care, only 4.7% of all patients required bladder catheterisation without permanent insertion of a UC [46].

Another population prone to intermittent catheterisation are patients with neurogenic bladders who were not identified as such in our study protocol [49,50]. Of note, our study involved acute care settings with the voluntary exclusion of long-term care facilities or homes where most patients with neurogenic bladders are usually

Table 3 Multivariate logistic regression models clustered on hospitals presenting independent factors associated with urinary tract infection stratified on gender, *Swiss-NOSO* Nationwide Prevalence Study, 2004

Variables	Male (n = 3703)			Female (n = 4171)		
	Odds ratio	95% CI	P value	Odds ratio	95% CI	P value
Age groups (%)			**0.01***			**0.10***
<70 years	1.00	-		1.00	-	-
> = 71 years	2.57	1.24-5.31		1.51	0.93-2.45	
Recent surgical intervention			0.78			0.43
No	1.00	-		1.00	-	
Yes	1.11	0.55-2.21		0.82	0.49-1.35	
ASA score (%)			0.30			0.47
<4 pts	1.00	-		1.00	-	-
4-5 pts	0.52	0.15-1.81		0.73	0.31-1.73	
Charlson group			0.50			0.89
0-3 pts	1.00	-		1.00	-	
> = 4 pts	1.44	0.50-4.11		0.94	0.39-2.28	
Length of stay			0.57			**<0.001***
<20 days	1.00	-	-	1.00	-	-
21-40 days	0.86	0.26-2.92	0.81	2.75	1.52-4.96	0.001
> = 41 days	1.75	0.59-5.17	0.31	2.89	1.41-5.92	0.004
Recent stay in intensive care			0.59			**0.04***
No	1.00	-		1.00	-	
Yes	0.79	0.35-1.81		1.83	1.03-3.24	
McCabe classification (%)			0.84			**0.14***
Non fatal	1.00	-	-	1.00	-	-
Fatal within 5 years	0.81	0.36-1.82	0.61	1.70	0.99-2.91	0.05
Fatal within 6 months	1.11	0.31-4.04	0.87	0.98	0.32-3.00	0.98
Prior exposure to urinary catheter			**<0.001***			**<0.001***
No	1.00	-		1.00	-	
Yes	6.77	3.20-14.35		3.04	1.83-5.04	
Hemiplegia			**0.08***			0.34
No	1.00	-		1.00	-	
Yes	2.04	0.93-4.46		1.36	0.73-2.54	
Immune suppression°			0.39			0.57
No	1.00	-		1.00	-	
Yes	1.55	0.57-4.18		1.24	0.58-2.65	

*Independent variables significantly (or slightly significantly) associated with urinary tract infection.
ASA American Society of Anesthesiologists; autoimmune disease, transplantation, hepatopathy, nephropathy, neoplasia.

housed. Thus, the prevalence of neurogenic bladders in acute care settings should be low. We consider that we have avoided a major bias by including paraplegic patients in the study population. Finally, the exact risk of symptomatic UTI after one single intermittent catheterisation is unknown. Most of the literature on intermittent catheterisation concerns individuals with repeated catheterisation due to neurologic problems [49,50]. Among these patients with intermittent self-catheterisation during several years or months, the cumulative risk of UTI is reported to be as high as 50% according to several surveys [50]. However, these patients cannot be compared with individuals with normal bladders who are only undergoing one single intermittent catheterisation for anaesthesiological or surgical reasons.

UTI can complicate urological interventions and be technically classified as surgical site infection. In a literature review, Slade reported approximately 19% UTI after urological surgery [48]. We are unable to provide information on the proportion of "official urological patients"

Table 4 Prevalence of urinary catheter use and/or symptomatic healthcare-associated urinary tract infection: reports in the peer-reviewed literature (January 1980-December 2012)

Author/s	Population	Methodology	Catheter use	Infection	Remarks
Jepsen et al. [19] 1982	40 hospitals in eight countries, n = 3899	Point prevalence	10.1% men, 11.8% women	6.5%	Conducted in 1980
Moro et al. [20] 1985	130 hospitals, n = 34,577	Point prevalence	9.4%	2.1%	National prevalence survey in Italy, 1983
Mertens et al. [21] 1987	106 hospitals, n = 8723	Point prevalence	15.7%	4.4%	National prevalence survey in Belgium 1984 70% surgery. Definition nosocomial: > 3rd day
Srámova et al. [22] 1988	23 hospitals, n = 12,260	Point prevalence		1.5%	Prevalence survey in Czechoslovakia, 1984
Emmerson et al. [23] 1996	157 centres, n = 37,111	Survey	-	2.4%	Prevalence survey in UK and Ireland, 1994
Gastmeier et al. [24] 1997	72 hospitals, n = 14,966	Point prevalence		1.1%	National prevalence survey in Germany, 1994
Scheel et al. [25] 1999	All acute care hospitals, n = 12,755	Point prevalence	-	2.2%	National prevalence survey in Norway, 1997
Vaqué et al. [26] 1999	n = 51,674 in 1997	Point prevalence	-	2.1%	National prevalence surveys in Spain, 1990-1997
French Prevalence Group [27] 2000	830 hospitals, n = 236,334	Point prevalence	9.6%	1.6%	National prevalence survey in France, 1996, including psychiatric and long-term care wards
Eriksen et al. [2] 2002	Acute care hospitals, n = 11,500-12,500	Point prevalence	-	1.7-2.0%	National prevalence surveys in Norway,2002 and 2003
Gikas et al. [28] 2002	n = 3925	Point prevalence	8.6%	2.1%	Survey in 14 Greek hospitals, 1999
Lizioli et al. [29] 2003	Public hospitals, n = 18,667	Point prevalence	-	1.6%	Prevalence survey in Lombardy, 2000
Klavs et al. [30] 2003	Acute care, n = 6695	Point prevalence	-	1.2%	National prevalence survey in Slovenia, 2001
Nicastri et al. [31] 2003	15 hospitals in Italy, n = 2165	Point prevalence	22.4%	1.7%	All participating hospitals have > 400 beds
Wald et al. [5] 2005	Surgery, n = 111,330 523 Medicare hospitals	Retrospective cohort study	32% at discharge day	-	Patients at discharge after hip replacement
Tammelin [32] 2005	31 hospitals, n = 6369		16.5%	1.65%	Acute hospitals and long-term care facilities in Sweden, 2002
Gravel et al. [33] 2007	n = 5750	Point prevalence	22%	3.4%	National prevalence survey in Canada, 2002
Hopmans et al. [34] 2007	2 tertiary Dutch hospitals, n = 2661	Point prevalence twice a year	-	2.3% (1.2%-3.4%)	2001-2004. Obstetric wards excluded
Kevens et al. [35] 2007	445 US hospitals, n = 33,726,611	Throughout the year 2002	-	1.3%	Estimations for the USA
Pelizzer et al. [36] 2008	21 Italian hospitals, n = 6352	Period prevalence	25.2%	2.2%	Prevalence study in Veneto region, Italy 2003
van den Broek et al. [37] 2011	10 hospitals, n = 16,495	Period prevalence	20.2%	2.6%	Netherlands, acute care hospitals
Cairns et al. [38] 2011	45 acute care hospitals, n = 11,090	Point prevalence	20.3%	2.0%	Scotland 2006, exclusion of obstetric patients
Cotter et al. [39] 2012	69 long-term care facilities, n = 4,170	Point prevalence	5.6%	1.5%	Long-term care facilities in Ireland, June 2010
Askarian et al. [40] 2012	8 university hospitals, n = 3450	Point prevalence	23.1%	1.4%	University hospitals in Shiraz, Iran
Health Protection Agency [41] 2012	103 healthcare facilities, n = 52,443	Point prevalence	18.8%	1.1%	English national point prevalence survey preliminary data
Present article	Acute care hospitals, n = 8169	Period prevalence Cluster-adapted	24%	1.5%	National prevalence survey in Switzerland, 2004

* Only reports including at least 2000 patients admitted to acute care facilities are included.

among all those undergoing surgery, because many Swiss surgical wards are mixed, especially in smaller hospitals, are mixed and care for urology and non-urology patients at the same time. Similarly, the same surgeons may often perform urologic and other surgical interventions during the same day. However, it is unlikely that these urologic patients represent a large group and that freshly-operated urological patients would have been exposed to UC for more than 24 h. Specialized, urology-only, surgical wards did not exist in Switzerland at the time of the study and urology patients constitute a maximum of 10% of all surgical patients in many university centres. As summarised in Table 4, few national prevalence studies further stratify or report surgical specialties in detail. In the studies by Emmerson et al. [23] and Sramova et al. [22], the proportion of patients hospitalised on urological wards was only 3.9% and 2.4%, respectively.

Our survey has several limitations. i) The study design was not targeted towards delineating the origin of UTI. The causal inference between exposure to UC and UTI seems logical, but is not proven *sensu strictu*. ii) Despite the large number of patients included, only 126 acquired UTI. Although positive in terms of infection control, these small numbers are associated with reduced statistical power that is recognized in the wide confidence intervals. iii) Results are limited to acute care sectors. Many patients exposed to UC in high-income countries live in nursing homes or other long-term care facilities where the prevalence is higher and UTI is one of the most frequent infections [1,10]. iv) Data related to antibiotic administration or urine acidification are lacking. This could be important as patients treated for other infections might be protected from UTI with antimicrobials covering Gram-negative rods, while antibiotic administration prior to hospital admission might equally have diminished the bacterial burden in the genitourinary system. To the best of our knowledge, no prevalence study has explored this theoretical relationship. Of note, in our study, symptomatic UTI occurred on average two weeks after hospital admission, but we ignore if patients already had asymptomatic urinary tract colonization before hospital admission. v) So far, only prevalence studies and personal clinical experience report a high proportion of UTI without prior exposure to UC. There are no prospective cohort studies or randomized trials to confirm this ubiquitous finding. We currently ignore if the ability to track the catheter as a risk factor for nosocomial UTI might be limited when using prevalence studies. vi) Our study protocol did not target differences in the clinical presentation between UTI with and without prior UC use. This may be a bias as the presence of UC may influence physicians in the work-up of fever, i.e., they might order urine cultures more often in patients with UC. This theoretical bias is likely to shift the proportion of UTI towards UC use.

In conclusion, exposure to UC is the most important risk factor for healthcare-associated UTI according to prevalence studies, but only for a proportion of all patients — at best two-thirds. This finding appears to be shared by other local or national prevalence studies. In our study, the separate analysis for UTI in the absence of prior UC use revealed only female gender [48], hemiplegia [5], and prolonged hospital stay as significant risk factors. The cumulative impact of other less inalienable risk factors should not be underestimated. Further research needs to place an emphasis on innovative strategies to address the specific issues of UTI in the absence of exposure to UC.

Competing interests
The authors declare that they have no competing interests.

Authors' contributions
The national prevalence study was designed by all authors. The study was primarily coordinated by HS and IU with support from all authors, including identifying patients and collecting data on cases. IU, HS and AG managed the data and performed the initial analysis of cases. IU, AG, and DP drafted the manuscript. All authors interpreted the results and revised the manuscript.

Financial support
This study was supported by the Swiss Federal Office for Public Health and unrestricted educational grants from Astra Zeneca, Bayer (Switzerland) AG, BBraun Medical AG, Beiersdorf AG, Ecolab GmBH, Mundipharma AG, and Schülke + Mayr AG.

Acknowledgments
We are indebted to Rosemary Sudan for editorial assistance, Nadia Colaizzi for help in data processing and study organisation, and François Eggimann for information technology support. We thank Pierre-Alain Raeber for help and Stephan Harbarth for critical reading of the manuscript.
Parts of the study were presented at the 50th Interscience Conference on Antimicrobial Agents and Chemotherapy Congress in Boston, USA, on 15 September 2010 (abstract #3192).

Author details
[1]Infection Control Programme and WHO Collaborating Centre on Patient Safety, University of Geneva Hospitals and Faculty of Medicine, 4 Rue Gabrielle Perret-Gentil, 1211, Geneva 14, Switzerland. [2]Orthopaedic Surgery Department, University of Geneva Hospitals and Faculty of Medicine, Geneva, Switzerland. [3]Department of Infectious Diseases, University of Geneva Hospitals and Faculty of Medicine, Geneva, Switzerland. [4]Division of Infectious Diseases, University Hospital of Zurich, Zurich, Switzerland. [5]Department of Infectious Diseases, University Hospital Bern, Bern, Switzerland. [6]Department of Infectious Diseases, Central Institute of the Valais Hospitals, Sion, Switzerland. [7]Department of Hospital Preventive Medicine, Centre Hospitalier Universitaire Vaudois and University of Lausanne, Lausanne, Switzerland. [8]Department of Infectious Diseases, Ospedale Civico, Lugano, Switzerland. [9]Division of Infectious Diseases, University of Basel Hospitals, Basel, Switzerland. [10]Swiss Federal Office of Public Health, Bern, Switzerland. [11]Current addresses: Department of Infectious Diseases and Hospital Hygiene, University of Zurich, Zurich, Switzerland. [12]Current addresses: Hirslanden Clinics, Zurich, Switzerland. [13]Current addresses: Public Health Service for the Canton of Vaud, Lausanne, Switzerland.

References
1. Nicolle LE: **Urinary tract infection in long-term-care facility residents.** *Clin Infect Dis* 2000, 31:757–761.
2. Eriksen HM, Iversen BG, Aavitsland P: **Prevalence of nosocomial infections in hospitals in Norway, 2002 and 2003.** *J Hosp Infect* 2005, 60:40–45.

3. Maki DG, Tambyah PA: Engineering out the risk for infection with urinary catheters. *Emerg Infect Dis* 2001, **7:**342–347.

4. Bouza E, San Juan R, Muñoz P, Voss A, Kluytmans J: Co-operative Group of the European Study Group on Nosocomial Infections II: A European perspective on nosocomial urinary tract infections I. *Clin Microbiol Infect* 2001, **7:**532–542.

5. Wald H, Epstein A, Kramer A: Extended use of indwelling urinary catheters in postoperative hip fracture patients. *Med Care* 2005, **43:**1009–1017.

6. Foxman B: Epidemiology of urinary tract infections: incidence, morbidity, and economic costs. *Dis Mon* 2003, **49:**53–70.

7. Tambyah PA, Knasinski V, Maki DG: The direct costs of nosocomial catheter-associated urinary tract infection in the era of managed care. *Infect Control Hosp Epidemiol* 2002, **23:**27–31.

8. Gardam MA, Amihod B, Orenstein P, Consolacion N, Miller MA: Overutilization of indwelling urinary catheters and the development of nosocomial urinary tract infections. *Clin Perform Qual Health Care* 1998, **6:**99–102.

9. Pittet D, Harbarth S, Ruef C, Francioli P, Sudre P, Pétignat C, Trampuz A, Widmer A: Prevalence and risk factors for nosocomial infections in four university hospitals in Switzerland. *Infect Control Hosp Epidemiol* 1999, **20:**37–42.

10. Sax H, Hugonnet S, Harbarth S, Herrault P, Pittet D: Variation in nosocomial infection prevalence according to patient care setting: a hospital-wide survey. *J Hosp Infect* 2001, **48:**27–32.

11. Sax H, Swiss-NOSO: Nationwide surveillance of nosocomial infections in Switzerland–methods and results of the Swiss Nosocomial Infection Prevalence Studies (SNIP) in 1999 and 2002. *Ther Umsch* 2004, **61:**197–203.

12. Sax H, Pittet D, Swiss-NOSO Network: Interhospital differences in nosocomial infection rates: importance of case-mix adjustment. *Arch Intern Med* 2002, **162:**2437–2442.

13. Owens WD, Felts JA, Spitznagel EL Jr: ASA physical status classifications: a study of consistency of ratings. *Anesthesiology* 1978, **49:**239–243.

14. McCabe WR, Jackson GG: Gram negative bacteremia I: etiology and ecology. *Arch Intern Med* 1962, **110:**847–855.

15. Charlson ME, Pompei P, Ales KL, MacKenzie CR: A new method of classifying prognostic comorbidity in longitudinal studies: development and validation. *J Chronic Dis* 1987, **40:**373–383.

16. Lambert P, Major L, Saint-Onge E, Saulnier D, Tilquin C, Vanderstraeten G: L'intégration de la planification des soins et de la mesure de la charge de travail au service des démarches scientifiques du soignant et du gestionnaire: la méthode PRN. In *Les systèmes de mesure de la charge de travail en soins infirmiers*. Edited by Thibault C. Montréal, Canada: Association des Hôpitaux du Québec; 1990:189–194.

17. Garner JS, Jarvis WR, Emori TG, Horan TC, Hughes JM: CDC definitions for nosocomial infections, 1988. *Am J Infect Control* 1988, **16:**128–140.

18. Warren JW: Catheter-associated urinary tract infections. *Int J Antimicrob Agents* 2001, **17:**299–303.

19. Jepsen OB, Larsen SO, Dankert J, Daschner F, Grönroos P, Meers PD, Nyström B, Sander J: Urinary-tract infection and bacteraemia in hospitalized medical patients - a European multicentre prevalence survey on nosocomial infection. *J Hosp Infect* 1982, **3:**241–252.

20. Moro ML, Stazi MA, Marasca G, Greco D, Zampieri A: National prevalence survey of hospital-acquired infections in Italy, 1983. *J Hosp Infect* 1986, **8:**72–85.

21. Mertens R, Kegels G, Stroobant A, Reybrouck G, Lamotte JM, Potvliege C, Van Casteren V, Lauwers S, Verschraegen S, Wauters G, *et al*: The national prevalence survey of nosocomial infections in Belgium, 1984. *J Hosp Infect* 1987, **9:**219–229.

22. Srámova H, Bartonova A, Bolek S, Krecmerova M, Subertova V: National prevalence survey of hospital-acquired infections in Czechoslovakia. *J Hosp Infect* 1988, **11:**328–334.

23. Emmerson AM, Enstone JE, Griffin M, Kelsey MC, Smyth ET: The Second National Prevalence Survey of infection in hospitals-overview of the results. *J Hosp Infect* 1996, **32:**175–190.

24. Gastmeier P, Kampf G, Wischnewski N, Schumacher M, Daschner F, Rüden H: Importance of the surveillance method: national prevalence studies on nosocomial infections and the limits of comparison. *Infect Control Hosp Epidemiol* 1999, **20:**124–127.

25. Scheel O, Stormark M: National prevalence survey on hospital infections in Norway. *J Hosp Infect* 1999, **41:**331–335.

26. Vaqué J, Rossello J, Arribas JL: Prevalence of nosocomial infections in Spain: EPINE study 1990–1997. *J Hosp Infect* 1999, **43:**105–111.

27. The French Prevalence Group: Prevalence of nosocomial infections in France: results of the nationwide survey in 1996. *J Hosp Infect* 2000, **46:**186–193.

28. Gikas A, Pediaditis J, Papadakis JA, Starakis J, Levidiotou S, Nikolaides P, Kioumis G, Maltezos E, Lazanas M, Anevlavis E, Roubelaki M, Tselentis Y, Greek Infection Control Network: Prevalence study of hospital-acquired infections in 14 Greek hospitals: planning from the local to the national surveillance level. *J Hosp Infect* 2002, **50:**269–275.

29. Lizioli A, Privitera G, Alliata E, Antonietta Banfi EM, Boselli L, Panceri ML, Perna MC, Porretta AD, Santini MG, Carreri V: Prevalence of nosocomial infections in Italy: result from the Lombardy survey in 2000. *J Hosp Infect* 2003, **54:**141–148.

30. Klavs I, Bufon Luznik T, Skerl M, Grgic-Vitek M, Lejko Zupanc T, Dolinsek M, Prodan V, Vegnuti M, Kraigher A, Arnez Z: Slovenian Hospital-Acquired Infections Survey Group: Prevalence of and risk factors for hospital-acquired infections in Slovenia - results of the first national survey, 2001. *J Hosp Infect* 2003, **54:**149–157.

31. Nicastri E, Petrosillo N, Martini L, Larosa M, Gesu GP, Ippolito G: Prevalence of nosocomial infections in 15 Italian hospitals: first point prevalence study for the INF-NOS project. *Infection* 2003, **31:**10–15.

32. Tammelin A: Urinary catheters and antibiotic treatment, Guidelines adherence could be better. *Lakartidningen* 2005, **102:**378–381.

33. Gravel D, Taylor G, Ofner M, Johnston L, Loeb M, Roth VR, Stegenga J, Bryce E: Canadian Nosocomial Infection Surveillance Program, Matlow A: Point prevalence survey for healthcare-associated infections within Canadian adult acute-care hospitals. *J Hosp Infect* 2007, **66:**243–248.

34. Hopmans TE, Blok HE, Troelstra A, Bonten MJ: Prevalence of hospital-acquired infections during successive surveillance surveys conducted at a university hospital in the Netherlands. *Infect Control Hosp Epidemiol* 2007, **28:**459–465.

35. Klevens RM, Edwards JR, Richards CL Jr, Horan TC, Gaynes RP, Pollock DA, Cardo DM: Estimating health care-associated infections and deaths in U. S. hospitals, 2002. *Public Health Rep* 2007, **122:**160–166.

36. Pellizzer G, Mantoan P, Timillero L, Allegranzi B, Fedeli U, Schievano E, Benedetti P, Saia M, Sax H, Spolaore P: Prevalence and risk factors for nosocomial infections in hospitals of the Veneto region, north-eastern Italy. *Infection* 2008, **36:**112–119.

37. van den Broek PJ, Wille JC, van Benthem BH, Perenboom RJ, van den Akker-van Marle ME, Niël-Weise BS: Urethral catheters: can we reduce use? *BMC Urol* 2011, **11:**10.

38. Cairns S, Reilly J, Stewart S, Tolson D, Godwin J, Knight P: The prevalence of health care-associated infection in older people in acute care hospitals. *Infect Control Hosp Epidemiol* 2011, **32:**763–767.

39. Cotter M, Donlon S, Roche F, Byrne H, Fitzpatrick F: Healthcare-associated infection in Irish long-term care facilities: results from the First National Prevalence Study. *J Hosp Infect* 2012, **80:**212–216.

40. Askarian M, Yadollahi M, Assadian O: Point prevalence and risk factors of hospital acquired infections in a cluster of university-affiliated hospitals in Shiraz Iran. *J Infect Public Health* 2012, **5:**169–176.

41. Hopkins S, Shaw K, Simpson L: *English national point prevalence survey on healthcare-associated infections and antimicrobial use*. London, UK: Health ProtectionAgency; 2011. http://www.hpa.org.uk/webc/HPAwebFile/HPAweb_C/1317134304594.

42. Kyrklund K, Taskinen S, Rintala RJ, Pakarinen MP: Lower urinary tract symptoms from childhood to adulthood: A population bases study of 594 Finnish individuals 4 to 26 years old. *J Urol* 2012, **188:**588–593.

43. Malmsten UGH, Milsom I, Molander U, Norlen LJ: Urinary incontinence and lower urinary tract symptoms: an epidemiological study of men aged 45 to 99 years. *J Urol* 1997, **158:**1733–1737.

44. Al-Rubeaan KA, Moharrem O, Al-Naqeb D, Hassan A, Rafiullah MRM: Prevalence of urinary tract infection and risk factors among Saudi patients with diabetes. *World J Urol* 2012, doi:10.10077s00345-012-0934-x.

45. Garibaldi RA, Mooney BR, Epstein BJ, Britt MR: An evaluation of daily bacteriologic monitoring to identify preventable episodes of catheter-associated urinary tract infection. *Infect Control* 1982, **3:**466–70.

46. Vieira FA: Nursing actions to prevent urinary tract infection associated with long-standing bladder catheter. *Einstein* 2009, **7:**372–375.

47. Stéphan F, Sax H, Wachsmuth M, Hoffmeyer P, Clergue F, Pittet D: **Reduction of urinary tract infection and antibiotic use after surgery: a controlled, prospective, before-after intervention study.** *Clin Infect Dis* 2006, **42:**1544–1551.

48. Slade N: **Postoperative urinary tract infections in urology and gynaecology: a review.** *J R Soc Med* 1980, **3:**739–743.

49. Newman DK, Willson MM: **Review of intermittent catheterization and current best practices.** *Urologic Nurs* 2011, **31:**12–28.

50. Wyndaele JJ: **Complications of intermittent catheterization: their prevention and treatment.** *Spinal Cord* 2002, **40:**536–541.

27

Estimating the burden of healthcare-associated infections caused by selected multidrug-resistant bacteria Finland, 2010

Mari Kanerva[1,2*], Jukka Ollgren[1], Antti J Hakanen[3] and Outi Lyytikäinen[1]

Abstract

Background: Knowledge of the burden of healthcare-associated infections (HAI) and antibiotic resistance is important for resource allocation in infection control. Although national surveillance networks do not routinely cover all HAIs due to multidrug-resistant bacteria, estimates are nevertheless possible: in the EU, 25,000 patients die from such infections annually. We assessed the burden of HAIs due to multidrug-resistant bacteria in Finland in 2010.

Methods: By combining data from the National Infectious Disease Registry on the numbers of bacteremias caused by *Staphylococcus aureus*, *Enterococcus faecium*, *Escherichia coli*, *Klebsiella pneumoniae*, *Enterobacter* spp., *Pseudomonas aeruginosa* and *Acinetobacter* spp., and susceptibility data from the National Antimicrobial Resistance Network and the Finnish Hospital Infection Program, we assessed the numbers of healthcare-associated bacteremias due to selected multidrug-resistant bacteria. We estimated the number of pneumonias, surgical site and urinary tract infections by applying the ratio of these infections in the first national prevalence survey for HAI in 2005. Attributable HAI mortality (3.2%) was also derived from the prevalence survey.

Results: The estimated annual number of the most common HAIs due to the selected multidrug-resistant bacteria was 2804 (530 HAIs per million), 6% of all HAIs in Finnish acute care hospitals. The number of attributable deaths was 89 (18 per million).

Conclusions: Resources for infection control should be allocated not only in screening and isolation of carriers of multidrug-resistant bacteria, even when they are causing a small proportion of all HAIs, but also in preventing all clinical infections.

Keywords: Multidrug-resistant microbes, Healthcare-associated infections, Burden of HAI, Infection control, Resource allocation

Introduction

According to the analysis of European Centre for Disease Prevention and Control (ECDC) and European Medicines Agency (EMEA) in 2007, an estimated number of deaths attributable to infections due to selected multidrug-resistant bacteria, *Staphylococcus aureus*, *Enterococcus* spp, *Escherichia coli*, *Klebsiella* spp., *Enterobacter* spp. or *Pseudomonas aeruginosa*, in the EU, Iceland and Norway was about 25,000 [1]. Approximately 37,000 patients die as a direct consequence of a hospital-acquired infection and an additional 111,000 die as an indirect consequence of the hospital-acquired infection annually [2]. As deaths due to resistant microbes are generally associated with healthcare-associated infections (HAI), antibacterial resistance could be responsible for up to half of HAI deaths. ECDC/EMEA analysis also reported the extra healthcare cost and productivity losses due to resistant bacteria in the EU and it was at least 1.5 billion each year [1].

These estimates give an overview of the magnitude of the problem of antibacterial resistance and HAI in

* Correspondence: mari.kanerva@hus.fi
[1]Epidemiologic Surveillance and Control Unit, Department of Infectious Disease Surveillance and Control, National Institute for Health and Welfare (THL), P.O. Box 30, FI-00271, Helsinki, Finland
[2]Helsinki University Central Hospital, Department of Medicine, Division of Infectious Diseases, POB 348, FIN-00029, HUS, FINLAND
Full list of author information is available at the end of the article

Europe and are important for policymakers and administrators who make resource allocation for infection control. However, the proportion of multidrug-resistant isolates among these bacteria varies between countries, and the data cannot be applied directly to different EU countries.

Earlier we estimated that annually approximately 6% of all patients in acute care hospitals in Finland get at least one HAI, and 3.2% of HAI patients die as a direct or indirect consequence of infection [3]. In the national prevalence survey in 2005, only 1.5% of microbiologically confirmed HAIs were due to tobramycin-resistant *Pseudomonas aeruginosa*, methicillin resistant *S. aureus* (MRSA) or extended spectrum β-lactamase (ESBL) producing *Enterobacteriacae* bacteria [4]. Thus most HAI deaths in Finland are most probably due to non-multidrug-resistant bacteria.

In Finland, several tools are available for the surveillance of antibacterial resistance, some of which are nationwide and others sentinel. However, these data sources cannot directly serve to assess the burden of HAI due to multidrug-resistant bacteria, since laboratory-based surveillance does not distinguish between colonisation and clinical infections, and since among clinical infections, only bacteremias are surveyed nationwide. By using various national surveillance and survey data, we estimated the number of HAIs and HAI mortality based on a set of the best surveyed multidrug-resistant bacteria in Finland in 2010.

Methods

Data sources included the following national and sentinel surveillance programmes. The National Infectious Disease Registry (NIDR) collects data on invasive bacterial isolates from blood and cerebrospinal fluid, all isolates of MRSA, vancomycin-resistant enterococci (VRE) and all isolates of *E. coli* and *Klebsiella pneumoniae* which are intermediately susceptible (I) or resistant (R) to third generation cephalosporins (potential ESBL producers). Since 2011, *Enterobacteriacae* isolates non-susceptible (I/R) to carbapenems were also surveilled; thus data for 2010 was unavailable. During 2011, however, notifications mainly entailed colonisations, rather than infections. The Finnish study group for antimicrobial Resistance (FiRe) is a network of 24 clinical microbiology laboratories (covering >95% of all clinical laboratories that process blood cultures in Finland) that collect susceptibility data on 15 bacteria. Of the 24 FiRe laboratories, 20 report susceptibility data on the invasive isolates of seven indicator pathogens to the European Antimicrobial Resistace Surveillance System (EARS-Net). The Finnish Hospital Infection Program (SIRO), a sentinel network of 15 hospitals, has surveilled HAI, including nosocomial bloodstream infections (BSI) and

surgical site infections (SSI) in selected surgical procedures since 1999. SIRO performed the first national prevalence survey of HAIs in 2005, which covered all HAI types and the outcomes of the study patients in 30 acute care hospitals [4].

The NIDR provided the total number of bacteremia cases caused by *S. aureus*, *Enterococcus faecium*, *E. coli*, *K. pneumoniae*, *Enterobacter* spp., *P. aeruginosa* and *Acinetobacter* spp. in 2010 [5]. Resistance percentages to antibiotics were identified as follows: from the NIDR, for MRSA and VRE as well as I/R for third generation cephalosporins in *E. coli* and *K. pneumonia*; from SIRO and FiRe, I/R for amikacin in *P. aeruginosa*, for third generation cephalosporins in *Enterobacter* spp. and for carbapenems in *Acinetobacter spp*. All these resistant bacteria were considered as multidrug-resistant isolates.

The national prevalence survey of HAIs in 2005 provided the number of pneumonias, SSI and urinary tract infections (UTI) in relation to BSI [4].

By applying the above mentioned resistance percentages to the numbers of bacteremias in the NIDR, we estimated the number of BSI cases due to these resistant bacteria. We estimated the number of other common types of HAIs (pneumonia, as well as SSI and UTI) due to these resistant bacteria by multiplying the number of bacteremias in the NIDR by their corresponding ratio in the national prevalence survey.

The dates and causes of death and 28-day attributable mortality due to HAI in the prevalence survey cohort were obtained from the National Population Information System by using the patient's national identity code, as described earlier [3]. We estimated the number of deaths from these infections by applying an average attributable mortality of 3.2% [3].

We calculated 95% Bayesian confidence intervals (credible intervals) using Markov Chain Monte Carlo simulations. We used coefficients 0.5 and 1.5 to describe uncertainty in the number of BSI due to resistant bacteria as well as in the proportion of other types of infection.

Results

Percentages of resistance to the antibiotics in blood isolates were: MRSA 1.9% (26/1370), VRE 1.1% (3/278), third generation cephalosporins for *E. coli* 3.4% (112/3211), and for *K. pneumoniae* 3.2% (16/504), and for *Enterobacter* spp. 34.0% of 259 isolates, amikacin for *P. aeruginosa* 5.0% of 318 isolates and carbapenems for *Acinetobacter* spp. 3.3% of 34 isolates (Table 1).

In the prevalence survey among all 753 infections, the numbers of the most common infection types were as follows: 44 (6%) primary BSIs, 110 (15%) pneumonias, 215 (29%) SSIs, 103 (15%) symptomatic UTIs and 281 (37%) other. In relation to BSIs, the corresponding ratio

Table 1 Observed* of estimated annual numbers of healthcare-associated infections due to multidrug-resistant bacteria

Type of HAI	Numbers of HAIs (95% confidence interval)						
	MRSA	VRE	Third gen ceph I/R			Amicacin I/R P. aeruginosa	Carbapenem I/R Acinetobacter spp.
			E. coli	K. pneumoniae	Enterobacter spp.		
Blood stream infection	26* (17–37)	3* (1-7)	112* (92–134)	16* (10–25)	88 (47–136)	16 (9–25)	1 (12)
Pneumonia	65 (29–114)	8 (1–20)	280 (142–440)	40 (16–75)	220 (87–415)	40 (16–75)	3 (1-5)
Surgical site infection	127 (58–22)	15 (3–40)	549 (278–862)	78 (33–147)	431 (172–814)	78 (32–147)	5 (2–10)
Urinary tract infection	60 (27–105)	7 (1–16)	258 (131–405)	37 (15–69)	202 (81–381)	37 (15–69)	2 (1-5)
All	278 (159–434)	33 (6–81)	1199 (795–1654)	171 (87–287)	941 (458–1584)	171 (86–287)	11 (5–19)

Footnote: HAI=healthcare-associated infection, MRSA=methicillin resistant Staphylococcus aureus, VRE=vancomycin resistant Enterococcus faecium, I/R = intermediately suscaptible or resistant.

of the other infection types were 110/44=2.5 for pneumonias, 4.9 (215/44) for SSIs and 2.3 (103/44) for UTIs. The estimated annual numbers of these four common types of HAIs due to the resistant bacteria were calculated by multiplying the number of the BSIs by these infection ratios. Thus for example, the estimated number of pneumonias due to MRSA was 26 x 2.5 = 65, and numbers of SSIs and UTIs due to MRSA were 26 x 4.9 = 127 and 26 x 2.3 = 60, respectively (Table 1).

The estimated total annual numbers of the four HAI types due to MRSA, VRE, third generation cephalosporin I/R E. coli and K. pneumoniae and Enterobacter spp., as well as amicacin I/R P. aeruginosa and carbapenem I/R Acinetobacter spp. were 278, 33, 1199, 171, 941, 171 and 11, respectively (Table 1), for a total of 2804 (530 HAIs caused by resistant bacteria per million population). The estimated total annual number of attributable deaths due to these infections was 89 (18 per million population).

Conclusions

This study represents the first attempt to estimate the burden of HAIs due to multidrug-resistant bacteria in Finland. The annual number of HAIs in acute care hospitals in Finland is at least 50 000 [3]. Here we show, that at approximately 2800 (6%) of them may be due to multidrug-resistant bacteria. The HAI morbidity and mortality due to multidrug-resistant bacteria is, in Finland, thus far relatively low and lower than the figures in the EU as a whole [1], but shows differences depending on the resistant bacterium. The methodology we used was based on the work presented by the ECDC/EMEA and might be applied also by other countries in their burden assessments [1].

The results we present here are a rough estimate. True figures of the burden of all HAIs due to all resistant microbes cannot directly be achieved through any national surveillance methods generally used. This data cannot easily be collected at a hospital level either: e.g.

prevalence surveys are vulnerable for chance, collection of full cover resistance data is laborious in prevalence survey, and often only half of HAIs are microbiologically confirmed. Therefore, an estimate of the burden is practically the best we can achieve to date. In the future, e.g. enhanced on line HAI reporting e.g. by using compulsory computerized reporting of antibiotic prescribing indications (HAI, community-acquired infection or prophylaxis) and automated combination of microbiological data of causative pathogens might improve the data coverage. To get the most applicable data now, we chose national data sources e.g. to cover estimates of HAIs and deaths. The national prevalence data were quite representative of Finnish acute care hospitals: over 8,000 adult inpatients in all five tertiary care hospitals, and all 15 secondary care hospitals as well as 10 (25% of all) other acute care hospitals took part in the voluntary survey. The resistance data from laboratories also well covered the whole country.

There are, however, several limitations in our estimates. Firstly, we included only seven microbes and four infection types. In the national prevalence survey data, the selected microbes, S. aureus, Enterococcus spp., E. coli, K. pneumoniae, Enterobacter spp., P. aeruginosa and Acinetobacter spp., caused 48% of all microbiologically conformed HAIs and comprised 34% of all causative microbes [4]. Selected infection types covered 63% of all HAIs. We excluded coagulase-negative staphylococci, as in the ECDC/EMEA report [1], due to its various resistance patterns and relatively low virulence, and pneumococci because a majority of these infections are community-acquired [6]. Rice et al. grouped E. faecalis and faecium, S. aureus, K. pneumoniae, A.baumannii, P. auruginosa and the Enterobacter species as the most common nosocomial pathogens that escape the effects of many antibiotics, and used the acronym ESKAPE [7].

Secondly, we used a prevalence survey, not incidence data, to estimate the HAI numbers and distribution. In the prevalence survey, because HAI prolongs the length of stay, severe HAIs, such as BSIs and pneumonias, are likely to be overrepresented in relation to mild infections, like UTIs. In addition, the prevalence data was from 2005, and lengths of stay may have shortened after that, also affecting the proportions of different HAI.

Thirdly, we applied the same ratio of other infections to BSIs for all microbes. In fact, *Enterobacteriaceae* are usually more prone to cause UTIs, and MRSA causes SSI. In addition, the NIDR surveillance data included both primary and secondary BSIs, but the prevalence survey included only primary BSI, which can affect the estimated distribution of infection types, leading to an overestimation of the number other infections by approximately 20%.

Fourthly, infections caused by ESBL producing gram-negatives, especially *E. coli* UTIs, can also be community-acquired, although severe and complicated infections, such as bacteremias [8], may more likely be healthcare-associated. In reports from different hospital settings from the years 1999–2007, the proportion of community-associated BSIs (i.e. in patients with no previous hospitalizations or healthcare-associated risk factors) among all BSIs due to ESBL producing *E. coli* has been low but variable: 1.6% in Italy, 3% in Finland, 19% in Spain but reached 42% in Canada [9-12]. This tendency of having the most bacteremic complications during hospital care also applies to MRSA, although community-acquired skin and soft tissue infections are common [13]. Infections due to other multidrug-resistant microbes in our study can mainly be considered healthcare-associated. We estimate that including all BSIs due to multidrug-resistant bacteria as HAIs leads to an overestimation of HAIs due to these bacteria by another 10%. Finally, the average attributable mortality of 3.2% from the Finnish prevalence survey reflects HAI mortality mostly due to sensitive bacteria, which may lead to underestimation of mortality due to multidrug-resistant pathogens even as much as 50%.

Estimates of the burden of HAI due to antibiotic-resistant microbes are important for those who allocate resources or prioritize the work of an infection control team. In countries with low prevalence of antibacterial resistance, a lot of resources of infection control are often allocated to prevent the spread of resistant microbes, i.e. contact tracing, screening patients for colonisation, applying isolation precautions and occasionally also on decolonization. The emergence of carbapenemase-producing *Enterobacteriaceae* is an example of the importance of timely identifying risk groups for screening and action. However, all infection control resources should not be focused on one microbe or resistance pattern only, such as MRSA or ESBL. Especially, if the prevalence of antibacterial resistance is high, these narrow spectrum interventions are

insufficient to prevent clinical complications. Infection control interventions including evidence-based guidelines, increasingly implemented as "care bundles" and "check lists", meticulous hand hygiene in all patient care, prudent use of antimicrobials are needed to reduce HAIs in general, along with those caused by multidrug-resistant bacteria. This approach has a greater impact on mortality, morbidity and costs than does screening alone [14,15].

As most HAIs are due to endogenous bacteria, and because e.g. in Finland, up to 94% of HAIs still stem from non-multidrug-resistant bacteria, we should not forget infection-type specific prevention when allocating resources in low prevalance countries either. This is especially important considering, for example ESBL producing bacteria, which are increasingly prevalent in the community and cause preventable catheter-associated bacteremic UTIs in hospital settings.

Abbreviations
(HAI): Healthcare-associated infection; (ECDC): European Centre for Disease Prevention and Control; (EMEA): European Medicines Agency; (NIDR): National Infectious Disease Registry; (MRSA): Methicillin-resistant *S. aureus*; (VRE): Vancomycin-resistant enterococci; (ESBL): Extended spectrum β-lactamase; (EARS-Net): European Antimicrobial Resistance Surveillance System; (SIRO): The Finnish Hospital Infection Program; (SSI): Bloodstream infection (BSI) and surgical site infection; (UTI): Urinary tract infection.

Competing interests
The author declares that they have no competing interests.

Authors' contributions
MK and OL have designed, analysed and interpreted the data, JO contributed to statistics and AH interpreted FiRe data. All authors read and approved the final manuscript.

Acknowledgements
This study has been conducted as a part of the Finnish Hospital Infection Program (SIRO), financed by the National Institute for Health and Welfare and by the Ministry of Social Affairs and Health.

Author details
[1]Epidemiologic Surveillance and Control Unit, Department of Infectious Disease Surveillance and Control, National Institute for Health and Welfare (THL), P.O. Box 30, FI-00271, Helsinki, Finland. [2]Helsinki University Central Hospital, Department of Medicine, Division of Infectious Diseases, POB 348, FIN-00029, HUS, FINLAND. [3]Unit of Antimicrobial Resistance, Department of Infectious Disease Surveillance and Contro, National Institute for Health and Welfare (THL), P.O. Box 57, FI-20521, Turku, Finland.

References
1. European Centre for Disease Prevention and Control ECDC/ European Medicines Agency: *EMEA Joint Technical Report: The bacterial challenge: time to react.* Stockholm Sweden: ECDC; 2009. Available from: http://www.ecdc.europa.eu/en/publications/Publications/0909_TER_The_Bacterial_Challenge_Time_to_React.pdf.
2. European Centre for Disease Prevention and Control (ECDC): *Annual Epidemiological Report on Communicable Diseases in Europe 2008.* Stockholm Sweden: ECDC; 2008. Available from: http://www.ecdc.europa.eu/en/publications/Publications/0812_SUR_Annual_Epidemiological_Report_2008.pdf.
3. Kanerva M, Ollgren J, Virtanen MJ, Lyytikäinen O: Prevalence Survey Study Group. **Estimating the annual burden of health care-associated**

infections in Finnish adult acute care hospitals. *Am J Infection Control* 2009, **7**:227–230.

4. Lyytikäinen O, Kanerva M, Agthe N, Möttönen T, Ruutu P: **Finnish Prevalence Survey Study Group. Healthcare-associated infections in Finnish acute care hospitals: a national prevalence survey, 2005.** *J Hosp Infect* 2008, **69**:288–294.

5. Infectious Diseases in Finland: **Annual Report of National Infectious Disease Registry.** In Edited by Hulkko T, Lyytikäinen O, Jaakola S, Kuusi M, Puumala J, Ruutu P. 2010. http://www.thl.fi/thl-client/pdfs/1d73f597-8188-4ff5-b33c-101d7e1c3e90.

6. Lyytikäinen O, Klements P, Ruutu P, *et al*: **Defining the population-based burden of nosocomial pneumococcal bacteremia.** *Arch Intern Med* 2007, **167**:1635–1640.

7. Rice LB: **Federal funding for the study of antimicrobial resistance in nosocmial pathogens: no ESKAPE.** *Infect Control Hospital Epidemiol* 2008, **197**:1079–1081.

8. Driex L, Brossier F, Duquesnoy O, *et al*: **Increase in hospital-acquired bloodstream infections caused by extended spectrum β-lactamase-producing *Escherichia coli* in a large French teaching hospital.** *Eur J Clin Microbiol Infect Dis* 2009, **28**:491–498.

9. Tumbarello M, Sali M, Trecarichi EM, *et al*: **Bloodstream infections caused by extended-sprectrum-b-lactamase-producing *Escherichia coli*: Risk factrs for inadequated intitial antimicrobial therapy.** *Antimicr Agents Chemother* 2008, **52**:3244–3252.

10. Forssten SD, Kolho E, Lauhio A, *et al*: **Emergence of extended-spectrum b-lactamase-producing *Escherichia coli* and *Klebsiella pneumoniae* during the years 2000–2004 in Helsinki, Finland.** *CMI* 2010, **16**:1155–1171.

11. Rodriques-Bano J, Navarro MD, Romero L, *et al*: **Bacteremia due to Extended-spectrum b-lactamase-producing *Escherichia coli* in the CTX-M era: anew clinical challenge.** *CID* 2006, **43**:1407–1414.

12. Pitout JDD, Gregson DB, Campbell L, Lauland KB: **Molecular characteristics of extended-spectrum-b-lactamase-producing *Escherichia coli* isolates causing bacteremia in the Calgary Health Region from 2000 to 2007: emergence of clones ST131 as a cause of community-acquired infections.** *Antimicr Agents and Chemotherapy* 2009, **53**:2846–2851.

13. Kanerva M, Salmenlinna S, Vuopio-Varkila J, *et al*: **Community-associated methicillin-resistant *Staphylococcus aureus* isolated in Finland in 2004 to 2006.** *J Clin Microbiol* 2009, **47**:2655–2657.

14. Wenzel R, Bearman G, Edmond M: **Screening for MRSA: a flawed hospital infection control intervention.** *Infect Control Hosp Epidemiol* 2008, **29**:1012–1018.

15. Wenzel RP, Edmond MB: **Infection control: the case for horizontal rather than vertical interventional programs.** *Int J Infect Dis* 2010, **14**(S4):S3–S5.

Permissions

The contributors of this book come from diverse backgrounds, making this book a truly international effort. This book will bring forth new frontiers with its revolutionizing research information and detailed analysis of the nascent developments around the world.

We would like to thank all the contributing authors for lending their expertise to make the book truly unique. They have played a crucial role in the development of this book. Without their invaluable contributions this book wouldn't have been possible. They have made vital efforts to compile up to date information on the varied aspects of this subject to make this book a valuable addition to the collection of many professionals and students.

This book was conceptualized with the vision of imparting up-to-date information and advanced data in this field. To ensure the same, a matchless editorial board was set up. Every individual on the board went through rigorous rounds of assessment to prove their worth. After which they invested a large part of their time researching and compiling the most relevant data for our readers.

The editorial board has been involved in producing this book since its inception. They have spent rigorous hours researching and exploring the diverse topics which have resulted in the successful publishing of this book. They have passed on their knowledge of decades through this book. To expedite this challenging task, the publisher supported the team at every step. A small team of assistant editors was also appointed to further simplify the editing procedure and attain best results for the readers.

Apart from the editorial board, the designing team has also invested a significant amount of their time in understanding the subject and creating the most relevant covers. They scrutinized every image to scout for the most suitable representation of the subject and create an appropriate cover for the book.

The publishing team has been an ardent support to the editorial, designing and production team. Their endless efforts to recruit the best for this project, has resulted in the accomplishment of this book. They are a veteran in the field of academics and their pool of knowledge is as vast as their experience in printing. Their expertise and guidance has proved useful at every step. Their uncompromising quality standards have made this book an exceptional effort. Their encouragement from time to time has been an inspiration for everyone.

The publisher and the editorial board hope that this book will prove to be a valuable piece of knowledge for researchers, students, practitioners and scholars across the globe.

List of Contributors

Sonja Hansen, Dorit Sohr, Christine Geffers and Petra Gastmeier
Institute for Hygiene and Environmental Medicine, Charité – University Medicine Berlin, Campus Benjamin Franklin, Hindenburgdamm 27, D-12203, Berlin, Germany

Pascal Astagneau
C-CLIN Nord - Département de santé publique, Université Pierre & Marie Curie, Paris, France

Alexander Blacky and Walter Koller
Clinical Institute for Hygiene and Medical Microbiology, Medical University of Vienna, Vienna, Austria

Ingrid Morales
National Surveillance of Infections in Hospitals - NSIH, Operational Direction Public Health and Surveillance, Scientific Institute of Public Health, Brussels, Belgium

Maria Luisa Moro
Agenzia Sanitaria e Sociale Regione Emilia Romagna, Area di Programma Rischio Infettivo, Bologna, Italy

Mercedes Palomar
Department of Intensive Care, Hospital Vall d'Hebron, Barcelona, Spain

Emese Szilagyi
National Centre for Epidemiology, Department of Hospital Epidemiology, Budapest, Hungary

Carl Suetens
European Centre for Disease Prevention and Control, Stockholm, Sweden

Sarah B. Doernberg
Department of Internal Medicine, Division of Infectious Diseases, University of California, San Francisco, 513 Parnassus Avenue, room S-380, San Francisco, CA 94143, USA

Victoria Dudas
UCSF Medical Center, 505 Parnassus Avenue, San Francisco, CA 94143, USA

Kavita K. Trivedi
Trivedi Consultants, 1563 Solano Avenue, #443, Berkeley, CA 94707, USA

Sanjeev Neupane and Megha Raj Banjara
Central Department of Microbiology, Tribhuvan University, Kirtipur, Kathmandu, Nepal

Narayan Dutt Pant
Department of Microbiology, Grande International Hospital, Dhapasi, Kathmandu, Nepal

Saroj Khatiwada
Department of biochemistry, CIST College, Kathmandu, Nepal

Raina Chaudhary
Shree Birendra Hospital, Chhauni, Kathmandu, Nepal

Bruce Alexander, Brice Beck and Kelly K. Richardson
Iowa City VA Health Care System, Iowa City, IA, USA

Daniel J. Livorsi and Michihiko Goto
Iowa City VA Health Care System, Iowa City, IA, USA
Division of Infectious Diseases, Department of Internal Medicine, University of Iowa Carver College of Medicine, 200 Hawkins Drive, Iowa City, IA 52242, USA

Jennifer McDanel
Iowa City VA Health Care System, Iowa City, IA, USA
Department of Epidemiology, College of Public Health, University of Iowa, Iowa City, IA, USA

Rajeshwari Nair and Eli N. Perencevich
Iowa City VA Health Care System, Iowa City, IA, USA
Division of General Internal Medicine, Department of Internal Medicine, University of Iowa Carver College of Medicine, Iowa City, IA, USA

Margaret Carrel
Department of Geographical and Sustainability Sciences, College of Liberal Arts and Sciences, University of Iowa, Iowa City, IA, USA

Makoto M. Jones
Salt Lake City VA Health Care System, Salt Lake City, UT, USA
University of Utah School of Medicine, Salt Lake City, UT, USA

Masoumeh Bagheri-Nesami, Mohammad Sadegh Rezai and Azin Hajalibeig
Infection Diseases Research Center with Focus on Nosocomial Infection, Mazandaran University of Medical Sciences, Sari, Iran

Alireza Rafiei
Molecular and Cell Biology Research Center, Department of Immunology, Faculty of Medicine, Mazandaran University of Medical Sciences, Sari, Iran

Gohar Eslami
Department of Clinical Pharmacy, Faculty of Pharmacy, Mazandaran University of Medical Sciences, Sari, Iran

Fatemeh Ahangarkani
Student Research Committee, Antimicrobial Resistance Research Center, Mazandaran University of Medical Sciences, Sari, Iran

Attieh Nikkhah
Traditional and Complementary Medicine Research Center, Mazandaran University of Medical Sciences, Sari, Iran

M. Colomb-Cotinat, J. Lacoste, B. Coignard and S. Vaux
Santé Publique France, The French Public Health Agency, F-94415 Saint-Maurice, France

C. Brun-Buisson
Assistance publique-hôpitaux de Paris, CHU Henri Mondor, F-94000 Créteil, France

V. Jarlier
Sorbonne Universités, UPMC Univ Paris 06, Inserm, Centre d'Immunologie et des Maladies Infectieuses, UMR 1135 & APHP, CHU Pitié-Salpêtrière, Laboratoire de Bactériologie-Hygiène, F-75013 Paris, France

Pooja Maharjan, Hridaya Parajuli, Govardhan Joshi and Deliya Paudel
Department of Clinical Laboratory Services, Manmohan Memorial Medical College and Teaching Hospital, Swayambhu, Kathmandu, Nepal

Narayan Prasad Parajuli
Department of Clinical Laboratory Services, Manmohan Memorial Medical College and Teaching Hospital, Swayambhu, Kathmandu, Nepal
Department of Laboratory Medicine, Manmohan Memorial Institute of Health Sciences, Kathmandu, Nepal

Sujan Sayami
Department of Pediatrics, Manmohan Memorial Medical College and Teaching Hospital, Kathmandu, Nepal

Puspa Raj Khanal
Department of Laboratory Medicine, Manmohan Memorial Institute of Health Sciences, Kathmandu, Nepal

Marya D. Zilberberg
EviMed Research Group, LLC, Goshen, MA 01032, USA

Brian H. Nathanson
OptiStatim, LLC, Longmeadow, MA, USA.

Kate Sulham and Weihong Fan
The Medicines Company, Parsippany, NJ, USA

Andrew F. Shorr
Washington Hospital Center, Washington, DC, USA

Yonas Alem Gessese, Mebratenesh Mengistu Amare, Yonas Hailesilassie Bahta and Assalif Demisew Shifera
Department of Medical Laboratory Sciences, Ambo University, College of Medicine and Health Sciences, Ambo, Ethiopia

Dereje Leta Damessa
West Shewa Health Bureau, Ambo District Health Office, Awaro Health Center, Ambo, Ethiopia

Fikreslasie Samuel Tasew
Ethiopian Public Health Institute, Addis Ababa, Ethiopia

Endrias Zewdu Gebremedhin
Department of VeterinaryLaboratory Technology, Ambo University, College of Agriculture and Veterinary Sciences, Ambo, Ethiopia

Yekaterina Khamzina, Byron Crape and Azliyati Azizan
Nazarbayev University School of Medicine (NUSOM), 5/1 Kerey and Zhanibek Khans Street, Astana, Kazakhstan010000

Dmitriy Viderman
Nazarbayev University School of Medicine (NUSOM), 5/1 Kerey and Zhanibek Khans Street, Astana, Kazakhstan010000
National Research Neurosurgery Center, Astana, Kazakhstan

Zhannur Kaligozhin, Makhira Khudaibergenova and Agzam Zhumadilov
National Research Center for Oncology and Transplantation, Astana, Kazakhstan

Lindsay E Nicolle
Departments of Internal Medicine and Medical Microbiology, University of Manitoba, Health Sciences Centre, Room GG443 – 820 Sherbrook Street, Winnipeg, MB R3A 1R9, Canada

Nahla O. Eltai, Eman Wehedy and Sara H. Al-Hadidi
Biomedical Research Center, Qatar University, Doha, Qatar

Asmaa A. Al Thani and Hadi M. Yassine
Biomedical Research Center, Qatar University, Doha, Qatar
College of Health Sciences, Qatar University, Doha, Qatar

Khalid Al-Ansari
Pediatrics Department, Hamad Medical Corporation, Doha, Qatar

Anand S. Deshmukh
Department of Laboratory Medicine and Pathology, Hamad Medical Corporation, Doha, Qatar

Ksenia Ershova
Center for Data-Intensive Biotechnology and Biomedicine, Skolkovo Institute of Science and Technology, Moscow, Russia

Vladimir Zelman
Center for Data-Intensive Biotechnology and Biomedicine, Skolkovo Institute of Science and Technology, Moscow, Russia
Department of Anesthesiology, Keck School of Medicine, University of Southern California, Los Angeles, USA

Ivan Savin, Nataliya Kurdyumova and Ekaterina Sokolova
Department of Intensive Care, Burdenko National Medical Research Center of Neurosurgery, Moscow, Russia

Darren Wong
Division of Infectious Diseases, Keck School of Medicine, University of Southern California, Los Angeles, USA

Gleb Danilov
Laboratory of Biomedical Informatics, Burdenko National Medical Research Center of Neurosurgery, Moscow, Russia

Michael Shifrin
IT Department, Burdenko National Medical Research Center of Neurosurgery, Moscow, Russia

Irina Alexandrova
Department of Microbiology, Burdenko National Medical Research Center of Neurosurgery, Moscow, Russia

Nadezhda Fursova
Federal Budget Institution of Science "State Research Center for Applied Microbiology & Biotechnology" (SRCAMB), Moscow, Russia

Olga Ershova
Department of Epidemiology and Infection Control, Burdenko National Medical Research Center of Neurosurgery, Moscow, Russia

Wen-Pin Tseng, Shang-Yu Chen and Shey-Ying Chen
Department of Emergency Medicine, National Taiwan University Hospital, College of Medicine, National Taiwan University, No. 7, Zhongshan S. Rd., Zhongzheng Dist., Taipei 100, Taiwan

Shan-Chwen Chang
Department of Internal Medicine,National Taiwan University Hospital, College of Medicine, National Taiwan University, No.7, Zhongshan S. Rd., Zhongzheng Dist., Taipei 100, Taiwan

Yee-Chun Chen
Department of Internal Medicine,National Taiwan University Hospital, College of Medicine, National Taiwan University, No. 7, Zhongshan S. Rd., Zhongzheng Dist., Taipei 100, Taiwan
Center for Infection Control, National Taiwan University Hospital, College of Medicine, National Taiwan University, No. 7, Zhongshan S. Rd., Zhongzheng Dist., Taipei 100, Taiwan

Giorgio Piccinelli, Francesca Caccuri, Arnaldo Caruso and Maria Antonia De Francesco
Institute of Microbiology, Department of Molecular and Translational Medicine, University of Brescia-Spedali Civili, P. le Spedali Civili 1, 25123 Brescia, Italy

Giovanni Lorenzin
Institute of Microbiology, Department of Molecular and Translational Medicine, University of Brescia-Spedali Civili, P. le Spedali Civili 1, 25123 Brescia, Italy
Institute of Microbiology and Virology, Department of Biomedical, Surgical and Dental Sciences, University of Milan, Milan, Italy

Lucrezia Carlassara and Francesco Scolari
Department of Nephrology, University of Brescia, Hospital of Montichiari, Brescia, Italy

Cho-Han Chiang and Tyan-Shin Yang
College of Medicine, National Taiwan University, Taipei, Taiwan

Shan-Chwen Chang
College of Medicine, National Taiwan University, Taipei, Taiwan
Department of Internal Medicine, National Taiwan University Hospital, Taipei, Taiwan

Jann-Tay Wang and Wang-Huei Sheng
College of Medicine, National Taiwan University, Taipei, Taiwan
Department of Internal Medicine, National Taiwan University Hospital, Taipei, Taiwan
Center for Infection Control, National Taiwan University Hospital, Taipei, Taiwan

Yee-Chun Chen
College of Medicine, National Taiwan University, Taipei, Taiwan
Department of Internal Medicine, National Taiwan University Hospital, Taipei, Taiwan
Center for Infection Control, National Taiwan University Hospital, Taipei, Taiwan
National Institute of Infectious Diseases and Vaccinology, National Health Research Institutes, Miaoli County, Taiwan

Sung-Ching Pan
Department of Internal Medicine, National Taiwan University Hospital, Taipei, Taiwan

Keisuke Matsuda
Faculty of Medicine, Osaka University, Osaka, Japan

Hong Bin Kim
Department of Internal Medicine, Seoul National University College of Medicine, Seoul, Republic of Korea
Division of Infectious Diseases, Seoul National University Bundang Hospital, Seongnam, Republic of Korea

Young Hwa Choi
Department of Infectious Diseases, Ajou University School of Medicine, Suwon, Republic of Korea

Satoshi Hori
Department of Infection Control Science, Juntendo University Faculty of Medicine, Tokyo, Japan

Feng-Yee Chang
Division of Infectious Diseases and Tropical Medicine, Department of Internal Medicine, Tri-Service General Hospital, National Defense Medical Center, Taipei, Taiwan

Yu Jin Park, Nguyen Le Phuong, Naina Adren Pinto, Mi Jeong Kwon, Jung-Hyun Byun and Dongeun Yong
Department of Laboratory Medicine and Research Institute of Bacterial Resistance, Severance Hospital, Yonsei University College of Medicine, 50-1 Yonsei-ro, Seodaemun-gu, Seoul 03722, Republic of Korea

Roshan D'Souza
Department of Laboratory Medicine and Research Institute of Bacterial Resistance, Severance Hospital, Yonsei University College of Medicine, 50-1 Yonsei-ro, Seodaemun-gu, Seoul 03722, Republic of Korea

J.Craig Venter Institute (JCVI), 9605 Medical Center Dr #150, Rockville, MD 20850, USA

Heungsup Sung
Department of Laboratory Medicine, Asan Medical Center, University of Ulsan College of Medicine, 88 Olympic-ro 43-gil, Songpa-gu, Seoul 05505,Republic of Korea

Anna M. Rohde
German Center for Infection Research (DZIF), Inhoffenstraße 7, 38124 Braunschweig, Germany
Charité – Universitätsmedizin Berlin, Institute of Hygiene and Environmental Medicine, Hindenburgstraße 27, 12203 Berlin, Germany

Janine Zweigner
German Center for Infection Research (DZIF), Inhoffenstraße 7, 38124 Braunschweig, Germany
Charité – Universitätsmedizin Berlin, Institute of Hygiene and Environmental Medicine, Hindenburgstraße 27, 12203 Berlin, Germany
Department of Infection Control and Hygiene, University Hospital Cologne, Kerpener Straße 62, 50937 Köln, Germany

Winfried V. Kern
German Center for Infection Research (DZIF), Inhoffenstraße 7, 38124 Braunschweig, Germany
Division of Infectious Diseases, Department of Medicine II, Medical Center and Faculty of Medicine, University of Freiburg, Hugstetter Strasse 55, 79106 Freiburg, Germany

Harald Seifert
German Center for Infection Research (DZIF), Inhoffenstraße 7, 38124 Braunschweig, Germany
Institute for Medical Microbiology, Immunology and Hygiene, University Hospital Cologne, 1Goldenfelsstrasse 19-21, 50935 Köln, Germany

Maria J. G. T. Vehreschild
German Center for Infection Research (DZIF), Inhoffenstraße 7, 38124 Braunschweig, Germany
Department I of Internal Medicine, University Hospital of Cologne, Herderstraße 52-54, 50931 Köln, Germany

Boudewijn Catry
Healthcare-associated infections & Antimicrobial resistance (https:// www.nsih.be), Sciensano, Ruy Juliette Wytsmanstraat 14, Brussels 1050, Belgium

Katrien Latour
Healthcare-associated infections & Antimicrobial resistance (https:// www.nsih.be), Sciensano, Ruy Juliette Wytsmanstraat 14, Brussels 1050, Belgium
Department of Public Health and Primary Care, KU Leuven - University of Leuven, Leuven, Belgium

Camellia Diba and Candida Geerdens
Interuniversity Institute for Biostatistics and statistical Bioinformatics (I-BIOSTAT), Hasselt University, Hasselt, Belgium

Robin Bruyndonckx
Interuniversity Institute for Biostatistics and statistical Bioinformatics (I-BIOSTAT), Hasselt University, Hasselt, Belgium
Laboratory of Medical Microbiology, Vaccine & Infectious Disease Institute (VAXINFECTIO), University of Antwerp, Antwerp, Belgium

Samuel Coenen
Laboratory of Medical Microbiology, Vaccine & Infectious Disease Institute (VAXINFECTIO), University of Antwerp, Antwerp, Belgium

Paola Algeri, Francesca Pelizzoni, Francesca Russo, Maddalena Incerti, Sabrina Cozzolino, Salvatore Andrea Mastrolia and Patrizia Vergani
Department of Obstetrics and Gynecology, University of Milano-Bicocca, S. Gerardo Hospital, MBBM Foundation, Via Pergolesi 33, Monza, 20900 Monza, Monza e Brianza, Italy

Davide Paolo Bernasconi
Department of Health Sciences, Center of Biostatistic for Clinical Epidemiology, University of Milan-Bicocca, Via Pergolesi 33, Monza, 20900 Monza, Monza e Brianza, Italy

Joseph T Spadafino
Department of Epidemiology, Columbia University Mailman School of Public Health, 722 West 168th Street, New York, NY 10032, USA

Bevin Cohen and Elaine Larson
Department of Epidemiology, Columbia University Mailman School of Public Health, 722 West 168th Street, New York, NY 10032, USA
Columbia University School of Nursing, 630 West 168th Street, New York, NY 10032, USA

Jianfang Liu
Columbia University School of Nursing, 630 West 168th Street, New York, NY 10032, USA

Setegn Eshetie
Department of Medicine, Debre Markos University, Debre Markos, Ethiopia

Chandrashekhar Unakal, Aschalew Gelaw, Mengistu Endris and Feleke Moges
Department of Microbiology, University of Gondar, Gondar, Ethiopia

Birhanu Ayelign
University of Gondar Hospital, Gondar, Ethiopia

Kamlesh Kumar Yadav, Nabaraj Adhikari and Rama Khadka
Department of Microbiology, Kantipur College of Medical Science, Sitapaila, Kathmandu, Nepal

Anil Dev Pant
Consultant pathologist, National Kidney Center, Vanasthali, Kathmandu, Nepal

Bibha Shah
Quality Control Department, Qmed Formulations Pvt. Ltd., Chhaling, Bhaktapur, Nepal

Steven Z Kassakian
Department of Medicine, Warren Alpert Medical School of Brown University, Providence, RI, USA

Leonard A Mermel
Department of Medicine, Warren Alpert Medical School of Brown University, Providence, RI, USA
Department of Epidemiology and Infection Control, Rhode Island Hospital, 593 Eddy Street, Providence RI 02903, USA
Division of Infectious Diseases, Rhode Island Hospital, 593 Eddy Street, Providence, RI 02903, USA

Odile Milan
Clinique Notre dame de Bon Secours, Chartres, France

Laurent Debroize
Laboratoire d'Analyses Médicales, Luisant, France

Xavier Bertrand
Service d'Hygiène, Centre Hospitalier Universitaire, Besançon, France
UMR 6249 Chrono-environnement, Université de Franche-Comté, Besançon, France

Patrick Plesiat
Centre National de référence, Centre Hospitalier Universitaire, Université de Franche-Comté, Besançon, France

Anne-Sophie Valentin and Roland Quentin
Service de Bactériologie et Hygiène, Tours, France

Nathalie Van der Mee-Marquet
Service de Bactériologie et Hygiène, Tours, France
Réseau des Hygiénistes du Centre, Hôpital Trousseau, Centre Hospitalier Universitaire, Tours, France

Angèle Gayet-Ageron
Infection Control Programme and WHO Collaborating Centre on Patient Safety, University of Geneva Hospitals and Faculty of Medicine, 4 Rue Gabrielle Perret-Gentil, 1211, Geneva 14, Switzerland

Ilker Uçkay
Infection Control Programme and WHO Collaborating Centre on Patient Safety, University of Geneva Hospitals and Faculty of Medicine, 4 Rue Gabrielle Perret-Gentil, 1211, Geneva 14, Switzerland
Orthopaedic Surgery Department, University of Geneva Hospitals and Faculty of Medicine, Geneva, Switzerland
Department of Infectious Diseases, University of Geneva Hospitals and Faculty of Medicine, Geneva, Switzerland

Hugo Sax
Infection Control Programme and WHO Collaborating Centre on Patient Safety, University of Geneva Hospitals and Faculty of Medicine, 4 Rue Gabrielle Perret-Gentil, 1211, Geneva 14, Switzerland
Current addresses: Department of Infectious Diseases and Hospital Hygiene, University of Zurich, Zurich, Switzerland

Carlo Balmelli
Department of Hospital Preventive Medicine,Centre Hospitalier Universitaire Vaudois and University of Lausanne, Lausanne, Switzerland

Enos Bernasconi
Department of Infectious Diseases, Ospedale Civico, Lugano, Switzerland

Andreas Widmer
Division of Infectious Diseases, University of Basel Hospitals, Basel, Switzerland

Jukka Ollgren and Outi Lyytikäinen
Epidemiologic Surveillance and Control Unit, Department of Infectious Disease Surveillance and Control, National Institute for Health and Welfare (THL), FI-00271, Helsinki, Finland

Mari Kanerva
Epidemiologic Surveillance and Control Unit, Department of Infectious Disease Surveillance and Control, National Institute for Health and Welfare (THL), FI-00271, Helsinki, Finland

Helsinki University Central Hospital, Department of Medicine, Division of Infectious Diseases, POB 348, FIN-00029, HUS, FINLAND

Antti J Hakanen
Unit of Antimicrobial Resistance, Department of Infectious Disease Surveillance and Contro, National Institute for Health and Welfare (THL), FI-20521, Turku, Finland

Index

www.ingramcontent.com/pod-product-compliance
Lightning Source LLC
Chambersburg PA
CBHW082041190326
41458CB00010B/3428